COLLINS
CHILDREN'S PILL GUIDE

- Is a complete and comprehensive guide to more than 400 brand-name and generic drugs

- Explains which medications have received extensive testing, and the questions surrounding those that have not

- Provides essential information on proper dosages, legitimate concerns, and possible side effects

- Presents detailed information on commonly recommended vaccines, including the benefits and risks of immunizations

- Is an invaluable consumer health guide that puts useful, important information for protecting your children at your fingertips

Collins
CHILDREN'S PILL GUIDE

DEBORAH MITCHELL
LISA E. DAVIS, Pharm.D., Consulting Editor

A Lynn Sonberg Book

HARPER

An Imprint of HarperCollins*Publishers*

This book contains advice and information relating to health care. It is not intended to replace medical advice and should be used to supplement rather than replace regular care by your doctor. It is recommended that you seek your physician's advice before embarking on any medical program or treatment. All efforts have been made to assure the accuracy of the information contained in this book as of the date of publication. The publisher and the author disclaim liability for any medical outcomes that may occur as a result of applying the methods suggested in this book.

HARPER

An Imprint of HarperCollins*Publishers*
10 East 53rd Street
New York, New York 10022-5299

CONTENTS

INTRODUCTION

You sat up all night with your sick child who was feverish, achy, and congested, then waited for hours in the doctor's office or the urgent care clinic the next day, and finally left with a prescription. Or perhaps you talked with a school counselor, child psychologist, or pediatrician about your child's lack of attention and disruptive behavior in school, and then were "strongly advised" to consider medication. You pondered the pros and cons of doing so, and found yourself in your doctor's office being handed a prescription for something that "should help."

Caring for a healthy child is challenging enough, but when your doctor recommends a prescription medication, you may have questions or concerns. Is this the right drug for my child? Is it safe to take with other medications? What side effects might it cause?

Most parents believe that any medicine recommended by a doctor has been well researched in children. However, the next time you pick up a prescription or an over-the-counter remedy, look carefully at the product information sheet that comes with the item. Chances are very good that you will see a statement that warns "safety and dosage have not been established for pediatric use." According to the American Academy of Pediatrics, only 25 percent of the prescription drugs marketed in the United States have specific, re-searched information about how to use the drug in children. That means only one fourth of the drugs have been adequately tested in children. The remaining 75 percent of drugs come with the disclaimer because they have been proven safe and effective only for adults.

1

So does this mean the drug your doctor prescribed for your child may not be safe? How does your doctor know which dosages are safe and effective for children if there is no scientific documentation to support them? Most experts think parents shouldn't be unduly alarmed by the way drugs are dispensed to children in the United States. Many, many drugs are prescribed for "off label" uses—that is, for uses that have not been approved by the U.S. Food and Drug Administration (FDA). They are prescribed for off-label use because extensive experience has shown doctors and other experts that the drugs are effective for these conditions or situations approved by the FDA.

You can feel confident that the dosing instructions your doctor gives you come from his or her experience as well as the experience of many other health-care practitioners who prescribe the drug and who have found them to be safe and beneficial for children.

The very low percentage of prescription drugs tested in children has concerned parents and health-care professionals for many years, but hopefully this situation will change soon. In November 2003, the U.S. House of Representatives approved legislation that requires pharmaceutical companies to test certain medicines that are used in children. The legistation won the approval of the American Academy of Pediatrics, whose 2003 president, Carden Johnston, MD, called the bill "just what the doctor ordered."

We'd like you to think of this book as "just what the doctor ordered." We hope it will help you maneuver your way around the wealth of data that surround the use of prescription and over-the-counter drugs your child may need. This book provides you with up-to-date information on more than 400 brand name and generic drugs that are prescribed for children *even though they may not have been tested in children.* The information within these pages is not a substitute for professional advice from your physician or pharmacist but a handy and reliable resource that can answer many of the questions you may have about the drugs prescribed for your child. As we know all too well, however, researchers are always uncovering new information about real and potential dangers associated with medications, so the information in this book is subject to change. Thus, you are strongly encouraged to question your physician or pharmacist about any drug you plan to give to your child.

How to Use This Book

That being said, we'd like to explain how you can use this book most effectively to find information about the medications your child may need to take now or in the future. Each drug entry in the book follows the same format and provides information in the following categories:

- **Generic Name (or Class Name).** All the entries are arranged alphabetically by generic name or, in a few cases, by class name. The generic name of a drug is its common, non-brand name. Ibuprofen, for example, is a generic name for several trade names, including Motrin and Advil. In a few instances, the name of the drug class or type, such as Penicillin Antibiotics, is listed along with the generic names in that class. This is done to avoid repetition in cases in which all the drugs within the class have similar qualities and side effects.
- **Brand Name(s).** We have included the most common brand (trade) names for each drug. Exclusion of any brand names is in no way an indication that the drugs are inferior to those listed.
- **Generic Available.** We let you know if a generic form of the drug is available. Such forms are typically much more inexpensive than the brand names.
- **About This Drug.** A brief description is given of how the drug is usually classified (e.g., muscle relaxant, antidepressant, or diuretic) as well as information that explains the most common medical conditions for which the drug is prescribed and a brief description of how it works in the body.
- **Side Effects.** The most common, less common, and/or rare side effects, if applicable, are listed.

- **How to Use This Drug.** The typical dosages for the most commonly prescribed forms of the drug are listed, as well as the forms available, how to take the drug (e.g., with or without food), and what to do if your child misses a dose.
- **Time Until It Takes Effect.** This information is especially helpful for parents, so you know what to expect once your child has taken the medication. The times given are averages, and in a few cases the time is unknown.
- **Possible Drug, Food, and/or Supplement Interactions.** Many medications interact in negative ways when taken along with other drugs or with specific foods or supplements. This section offers warnings about possible interactions. You will note that it often includes names of drugs that are not typically recommended for use in children. We include them, however, because your child may be taking one of these drugs along with the drug in the entry, and it is important for you to know there may be serious consequences of such a combination.
- **Symptoms of Overdose.** Signs and symptoms associated with a drug overdose are given, along with information on what to do if an overdose does occur.
- **Things to Tell Your Doctor.** This section includes information you should provide to your doctor about your child, as well as items your doctor may ask you about your child that may have an impact on how your child reacts to the prescribed drug. Examples of information included here may be any allergies your child has, other medical conditions that may place your child at risk if he or she takes the drug, and special conditions under which the drug should not be used.
- **Important Precautions.** Information in this section includes storage instructions and any special warnings from the FDA or pharmaceutical manufacturers about the drug, such as the "black box warnings" now mandatory on antidepressant drugs.

Also included at the back of the book is a handy appendix that lists both generic and brand names, cross-referenced so you can quickly find the drug you want to research.

The bulk of the book is made up of drug "profiles." The remainder of this introductory material is devoted to discussion of medication-related topics that are of special interest to parents and, in some cases, are controversial: the safety and usefulness of vaccinations, psychiatric medications (including those for attention deficit/hyperactivity disorder [ADHD]), herbal remedies, cold and flu remedies, and safety guidelines for drug use in children.

VACCINATIONS

I'm willing to bet you remember getting vaccinated as a child. Perhaps you stood in a school auditorium with hundreds of other children as you all nervously waited to be stuck in the arm. Maybe your parents took you to a doctor's office or a clinic where you sat in a waiting room and listened for the cries of the kids that went into the examination rooms ahead of you. Your mother or father may have tried to reassure you or bribe you with candy or another treat. Or perhaps you've managed not to remember or think about those experiences at all.

But now that you're a parent, the issue of vaccinations has come back, and it is now one of the most hotly debated issues about children's health in the United States. By age 5 years, most children in the United States have been immunized with about 33 doses of 10 different vaccines. Vaccinations are a source of comfort to many parents but a significant concern to others, as some studies indicate that some vaccines may have the potential to cause serious and even deadly harm to children. **Thus,** it is critical that you learn all you can about the benefits and risks associated with vaccinations so you can make informed decisions when it comes time to vaccinate your children.

The Ten Vaccines

As of 2005, the ten vaccines recommended by the federal government and mandated by the states for children were as follows. (Note that there are many other vaccinations available on an as-needed basis for other medical conditions).

- Hepatitis B: Typically, this is the first vaccine children are given, with the first injection administered shortly after birth, the second within 1 to 4 months of age, and the third between 6 and 18 months of age.
- DTaP: Diphtheria, tetanus, and acellular pertussis (whooping cough), a revision of the original DTP vaccine. A total of 5 injections are administered over a period beginning at 2 months of age and continuing until age 4 to 6 years.
- Hib: *Haemophilus influenzae* type B, 4 injections given at 2, 4, 6, and 12 to 15 months of age.
- Polio: The injectable form of the polio vaccine, IPV (inactivated polio vaccine) has been recommended over the oral polio vaccine since January 1, 2000. It is given at 2, 4, and 6 to 18 months of age, followed by a booster dose at 4 to 6 years.
- MMR: A combination of measles, mumps, and rubella vaccine, given at 12 to 15 months of age, with a second dose at 4 to 6 years of age.
- Varicella: Chicken pox, given as a single dose between the ages of 12 months and 12 years.

(Note: You can see the list of vaccines recommended by the U.S. government and required by the states at *www.aap.org/family/parents/immunize.htm*. See also information about the flu vaccine below.)

When a child receives a mandated childhood vaccine, the administering doctor is required by law to give the parent(s) or guardian(s) a Vaccine Information Statement (VIS), which is produced by the Centers for Disease Control and Prevention (CDC), for each different vaccine. The best time for you to get this information is *before* the scheduled immunization, so you have time to learn all you can about the vaccine, ask questions, and seek out additional information. You can get Vaccine Information Statements from:

- Your doctor
- Your local or state health department
- The Centers for Disease Control and Prevention: download them at *www.cdc.gov/nip/publications/vis*
- Immunization Action Coalition: *www.immunize.org/vis*, which allows you to download them in English or dozens of other languages

What Are Vaccines?

Vaccines are substances designed to protect people against disease by helping the body develop immunity against certain pathogens (germs). To do this, vaccines are made from the virus or pathogen that causes the disease you wish to fight. When a minute amount of the pathogen or virus is introduced into the body (either via injection or by mouth), the immune system responds by producing substances called antibodies, which fight against (anti) disease-causing bodies (bacteria, viruses). The goal is to stimulate the development of enough antibodies to stop the pathogens from causing disease.

There are three basic types of vaccines: live, killed, and recombinant DNA. Most are given via injection under the skin or into muscle, and a few can be taken orally or intranasally. In a few cases, both live and killed vaccines can be given to treat the same disease.

Live vaccines are made in a laboratory from the germ (usually a virus) that causes the disease. Live vaccines are weakened (attenuated) with the intention of triggering the body's immune system to generate an immune response without causing the disease. Occasionally, however, individuals react to a vaccination by developing symptoms of the disease, although the reaction is usually mild. Attenuated viruses include chicken pox, measles, mumps, polio (oral dose), rubella, and yellow fever, whereas attenuated bacter-

ial vaccines include typhoid fever and bacillus-Calmette-
Guérin (used for tuberculosis).

The controversy over live vaccines includes questions
about whether they should be given to infants, who do not
have a fully developed immune system. Some experts say
these vaccines have the potential to cause autism and autoimmune diseases; others dismiss this claim. Hopefully
further research will soon answer this critical question.

Killed vaccines, also referred to as inactivated vaccines,
are composed of all or a portion of a disease-causing organ-
ism that has been killed, which means it no longer can reproduce and cause disease. For this reason, they trigger a
weaker response by the immune system than do live vaccines and thus also tend to be safer, especially for children
younger than one year, whose immune systems are not fully
developed.

Killed vaccines have been developed for the following
diseases: cholera, hepatitis A, hepatitis B, influenza, Lyme
disease, pertussis (whooping cough), polio (injection), ra-
bies, and typhoid. Another type of killed vaccine is a toxoid,
which is made by inactivating the poisons (toxins) that are
produced by bacteria and viruses. Vaccines against diphtheria and tetanus are made in this way.

Recombinant DNA vaccines are genetically engineered,
which means researchers manipulate the genes to create the
vaccine. An example of a recombinant DNA vaccine is the
hepatitis B vaccine. To make this vaccine, researchers take
specific genes from the hepatitis B virus and add them to a
culture (baker's yeast) and allow them to reproduce. Once
the virus has reproduced, miniscule amounts can be mixed
with solution and injected. Some experts say recombinant
DNA vaccines are safer and more effective than live or
killed vaccines because they contain only a portion of the infectious agent and so cannot cause an infection. However,
some scientists argue that these vaccines may trigger the immune system to produce antibodies, which will attack the
body and cause various health problems. As yet, researchers
are not certain about the effects recombinant DNA vaccines
can have on the body.

Booster Shots: What's the Story?

As you see in the list of ten different vaccinations given to children, most require more than one dose. The one or more additional doses of a vaccine given to help ensure the immunity that is supposed to be provided by the original dose(s) are called *boosters*. Booster doses are administered months or even years after the original dose. It's important to know that an "original dose" may actually include up to three injections. This is the case with DTaP shots, in which the first three shots are considered the original doses, as they are needed to establish immunity, and the next two shots, given at 12 to 18 months and then again at 4 to 6 years, are the boosters.

Some experts say that boosters are not always necessary and should not be given automatically to all children. But how do you know if your child needs a booster injection? You can ask your doctor to check your child's titers, which is a measurement of the concentration of a substance (in this case, the concentration of antibodies) in a solution (your child's blood). If the antibody titer is at a level high enough to make your child immune to a specific disease, then he or she doesn't need the booster. You have the right to ask your doctor to check your child's titers before a booster is given, and thus eliminate exposing your child to possible adverse reactions.

Natural Immunity and Acquired Immunity

When infants are born, they already have antibodies that they received through the placenta from their mother. These antibodies help them develop immunity against a wide variety of illnesses. Infants who are breastfed keep receiving important antibodies, from both colostrum (the thick premilk a woman secretes during the first few days after giving birth) and breast milk. By the end of the first year of life, however, the immunity the infant received from its mother wears off, and the ability to ward off many diseases fades as well. On average, an infant has natural immunity against diphtheria, tetanus, whooping cough, polio, and the Hib form of meningitis for only 2 to 3 months after birth, and for measles and mumps for about 1 year. Administering vaccines is an attempt to protect children against certain diseases known to be potentially dangerous and against which they have little or no natural immunity.

Humans can attain acquired immunity against certain diseases when they allow the immune system to "do what it does naturally," which is heal the body. Here's how it works: The immune system makes billions of special cells designed to fight and destroy germs as soon as they enter the body. This is the natural or inborn immunity newborns receive from their mother. If an infection begins to take hold in the body, the immune system fights back by producing even more of the special cells. In fact, the system is so sophisticated that different groups of cells are tailored to target different germs. The selected cells not only reproduce quickly and fight the infection, they also "remember" the germ that caused the infection, thus making an individual immune to another attack by the same type of germ. This is acquired immunity.

Vaccinations are given to trigger acquired immunity and provide long-lasting protection against certain diseases. Some people argue that it is better to allow acquired immunity to occur naturally; that is, if a child becomes infected with measles, for example, the immune system should be allowed to develop acquired immunity against the germ rather than risk exposing the child to a vaccine and any possible adverse reactions.

Weighing the Benefits and Risks of Immunization

Although experience has shown us that in most cases vaccines prevent more disease and serious symptoms than ones they may cause or fail to block, parents need to know that immunization is no guarantee that their child will not get the disease against which he or she is being immunized. Proof of the effectiveness of various vaccines can be seen in the statistics. For example, in 1920 there were more than

469,000 cases of measles and 7,575 deaths associated with the disease. From 1958 to 1962, an average of more than 503,000 cases of measles were reported in the United States. But when the measles vaccine was first introduced to the world in 1963, the number of measles cases began to decline. By 1995, deaths from measles had decreased 95 percent worldwide and 99 percent in Latin America. In 1998, the incidence of measles in the United States reached a new low: 89 cases and no deaths. Similar dramatic declines were seen after the introduction of other vaccines.

Some parents and experts question whether giving children several vaccines at the same time, a practice called *multiple dosing,* is safe. In fact, the MMR vaccine—measles, mumps, and rubella—an example of one vaccine that contains multiple doses, has been named as a possible cause of autism and gastrointestinal problems in children. Multiple dosing also is practiced when some doctors play "catch up," giving a child two, three, or more shots in one day because the child missed an earlier scheduled vaccination. The CDC insists that multiple dosing is safe, saves time and money for parents, and reduces trauma for the child. But other experts say the practice is dangerous. Marcel Kinsbourne, MD, a pediatric neurologist and research professor at the Center for Cognitive Studies at Tufts University, told the U.S. House Committee on Government Reform that giving multiple doses at the same time "may have adverse effects that none of the individual vaccines have when they are given by themselves."

Stephanie Cave, MD, author of *What Your Doctor May Not Tell You about Children's Vaccinations*, agrees, and also is concerned that researchers are developing even more combination vaccines, which may contain a dozen or more disease-causing organisms in one vaccine to be given at birth. Clearly, multiple dosing is yet another aspect of children's vaccinations that is controversial and one that parents need to consider. If you are concerned about multiple dosing but want to vaccinate your child, one step you can take is to ask your doctor to administer the individual components of the MMR vaccine at different times. You can also stay as close to the recommended vaccine schedule as possible and not allow your child to be given "catch up" shots.

The Thimerosal/Mercury Dilemma

Vaccines are not without potential risks, some of which can be very serious and even deadly. Part of the reason for some of these risks may be the presence of thimerosal/mercury in childhood vaccines. For many years, vaccine manufacturers matter-of-factly included thimerosal, a mercury-based preservative, in their products. Mercury is a known neurotoxin, which means it can poison the nervous system, causing symptoms such as muscle weakness, memory loss, attention deficit, impaired speech and hearing, and rash. Children who are exposed to mercury early in life can develop neurological difficulties that may appear as subtle learning disabilities, speech impairment, muscle weakness, incoordination, and behavioral problems.

Some experts believe that injecting mercury into the bodies of infants and children, whose nervous systems have not yet fully developed, is a cause or contributing factor in autism, attention deficit/hyperactivity disorder, mental retardation, obsessive-compulsive disorder, seizure disorders, and other psychiatric, neurologic, and/or behavior problems. Vaccine-based mercury is also believed to have a role in causing asthma and autoimmune disorders, such as thyroid disorders, lupus, and juvenile rheumatoid arthritis. A link between thimerosal and autism or any other of these conditions is still a point of debate among medical professionals. In the case of autism, in particular, some researchers have said such a connection is "improbable" whereas others have urged more investigation and are cautious about flatly stating that thimerosal has no role in autism or other medical conditions. Clearly, the jury is still out on this issue, and it is a topic parents need to follow as studies continue.

How do you know if the vaccine your child receives contains thimerosal? You should ask your doctor. Better yet, request a thimerosal-free vaccine, as there is at least one version of all childhood vaccines that are completely or nearly mercury-free. (Your doctor may have vaccines for flu that may still contain thimerosal, but you can request a mercury-free version.) You can see a list of thimerosal contents in U.S. licensed vaccines (provided by Johns Hopkins Bloomberg School of Public Health) at *www.vaccinesafety.edu/thi-table.htm*.

The Influenza Vaccine

Headache, cough, chills, muscle aches, fever—yes, it sounds like the flu. Every year, right around the time your kids are donning their backpacks and going back to school, the threat of flu returns. Then, just as your kids gear up for the December holiday season, flu season is in full force, typically going strong until April. In other words, much of the school season coincides with the flu season, which means your kids could have a good excuse to miss at least several days of classes if they catch the flu. So should you be thinking about a flu vaccine?

There are several things you need to consider. One, unlike vaccines designed to protect your child against most other organisms, the influenza (flu) vaccine is new each year in an attempt to keep up with the most common strains of the flu virus that are in the environment. There is no guarantee, however, that the strains chosen for each year's vaccine will be the ones to which you and your child will be exposed.

Two, the flu vaccine is recommended for only certain high-risk groups of children and adolescents, based on age and/or medical conditions. For example, beginning in 2005 the flu vaccine was formally recommended for all children ages 6 to 23 months and their close contacts (e.g., siblings). Any child who has a chronic medical condition, such as asthma, other airway disease, or cancer, also should receive the vaccine. To get the best response to the vaccine, experts recommend that children younger than 9 years who are at high risk receive 2 doses of the vaccine administered at least one month apart. Children older than 9 years and younger children who have had a flu shot previously need only a single injection each year.

If your child needs a flu shot, the best time to get it is during October or November, especially if your child will need 2 shots, as the flu usually begins its peak in December. It takes about 2 weeks for the vaccine to offer protection against the flu. Side effects from the shot are usually mild and may include redness, soreness, or swelling at the vaccination site, as well as fever or general body aches. These should disappear within a day or two. If your child is younger than 12 years, ask for the "split virus" shot, which usually causes fewer side effects than the "whole virus" vaccine. In very rare cases, a life-threatening allergic reaction occurs, characterized by swelling of the tongue and throat, severe difficulty breathing, and loss of consciousness. If such a reaction occurs, seek immediate medical assistance.

If you and your child want to avoid a shot, you can ask your doctor for a prescription for FluMist, a live intranasal flu vaccine approved by the FDA. Children ages 5 to 8 years need two treatments at least 6 weeks apart the first year they take this vaccine. FluMist should not be given to children who are younger than 5 years old or to those who have asthma, any other airway disease, any problems with immune system suppression (e.g., AIDS, cancer), or who are receiving drugs that cause immunosuppression. Children who are allergic to eggs also should not receive this vaccine.

FluMist has the advantage of not containing the preservative mercury/thimerosal (see earlier, "Weighing the Benefits and Risks of Immunization"), which prevents the growth of microorganisms in many multidose containers of flu vaccine. Not all flu shots contain this preservative, however. Make sure you ask your doctor for a mercury-free vaccine if you chose to have your child vaccinated. If you would like more information about this intranasal flu vaccine, you can read the package insert at the FDA website (*www.fda.gov/cber/label/inflmed061703LB.pdf*).

How to Be a Proactive Parent

In today's confusing and complex health-care environment, it's more important than ever for you to be informed and involved in your children's health care. Fortunately, many parents realize this is true, and so there are many citizen-based groups and sources of reliable information you can access. Before you can make any decisions about whether your child should get vaccinated and which vaccines he or she should get, you need to find out all you can about the benefits and risks of vaccinations from the research and from doctors and other professionals on both sides of the issue. Only then will you able to make an informed decision. To help you get started, we've provided a list of resources that looks at all sides of the issue (see below, "Resources for Parents").

You can also take steps to help prevent your child from having a reaction to a vaccine. Some children are at greater risk of reacting to vaccines. Your child may have a reaction if he or she:

- Reacted to a vaccine in the past
- Has a sibling or other family member who reacted to a vaccine
- Was born prematurely or with a low birth weight
- Has a personal or family history of an immune disease disorder, neurological disorder, convulsions, allergies, asthma, eczema, or allergy to cow's milk
- Is experiencing an illness, including a cold, ear infection, diarrhea, or flu, or is recovering from an illness within 1 month before the vaccination
- Has ever experienced brain trauma or irritation, such as meningitis or head trauma during delivery

Resources for Parents

Coalition for SafeMinds
Sensible Action for Ending Mercury-Induced
   Neurological Disorders
14 Commerce Drive, 3rd Floor
Cranford NJ 07016
908-276-8032
www.safeminds.org

Every Child By Two
666 11th Street NW, Suite 202
Washington DC 20001
202-783-7035
http://www.ecbt.org

Global Vaccine Awareness League
PO Box 846
Lake Forest CA 92630
949-929-1191
www.gval.com

Institute for Vaccine Safety
Johns Hopkins Bloomberg School of Public Health
615 N Wolfe Street, Room W5041
Baltimore MD 21205
410-995-2955
www.vaccinesafety.edu

National Childhood Vaccine Injury Compensation
    Program
Parklawn Building, Room 8A-46
5600 Fishers Lane
Rockville MD 20857
301-443-6593
www.hrsa.gov/vaccinecompensation

National Network for Immunization Information
301 University Blvd, CH 2.218
Galveston TX 77555
409-772-0199
www.immunizationinfo.org

National Vaccine Information Center (NVIC)
204 Mill Street, Suite B1
Vienna VA 22180
800-909-SHOT
www.909shot.com

Parents of Kids with Infectious Diseases (PKIDs)
PO Box 5666
Vancouver WA 98668
360-695-0293
www.pkids.org

People Advocating Vaccine Education (PAVE)
PO Box 36701
Charlotte NC 28236
www.vaccines.bizland.com

ThinkTwice Global Vaccine Institute
PO Box 9638
Santa Fe NM 87504
505-983-1856
http://www.thinktwice.com

Vaccine Adverse Events Reporting System (VAERS)
800-833-7967
www.fda.gov/cber/vaers/vaers.htm

The Vaccine Page: Vaccine News & Database
www.vaccines.com

Reporting Adverse Reactions

If your child has a serious adverse reaction after he or she
has received a vaccine, you should report it as soon as possible. There are two places to report this information. One is
the health-care professional who administered the vaccine.
He or she is required by law to report adverse reactions that
arise within 30 days of vaccination to the Vaccine Adverse
Event Reporting System (VAERS), a program run by the federal government. If the individual refuses or fails to do so,
you can make the report yourself or ask another organization,
the National Vaccine Information Center (NVIC), to help you
file a report. (Even if your health-care practitioner has filed
with VAERS, you should also report to the NVIC). The

NVIC is a nonprofit organization that maintains a database on vaccine adverse events. By reporting an adverse event to the NVIC, you can help experts find ways to prevent other children from experiencing the same vaccine-related response your child has had, as well as help contribute to the development of ways to avoid vaccine damage.

The Right to Say No

Many parents are unaware that they have a right to refuse vaccinations for their child. In fact, each state has its own process by which parents can get an exemption from vaccinating their child based on philosophical, medical, and/or religious reasons. Because states require children to meet state vaccination criteria before they enter school, parents need to seek an exemption before their child starts classes. In some cases, children have been removed from school or parents have been charged with neglect for failing to meet state standards for vaccinations.

If you are considering not vaccinating your child, you can get information at the following sites on how to file for an exemption:

www.909shot.com/state-site/legal-exemptions.htm
www.909shot.com/state-site/state-exemptions.htm
www.unhinderedliving.com/statevaccexemp.html

Vaccines provide peace of mind for a great many parents and help ensure the current health of our children and their healthier future. But each vaccine also carries an element of risk—more for some children than for others—and so the advantages and dangers of each and every immunization should be weighed before a decision of whether to vaccinate is made.

The Future of Vaccines

The CDC and other health agencies are contemplating the addition of more immunizations for children. In 1996, for example, the Advisory Committee on Immunization Practices recommended giving hepatitis A vaccinations to high-risk populations and routine vaccinations to children who live in areas that have the highest hepatitis A rates. In 1999, this committee expanded its recommendations for routine vaccination of children to include those who live in seventeen states that had consistently high rates of this disease. As of this writing, hepatitis A vaccines have not been added to the routine immunization schedule for children, but the possibility exists for that addition in the future.

Yet another example arose in summer 2005, when the CDC and the American Academy of Pediatrics released policy statements recommending a routine meningococcal vaccination for certain children and young adults—children 11 to 12 years of age, or adolescents 15 years of age who have not been vaccinated previously. Also included in the recommendation is all college freshmen who live in dormitories.

As with the vaccinations that are currently part of the recommended immunization schedule, parents should educate themselves about any new vaccines that may or will be added to this schedule.

PSYCHIATRIC DRUGS

Fourteen-year-old Emma seems depressed and withdrawn, and her once honor roll grades have slipped to Cs. Ten-year-old Scott has become a major discipline problem at school and at home, and his teacher has said "something must be done" or else he can't remain in the classroom. Eight-year-old Raymond has begun bullying his five-year-old sister and recently started to abuse the family dog. Eleven-year-old Constance can't pay attention in class and is always either looking out the window with a blank expression in her eyes or hopping out of her seat every few minutes. Is your child anywhere in this picture? Millions of parents can say yes, and at the same time they are asking, "Will he/she grow out of it? Is it just a phase? Should I/we be worried about this behavior? Does my child need medication?"

According to the Department of Health and Human Services, mental health problems affect 20 percent of young people at any given time, with an estimated 7.7 to 12.8 million children being affected. And there's more:

- As many as 3 percent of children and 12 percent of adolescents may have clinical depression.
- Attention deficit/hyperactivity disorder (ADHD), which is the most common psychiatric condition affecting children, is estimated to impact 5 to 10 percent of young people. Yet as many as half of children with ADHD are never diagnosed.
- Nearly one third of children ages 6 to 12 years who have been diagnosed with major depression will develop bipolar disorders within a few years.
- As many as 4 percent of children and adolescents may have conduct disorder.

Treatment of young people who are depressed or who have ADHD or similar conditions has become increasingly controversial in recent years, especially when it comes to prescription medications—antidepressants and stimulants, in particular. Antidepressants are used primarily for prevention and treatment of depression, as well as anxiety, obsessive-compulsive disorder, attention deficit/hyperactivity disorder, and other psychiatric and behavioral disorders, and often along with other medications as well. Stimulants (e.g., methylphenidate and amphetamines) are prescribed to treat ADHD and children who have educational, psychological, and social disorders.

Sharp Increase in Antidepressant and Stimulant Use

In recent years, there has been a surge in the use of antidepressants and similar drugs to treat psychiatric and behavioral conditions. A study of more than 900,000 children, published in the *Archives of Adolescent and Pediatric Medicine,* noted that prescriptions for children and adolescents who have behavioral and/or mood disorders doubled and in some cases tripled from 1987 through 1996. This trend continued in subsequent years: according to IMS Health, a respected source for pharmaceutical market information, the use of Prozac-like drugs for young people increased 74 percent between 1995 and 1999, prescriptions for newer antipsychotic drugs increased nearly 300 percent, and use of mood stabilizers (not including lithium) soared 4,000 percent.

Notice that we mention "Prozac-like drugs" when we talk about use of antidepressants in young people. That's because Prozac (fluoxetine) is the only antidepressant formally approved by the FDA for the treatment of major depressive disorder in pediatric patients. (Prozac, Zoloft, Luvox, and Anafranil have FDA approval for treatment of obsessive-compulsive disorder in pediatric patients.) That does not mean, however, that fluoxetine is the only antidepressant being prescribed for children: off-label prescribing—when a health-care provider prescribes a drug that has not been formally approved by the FDA for treatment of a specific condition—has been and continues to be a very common practice. But is it safe?

The same question can be asked about drugs given to treat ADHD. Chronic use of methylphenidate for example, the most widely used drug in the treatment of ADHD, and its different formulations (e.g., Ritalin, Concerta, Metadate) can result in tolerance and/or physical or mental dependence. Some experts warn that the drugs are being overprescribed, but others say they are underutilized. One major problem that is fueling this widely differing view of stimulant use among children is the difficulty in getting an accurate diagnosis. A recent review (*British Journal of Psychiatry*, 2003) of ADHD research studies concluded that "the number of young people being treated in the USA with stimulants . . . and who do not have ADHD is unacceptably high."

Contributing to this problem are the various and inconsistent guidelines for the treatment of ADHD, which leave much room for interpretation. One result is that some children are being treated with drugs simply because they are "behavior problems," despite never having been diagnosed with ADHD. Improved diagnostic guidelines and a clearer understanding of the cause and effects of ADHD and related conditions are needed. Another factor parents should be aware of is that **schools are given additional money by the state and federal government for every child it enrolls that has been diagnosed and medicated.** Therefore, schools have a financial incentive to demand that parents medicate any child who may display some behavior or attention problems. The dramatic increase in the number of children diagnosed with ADHD and similar conditions in the last few years coincides with this financial incentive. You should also know, however, that as of December 3, 2004, schools are prohibited from recommending or requiring that a child take a controlled substance (e.g., methylphenidate, amphetamines) in order to attend school. This right was extended to parents and guardians in the Prohibition on Mandatory Medication Amendment, which is part of the Individuals with Disabilities Education Improvement Act (IDEA).

How Safe Are Psychiatric Drugs?

This is a question parents are asking themselves and their doctors, especially since reports of an increased risk of suicide among children and adolescents who are taking antidepressants. This is how events unfolded. In 2004, the FDA reviewed the results of 23 clinical trials that included more than 4,400 children and adolescents who received any of nine different antidepressants for treatment of major depressive disorder, obsessive-compulsive disorder, and other psychiatric disorders. It found that 4 percent of patients shared thoughts about suicide or potentially dangerous behavior (referred to collectively as "suicidality") compared with 2 percent of patients who were taking placebo who had the same thoughts. No suicides occurred during any of these trials.

As a result of these findings, the FDA issued a "black box warning" for antidepressant medications used to treat depression and related disorders in children and adolescents, as well as adults. The warning appears on the label of all antidepressants (see list below) and makes the following points:

- Use of antidepressants increases the risk of suicidality in children and adolescents who have major depressive disorder or other psychiatric disorders.
- Individuals who start treatment with antidepressants should be observed closely for suicidality, unusual behavior changes, and any worsening of depressive symptoms.
- Anyone who is considering giving an antidepressant to a child or adolescent should carefully consider the risk of increased suicidality with the severity of need.
- Parents, family members, and caregivers should carefully observe the patient once he or she begins antidepressant treatment and report any unusual reactions to the doctor.

In June and July 2005, the FDA began issuing FDA Alerts for the antidepressants in the list, which stated in part that "suicidal thinking or behavior may increase in pediatric patients treated with any type of antidepressant, especially early in treatment," and that such thinking or behavior "can be expected in about 1 out of 50 treated pediatric patients." If your child is prescribed an antidepressant, you can also expect to receive information about the drug and possible effects in the form of a MedGuide, a publication distributed by the pharmacist with each prescription or refill of the medication. MedGuides are designed to inform consumers about the risk of suicidality in children and adolescents who are taking antidepressants. Drugs that have a black box warning and for which MedGuides have been prepared include the following:

Anafranil (clomipramine)
Asendin (amoxapine)
Aventyl (nortriptyline)
Celexa (citalopram)

Cymbalta (duloxetine)
Desyrel (trazodone)
Effexor (venlafaxine)
Elavil (amitriptyline)
Lexapro (escitalopram)
Limbitrol (chloridazepoxide/amitriptyline)
Ludiomil (maprotiline)
Luvox (fluvoxamine)
Nardil (phenelzine)
Norpramin (desipramine)
Pamelor (nortriptyline)
Parnate (tranylcypromine)
Paxil, Pexeva (paroxetine)
Prozac (fluoxetine)
Remeron (mirtazapine)
Sarafem (fluoxetine)
Serzone (nefazodone)
Sinequan (doxepin)
Surmontil (trimipramine)
Symbyax (olanzapine/fluoxetine)
Tofranil (imipramine)
Tofranil-PM (imipramine pamoate)
Wellbutrin (bupropion)
Zoloft (sertraline)
Zyban (bupropion)

Atypical Antipsychotic Drugs

During recent years, more and more physicians have prescribed atypical antipsychotic drugs (second generation antipsychotics) for children who have bipolar disorder or ADHD. Although mood stabilizers such as lithium and valproic acid have been the main drugs used to treat these children, mood stabilization is often very difficult to achieve using these drugs alone. Now, atypical antipsychotics, such as risperidone, clozapine, and olanzapine, among others, are being prescribed along with the standard mood stabilizers to help achieve stabilization. It is important for you to know several things about the use of atypical antipsychotics in children.

One is that there is limited data from controlled trials on the use of these medications in children and adolescents who have bipolar disorder or ADHD. Therefore, in most cases physicians base their treatment decisions on data from whatever studies are available and the specific needs of your child. The good news, however, is that more controlled studies in children and adolescents are being done.

Another critical point is that these drugs are associated with significant and even deadly side effects. FDA data from 2000 to 2004 show there were 45 deaths in children in which an atypical antipsychotic was the "primary suspect." During the same time period, more than 1,300 cases of serious side effects, some of them life-threatening, were also reported. The more common side effects included dystonia (neurological disorder characterized by involuntary muscle contractions), tremors, and significant weight gain. Research suggests that only 1 to 10 percent of deaths and side effects are reported to the FDA—although drug companies are required to make such reports, doctors and consumers are not—and so the actual number of affected children is much greater. The overall message, therefore, is that you need to be very cautious when it comes to use of atypical antipsychotics: talk with your physician and learn all you can about these drugs before you decide whether they are right for your child.

Stopping Antidepressants

Withdrawing from antidepressant treatment should be done under the supervision of your physician, as troublesome symptoms may occur. Despite gradual tapering of doses, however, symptoms may still appear. These symptoms are especially evident in patients taking selective serotonin reuptake inhibitors (SSRIs). The incidence of symptoms upon withdrawal is between 17 and 30 percent with two medications, paroxetine (Paxil) and fluvoxamine (Luvox), but less than 5 percent with other SSRIs. Symptoms include dizziness, irritability, nausea, poor mood, tingling of the extremities, and vivid dreams, any or all of which may appear within a few days of discontinuing medication. They generally last for about 12 days, but may persist for up to 3 weeks.

Safety of Stimulant Use

Between 1990 and 2000, there were 186 deaths from methylphenidate reported to the FDA's MedWatch program. It is generally acknowledged that the number of deaths and other adverse events filed with this voluntary report program is no more than 10 to 20 percent of the actual incidence. But even if the number were "only" 186, most people would likely agree that the deaths of 186 children because of a drug are 186 deaths too many.

The truth is, the impact of long-term use of stimulants in children is unknown. A few studies have looked at the use of methylphenidate in children for up to 24 months, but in reality, many children have been taking this and other stimulants for many more years. Because ADHD often extends into adulthood, millions of children may be taking these drugs for a period of decades. No one knows for sure what the consequences of such prolonged drug use will be, although there has been some research indicating these children are much more susceptible to addiction and drug abuse in later years. We do know that chronic or abusive use of methylphenidate and/or amphetamines and amphetamine-type drugs has the potential to result in mental or physical dependence. These drugs should always be used with caution in anyone who has a history of drug or alcohol abuse or mental illness.

Aside from the possible fatal effects of methylphenidate, the most common side effects include headache, insomnia, decreased appetite, nausea, vomiting, dizziness, nervousness, tics, and psychosis (abnormal thinking or hallucinations). Ritalin users may experience fever, rash, and various other skin reactions, as well as possible heart problems, including changes in blood pressure, angina, and cardiac arrhythmia. Amphetamines are more likely to cause restlessness, tremor, anxiety, nervousness, headache, dizziness, insomnia, dry mouth, diarrhea, or constipation.

COMBINATION COLD/FLU MEDICATIONS FOR CHILDREN

If you've walked into the cold medication aisle of a drugstore recently, you may have been overwhelmed by the number of choices. You would not be alone: many parents are confused by the variety, forms, and flavors of cold and flu medications with their promises to relieve from one to nearly a dozen symptoms. How do you choose the best medication for your child?

The first question should be, Does my child really need any of these medications? None of the medications will make your child get better faster than taking no medicine at all. What they *can* do is make your child feel more comfortable while the cold or flu runs its course. Beware, however, of overmedicating. Many cold and flu formulas are designed to treat multiple symptoms, some of which your child may not have. Such multisymptom formulas can expose your child to medications he or she does not need and, at the same time, a risk of side effects. It is wise, therefore, to select a formula that can address your child's specific symptoms or, if your child's symptoms are not especially bothersome or causing curtailment of activities, to forego any drug treatment at all.

If you do choose to medicate your child, here are a few things you should know:

- Expectorants are supposed to help loosen mucus, but their effectiveness in children is questionable. The drug typically included for this purpose in cold formulas is guaifenesin.
- Decongestants help relieve a stuffy, runny nose. Two ingredients, phenylephrine and pseudoephedrine, may be used for this purpose. A third substance, phenylpropanolamine (PPA) was removed from the market in 2000. Some children become irritable and hyperactive when taking a decongestant.
- Antihistamines can help dry up a runny nose and, because they cause drowsiness, also help your child

sleep. For that reason antihistamines are best given before bedtime. Common antihistamines in children's formulas include brompheniramine, chlorpheniramine, and diphenhydramine.

- In rare cases, children become highly excitable, rather than drowsy, when taking antihistamines.
- Antitussives (cough suppressants) include dextromethorphan (in over-the-counter formulas) or codeine or hydrocodone (prescription). The latter two drugs may cause drowsiness.
- When treating flu symptoms, avoid giving your child aspirin or any product that contains aspirin, as aspirin can cause an often fatal condition called Reye's syndrome.
- If you are giving your child more than one medication, read the ingredient information carefully to make sure your child is not getting an excessive amount of acetaminophen (see *Acetaminophen* entry for dosing information). Many cold and flu products contain acetaminophen, and it is not uncommon to inadvertently give your child an excessive amount of the drug.

Before you make your purchase, weigh the risks and benefits of giving the medication to your child. You can read about the potential side effects and other precautions for the individual drugs noted above in their respective entries, or talk to your doctor or pharmacist. In many cases, the best medicine for a bout of cold or flu is hot soup, plenty of fluids, and rest.

HERBAL SUPPLEMENTS FOR CHILDREN

As the use of herbal remedies increases among adults, especially women, it is no surprise that more and more parents are considering these remedies for their children. Unfortunately, many commonly used herbal supplements have not been evaluated in controlled, systematic studies, although in many cases there is much anecdotal evidence of effectiveness and safety. Some parents may be willing to "take a chance" themselves with an herbal remedy that hasn't been thoroughly investigated, but not willing to do so for their child. Therefore, any evidence that certain herbal remedies are safe and effective for children would be welcome news to these parents.

Study results published in March 2005 in *The Journal of Pediatrics* by Andrea Hrastinger, PhD, and her colleagues noted the effectiveness of several common herbal supplements for children, including evening primrose oil, ivy leaf, and valerian.

When it comes to treating asthma and chronic bronchitis, studies suggest that ivy leaf may increase airway resistance in the former and decrease symptoms in the latter. In fact, one third of children with bronchitis who took ivy leaf reported freedom from symptoms.

Evening primrose oil has proven effective in reducing the severity of dermatitis in children, as well as improving the performance of certain activities by children who have been diagnosed with hyperactivity disorders. Another herbal remedy useful for hyperactivity is valerian, which is also helpful for treating sleep disorders. One study found that boys with developmental deficiencies and hyperactivity experienced better sleep quality and improved sleep time after taking valerian nightly for 2 weeks.

While some herbal remedies have been shown to be safe and effective in adults, they often have not been appropriately tested in children. Therefore, you should consult your pediatrician before giving any herbal supplement to your children.

GUIDELINES FOR SAFE PEDIATRIC DRUG USE

In an ideal world, children would never need to take a drug: either they would never get ill, or there would be a perfect substance that would cure all maladies. Until that day comes, parents must face a world of pharmaceuticals that is fraught with side effects and warnings about possible drug interactions and other dangers that could harm their children, perhaps irreparably. To help you maneuver your way around this world, we offer guidelines on safe and effective drug purchase, use, and storage, as well as questions you should ask about your child's medication.

Questions You Should Ask about Your Child's Medication

Whether your child is taking an over-the-counter or prescription medication, you need to know all you can about that drug *before* your child uses it. Here is a list of questions you should be prepared to ask your doctor and/or pharmacist:

- What is the drug used for?
- Will the drug interact with any other drugs my child is taking? (Have a list handy to show your doctor/pharmacist.)
- How long will my child need to take the drug?
- What is the dosing schedule for this drug?
- What side effects might my child experience?
- How should this drug be stored?
- How soon until the medication begins to work?
- What should I do if my child misses a dose?

Over-the-Counter Medications

Although this book focuses on prescription medications, there likely will be many times you will give your child an over-the-counter (OTC) medication. In fact, some of the drugs your doctor will prescribe are available without a prescription as well. Just because a drug is available without a prescription does not mean it can't cause side effects or more serious consequences. Therefore, you should proceed with caution whenever you decide to give your child an OTC drug.

- Never give a child younger than 2 years an OTC drug without first consulting with his or her doctor.
- Make sure the safety seal is intact on OTC drugs.

- Read the label carefully. If the label doesn't have information on pediatric doses, consult with your physician or pharmacist before giving it to your child, especially if he or she is younger than 12 years of age.
- Many drugs, especially cold medications, contain alcohol and/or antihistamines, which can cause adverse reactions in young children, such as excessive drowsiness or excitability. Talk to your doctor before giving such medications to your child.
- Before you give your child an OTC drug, stop and consider whether it's truly necessary. The common cold and other common viruses run their course in 7 to 10 days with or without medication. Although some OTC drugs can relieve some symptoms, they may also cause allergic reactions or trigger problems with eating, sleeping, or behavior. In such cases, lots of fluids and rest, along with optimal nutrition may be the best medicine. Consult with your physician before running to the medicine cabinet.
- Never give your child aspirin or aspirin-containing products for fever or pain, as it can cause an often fatal condition called Reye's syndrome.

How to Read a Prescription Label

A prescription label should contain a lot of important information about your child and the drug he or she is supposed to take. Look for the following: your child's full name, the name of the prescriber, the drug name (trade and/or generic), the pharmacy's address and telephone number, a prescription number, instructions on how to use the drug, the number of refills allowed, the date it was dispensed, and a drug expiration date. Make sure all of this information is on the label before you leave the pharmacy.

Instructions on how to use the drug are typically in a type of shorthand that can be very difficult to decipher. It is best to ask the pharmacist to review these instructions with you. The table "How to Read Abbreviations on a Prescription Label" provides an explanation of the instructions you may encounter.

HOW TO READ ABBREVIATIONS ON A PRESCRIPTION LABEL		
Abbreviation	*Latin for*	*What It Means*
ac	ante cibum	before meals
bid	bis in die	twice a day
hs	hora somni	at bedtime
od	oculus dexter	right eye
os	oculus sinister	left eye
pc	post cibum	after meals
po	per os	by mouth (orally)
prn	pro re nata	as needed
q3h	quaque 3 hora	every three hours
qd	quaque die	every day (daily)
qid	quarter in die	four times a day
tid	ter in die	three times a day

How to Take and Stop Taking Medications

The vast majority of people don't ask their doctor or pharmacist any questions about the medications they've been prescribed. Although this can result in significant problems with people of any age, it is especially critical when the prescription is for children, as in most cases they must depend on a parent or other caregiver to make sure the right drug is prescribed and dispensed properly.

Once you have the proper drug in hand, it's important to understand exactly how the drug should be given. Timing is everything. If the instructions say to give the drug 3 times a day, does that mean every 8 hours, 3 times during waking hours, or with each meal? If it means every 8 hours, does that mean you will need to wake your child at midnight to administer the last dose of the day? If it means during waking hours, how far apart should the drug be given? Be sure you have specific instructions from your doctor or pharmacist. It is also critical to tell your doctor whether your child is taking any other medication (prescription or over-the-counter), supplements, or herbal remedies, as they may interact with the prescription drug.

If at any time you want to stop giving a particular drug to your child, do not do so without first consulting with your physician, as adverse reactions can occur. Narcotics, including codeine and morphine for pain or chronic cough, and antianxiety drugs, for example, can cause severe withdrawal symptoms, such as vomiting, hallucinations, and tremors, if they are stopped abruptly, whereas certain antidepressants and sedatives can cause nausea and vomiting.

How to Prevent Overdoses and Poisonings

Children are naturally curious, so it's important to handle medications responsibly in your home. Here are some tips on how to prevent overdoses and poisonings.

- Child-resistant caps only work if they are put on properly. Make sure you replace caps on medication containers correctly.
- Always give medications in adequate light. If you need to dose your child in the middle of the night, make sure you have sufficient light to see the label clearly. Giving medication in poor light increases the chance of administering a wrong dose.
- If you need to measure out a liquid medication, it is very important that you use the measuring device provided with the medicine. Do *not* use regular kitchen utensils; they are not accurate measuring tools. If the medication does not come with the proper measuring instrument, ask your pharmacist for one. For reference: 1 teaspoon (tsp) = 5 mL (milliliters); 1 tablespoon (Tbs) = 3 tsp = 15 mL; 1 ounce (oz) = 30 mL.
- Keep all medications out of reach and sight of children. There are so many look-alike medications on the market, children are easily fooled into thinking a medication is candy or something else to eat or drink. There is also always the chance that children will put anything they find into their mouth, just out of curiosity or because they are hungry or thirsty.
- When giving your child medication, put it away immediately after you administer it.
- Never tell your child that a medication is like candy or soda or that it "tastes good."

- Throw away any unneeded or unwanted medications by emptying the containers, crushing the contents, and flushing them down the toilet. Liquid medications can be poured down the sink.
- Keep the telephone numbers for your doctor and the Poison Control Center next to every phone in the house. The Poison Control Center number is 1-800-222-1222.
- If you leave your children with a babysitter, make sure he or she knows how to reach the doctor and Poison Control Center.
- The American Academy of Pediatrics no longer recommends that syrup of ipecac be used in cases of accidental poisoning, as it can cause serious damage if used incorrectly, and more effective treatments are now available. However, if you live more than 30 minutes away from a hospital, your doctor may recommend you keep ipecac on hand. It's important that you never use ipecac unless you have been told to do so by your physician or the Poison Control Center.
- Activated charcoal is now often used in poisoning cases because it binds to certain poisons and allows them to leave the body safely through the intestinal tract. You can purchase activated charcoal at pharmacies. Do not use it, however, unless instructed to do so by a physician or the Poison Control Center.

DRUG PROFILES

ACETAMINOPHEN

BRAND NAMES
Acephen, Anacin-3, Datril, Feverall Suppositories, Jr. Strength Tylenol Caplets, Liquiprin, Phenaphen, St. Joseph Aspirin-Free, Suppap, Tempra, Tylenol Chewable Tablets, Tylenol Drops, Tylenol Elixir
Generic Available/Over-the-Counter Available

ABOUT THIS DRUG
Acetaminophen is an analgesic (painkiller) and antipyretic (antifever). It relieves pain and fever by reducing production of substances in the body that cause these symptoms.

SIDE EFFECTS
Acetaminophen rarely causes side effects if it is used as directed. However, contact your physician if your child experiences any side effects that are persistent or troubling, including any that are not listed here.

- *Less common:* anemia, rash. Contact your physician if your child has fever or yellowing of the eyes or skin.

HOW TO USE THIS DRUG
Acetaminophen is available in chewable tablets, regular tablets, capsules, liquid/elixir, drops, and suppositories. The dosages given here are ones that are usually recommended. However, you should consult your doctor about the specific brand or prescription of acetaminophen you have for your child and allow him or her to determine the most appropriate dose and schedule.

- Children younger than 4 months: 40 mg given 4 to 5 times daily
- Children 4 to 11 months: 80 mg given 4 to 5 times daily

- Children 1 to 2 years: 120 mg given 4 to 5 times daily
- Children 3 years: 160 mg given 4 to 5 times daily
- Children 4 to 5 years: 240 mg given 4 to 5 times daily
- Children 6 to 8 years: 320 mg given 4 to 5 times daily
- Children 9 to 10 years: 400 mg given 4 to 5 times daily
- Children 11 years: 480 mg given 4 to 5 times daily
- Children 12 years and older: 300 to 600 mg given 4 to 6 times daily; or 1,000 mg given 3 to 4 times daily.

Do not give acetaminophen to your child for more than three consecutive days without consulting your doctor. If you use acetaminophen to treat fever, do not wake your child to give the medication, as it is important for your child to sleep. If your child misses a dose, give it as soon as you remember. However, if it is within an hour of the next dose, do not give the skipped dose and continue with the regular dosing schedule.

TIME UNTIL IT TAKES EFFECT
Typically provides results within 30 minutes to 2 hours.

POSSIBLE DRUG, FOOD, AND/OR SUPPLEMENT INTERACTIONS
Tell your doctor if your child is taking any prescription or over-the-counter medications or any vitamins, herbs, or other supplements. Possible interactions with acetaminophen may include the following:

- Use of barbiturates (e.g., phenobarbital, carbamazepine, phenytoin, rifampin) can increase the risk of liver damage.
- Do not give your child acetaminophen with any of the following drugs for more than a few days unless your physician is supervising: aspirin or other salicylates, diclofenac, diflunisal, etodolac, fenoprofen, ibuprofen, indomethacin, ketoprofen, ketorolac, meclofenamate, mefenamic acid, naproxen, oxaprozin, phenylbutazone, piroxicam, sulindac, tenoxicam, and tolmetin.

SYMPTOMS OF OVERDOSE

Symptoms include nausea, vomiting, sweating, and loss of appetite. Acetaminophen overdose can cause significant liver damage. If an overdose occurs, seek immediate medical attention and bring the drug container(s) with you.

THINGS TO TELL YOUR DOCTOR

- Tell your physician if your child has had allergic reactions to any medications in the past, if he or she is taking any medications now, or if your child has any disease or medical condition.
- Contact your physician immediately if your child has a fever of 105° F or higher.
- If your child is taking acetaminophen to relieve pain and the pain lasts for more than 5 days, the pain gets worse, or new symptoms develop, consult your doctor as soon as possible, as these are signs of a serious condition.
- Consult your doctor if your child becomes pregnant while taking acetaminophen.

IMPORTANT PRECAUTIONS

- If your child is taking any other medication—prescription or over-the-counter drugs—check to see if they contain acetaminophen, as taking such medications along with acetaminophen may cause an overdose.
- Store acetaminophen in a tightly closed container and keep at room temperature away from excess heat and moisture (e.g., the bathroom, near a stove or sink).
- Do not allow the liquid and suppository forms of acetaminophen to freeze.

ACETAMINOPHEN PLUS CODEINE

BRAND NAMES

APAP with Codeine, Capital with Codeine, Codaphen, Margesic, Myapap with Codeine, Phenaphen with Codeine,

Proval, Ty-Pap with Codeine, Ty-Tab with Codeine, Tylenol with Codeine
Generic Available

ABOUT THIS DRUG

Acetaminophen + codeine is a narcotic analgesic (pain-killer) used to treat mildly to moderately severe pain. The acetaminophen component helps reduce pain and fever, and the codeine portion helps reduce moderate to severe pain, suppresses cough, and induces a calming effect. Both of these drugs suppress certain brain functions that are associated with pain perception and emotional response to pain. Codeine also has an effect on the cough reflex.

SIDE EFFECTS

Contact your doctor if your child experiences any side effects that are persistent or troubling, including any that are not listed here.

- *Most common:* constipation, dizziness, drowsiness, dry mouth, lightheadedness, nausea, sedation, shortness of breath, urinary retention, vomiting
- *Less common/rare:* abdominal pain, rash, allergic reactions (difficulty breathing, hives, swelling), depression, itching. Seek immediate medical help if your child suffers an allergic reaction.

HOW TO USE THIS DRUG

Acetaminophen + codeine is available as capsules, elixir, oral suspension, and tablets. Generally, children are given the elixir or oral suspension rather than the capsules or tablets. The dosages given here are ones that are usually recommended for children. However, your doctor may provide different dosing instructions, which should be followed.

- Children 3 to 6 years: 1 teaspoon elixir 3 or 4 times daily
- Children 7 to 12 years: 2 teaspoons elixir 3 or 4 times daily

- Children 13 years and older: 1 tablespoon every 4 hours as needed. For tablets, 15 to 60 mg of codeine and 300 to 1,000 mg acetaminophen per dose.

Give your child this medicine with food to reduce the risk of stomach upset. If your child has difficulty swallowing the tablet, it can be crushed and placed in a small amount of soft food, such as applesauce or pudding, which should be swallowed, not chewed.

If your child misses a dose, give it as soon as you remember. If it is nearly time for the next dose, skip the missed dose and continue with the regular dosing schedule. Never give a double dose.

TIME UNTIL IT TAKES EFFECT
30 to 60 minutes

POSSIBLE DRUG, FOOD, AND/OR SUPPLEMENT INTERACTIONS
Tell your doctor if your child is taking any prescription or over-the-counter medications or any vitamins, herbs, or other supplements. Possible interactions with acetaminophen plus codeine may include the following:

- Cimetidine may increase the risk of breathing problems and suppression of the central nervous system.
- This drug combination may increase the effects of antianxiety medications (e.g., diazepam), antidepressants (e.g., amitriptyline), tranquilizers (e.g., haloperidol), antihistamines (e.g., chlorpheniramine), other narcotic painkillers (e.g., meperidine), anticonvulsants (e.g., benztropine), and other drugs that suppress the central nervous system.
- Use of antihistamine-like drugs increases the risk of urinary retention and constipation.
- Any herb that produces a sedative effect (e.g., capsicum, catnip, goldenseal, gotu kola, hops, kava, passionflower, sage, Siberian ginseng, St. John's wort, and valerian, among others) should be avoided, as

they may cause potentially serious excessive sedation.

SYMPTOMS OF OVERDOSE
Symptoms include bluish skin, cold and clammy skin, extreme sleepiness, heart problems, excessive sweating, kidney problems, limp muscles, liver failure, low blood pressure, nausea, slow heartbeat, and vomiting. If overdose occurs, seek immediate medical attention and bring the drug container(s) with you.

THINGS TO TELL YOUR DOCTOR
- Tell your doctor if your child has had allergic reactions to any medications in the past or if he or she is taking any medications now.
- Let your doctor know if your child has any of the following medical conditions: adrenal, kidney, liver, or thyroid disease, difficulty urinating, stomach disorders.
- Before your child takes this drug, tell your doctor if your child has ever suffered a head injury.
- Use of acetaminophen + codeine during pregnancy can result in physical dependence and withdrawal symptoms, and may cause breathing problems in newborns if taken during or before delivery. Consult your doctor if your child is pregnant and taking this drug.

IMPORTANT PRECAUTIONS
- Acetaminophen + codeine should not be used for more than 2 weeks and may become less effective before that time.
- Because this drug can cause drowsiness, dizziness, lightheadedness, and/or sedation, monitor your child carefully when he or she takes it and do not let your child participate in potentially dangerous activities, such as riding a bike, driving a car, or operating machinery.
- Store acetaminophen + codeine in a tightly closed container and keep at room temperature away from excess heat and moisture (e.g., the bathroom, near a stove or sink). Do not allow the oral solution or elixir to freeze.

ACETAZOLAMIDE

BRAND NAMES
Ak-Zol, Dazamide, Diamox, Diamox Sequels
Generic Available

ABOUT THIS DRUG
Acetazolamide is an anticonvulsant medication prescribed
for several conditions, including seizures and glaucoma. For
seizures, acetazolamide is believed to reduce the firing of
neurons in the brain. When given for glaucoma, it blocks the
enzyme carbonic anhydrase, which in turn reduces the se-
cretion of fluid inside the eyeball.

SIDE EFFECTS
Contact your physician if your child experiences any side effects that are persistent or troubling, including any that are
not listed here.

- *Most common:* diarrhea, increased urination, loss of
  appetite, metallic taste, nausea, ringing in the ears, tingling ("pins and needles") in the extremities, mouth, or
  anus; vomiting
- *Less common or rare:* anemia, bloody or black stools,
  blood in urine, confusion, convulsions, drowsiness,
  fever, hives, liver problems, nearsightedness, paralysis,
  peeling skin, photosensitivity, rash

HOW TO USE THIS DRUG
Acetazolamide is available in extended-release capsules and
regular tablets. The dosages given here are ones that are usually recommended. However, your doctor will determine the
most appropriate dose and schedule for your child.

- For seizures, tablets only: 4.5 mg per lb of body weight
  daily, in divided doses
- For glaucoma, tablets only: 4.5 to 6.8 mg per lb of
  body weight daily, in divided doses

Acetazolamide can be taken with food to help reduce the risk of stomach upset. If your child has difficulty swallowing the tablets, they can be crushed and mixed with 2 teaspoons of honey (do not give honey to a child younger than 1 year old) and 2 teaspoons of water. If your child misses a dose, give it as soon as you remember. However, if it is nearly time for the next scheduled dose, do not give the missed dose. Continue with the prescribed dosing schedule.

TIME UNTIL IT TAKES EFFECT
Capsules: 2 hours; tablets: 1 to 1.5 hours.

POSSIBLE DRUG, FOOD, AND/OR SUPPLEMENT INTERACTIONS
Tell your doctor if your child is taking any prescription or over-the-counter medications or any vitamins, herbs, or other supplements. Possible interactions with acetazolamide may include the following:

- Acetazolamide causes a loss of potassium, so it should be taken with potassium-rich foods, such as bananas, citrus, or melon.
- When used with carbamazepine, phenobarbital, phenytoin, or primidone, acetazolamide can cause anemia, increased softening of the bones, and blood abnormalities.
- Use of acetazolamide with amphetamines, ephedrine, flecainide, mexiletine, pseudoephedrine, tocainide, or quinidine can result in an increased risk of side effects with these drugs.
- Acetazolamide may reduce the response to insulin or oral antidiabetic medications.
- Use of acetazolamide along with diflunisal may cause excessive reduction of eye pressure.
- Use of acetazolamide along with primidone may delay or prevent absorption of the latter drug.
- Use of adrenocorticoids with acetazolamide may increase the risk of edema or hypernatremia.

SYMPTOMS OF OVERDOSE

Symptoms include decreased appetite, dizziness, drowsiness, nausea, numbness or tingling in the extremities, ringing in the ears, tremors, and vomiting. If an overdose occurs, seek medical attention immediately and bring the prescription container(s) with you.

THINGS TO TELL YOUR DOCTOR

• Tell your physician if your child has had allergic reactions to any medications in the past or if he or she is taking any medications now.

• Let your doctor know if your child has any of the following medical conditions, as use of acetazolamide may cause complications: diabetes, emphysema, low potassium levels, kidney disease, kidney stones, liver disease, or Addison's disease.

IMPORTANT PRECAUTIONS

• If your child becomes pregnant while taking acetazolamide, inform your physician immediately. No studies have adequately studied the impact of acetazolamide during pregnancy or breastfeeding.

• Store acetazolamide at room temperature in a tightly closed, light-resistant container away from excess heat or moisture (e.g., in a bathroom, near a sink).

ACYCLOVIR

BRAND NAME

Zovirax
Generic Available

ABOUT THIS DRUG

Acyclovir is an antiviral drug used to treat various herpes viral infections, including chicken pox. It works by interfering with the reproduction of DNA in the herpes viruses and hinders the growth of existing viruses.

SIDE EFFECTS
Contact your physician if your child experiences any side effects that are persistent or troubling, including any that are not listed here.

- *Most common (oral doses):* diarrhea, nausea, overall bodily discomfort, vomiting
- *Less common and rare (oral doses):* constipation, fever, headache, loss of appetite, leg pain, sleeplessness, sore throat

HOW TO USE THIS DRUG
Acyclovir is available in tablets and capsules, as an oral suspension, and via injection. (Information on the injectable form is not provided here.) The dosages given here are ones that are usually recommended for children. However, your doctor will determine the most appropriate dose and schedule for your child.

For Chicken Pox
- Children who weigh more than 88 lbs: 800 mg 4 times a day for 5 days
- Children 2 years and older who weigh 88 lbs or less: Dose is based on body weight and should be determined by your doctor. The typical dose is 9 mg per lb of body weight, up to 800 mg, 4 times a day for 5 days

Acyclovir can be taken with food to reduce the chance of stomach upset. If your child does not take acyclovir with food, he or she should take it with a full glass of water. Your child should take all the acyclovir that has been prescribed, even if he or she feels better before the prescription has been completed.

If your child misses a dose, give it unless it is near the time for the next dose, in which case you should skip the missed dose and continue with the regular dosing schedule. Never give a double dose.

TIME UNTIL IT TAKES EFFECT
It may take several days for it to affect the infection.

POSSIBLE DRUG, FOOD, AND/OR SUPPLEMENT INTERACTIONS
Tell your doctor if your child is taking any prescription or over-the-counter medications or any vitamins, herbs, or other supplements. Possible interactions with acyclovir may include the following:

- Use of cyclosporine may increase the risk of kidney toxicity.
- Meperidine may cause neurological problems.
- Use of phenytoin or valproic acid may cause a loss of control with seizures.
- Use of herbal remedies such as ephedra, ginseng, saw palmetto, or licorice may cause blood pressure to rise and reduce the effects of acyclovir.

SYMPTOMS OF OVERDOSE
Symptoms include hallucinations, kidney damage (reduction in urine output), and seizures. If overdose occurs, seek immediate medical attention and bring the drug container(s) with you.

THINGS TO TELL YOUR DOCTOR
- Tell your physician if your child has had allergic reactions to any medications in the past, if he or she is taking any medications now, or if your child has any disease or medical condition.
- If your child develops unusual bruising or bleeding under the skin while using this drug, tell your doctor immediately.
- Although use of acyclovir appears to be safe during pregnancy, tell your doctor if your child becomes pregnant while taking this drug.

SPECIAL PRECAUTIONS

- It is important for your child to drink a lot of liquids while taking acyclovir. Talk to your doctor about the proper amount for your child.
- Store acyclovir at room temperature in a tightly closed, light-resistant container away from excess heat and moisture (e.g., in a bathroom, near a stove or sink). The liquid form can be refrigerated, but do not allow it to freeze.

ALBUTEROL

BRAND NAMES
Proventil, Proventil HFA, Ventolin, Volmax
Generic Available

ABOUT THIS DRUG
Albuterol is a bronchodilator that is prescribed to relieve shortness of breath and wheezing associated with lung conditions such as asthma, bronchitis, and emphysema. It works by relaxing constricted airways.

SIDE EFFECTS
Contact your doctor if your child experiences any side effects that are persistent or troubling, including any that are not listed here.

- *Common:* aggression, agitation, appetite changes, cough, diarrhea, dizziness, general discomfort, headache, increased difficulty breathing, muscle cramps, nausea, nightmares, nosebleed, palpitations, rash, ringing in the ears, sleeplessness, sore throat, stuffy nose, tremors, vomiting, wheezing
- *Common for Proventil HFA:* allergic reaction, back pain, fever, inflamed nasal passages, respiratory infection, urinary difficulties

On very rare occasions, albuterol has caused life-threatening allergic reactions with symptoms that include swelling of the tongue and throat, rapid heartbeat, and hives. If such a reaction occurs, seek immediate medical attention.

HOW TO USE THIS DRUG

Albuterol is available in forms to be used in a nebulizer or metered-dose inhaler (inhalation capsules, inhalation solution, inhalation aerosol), as well as tablets and syrup. The dosages given here are ones that are usually recommended. However, your doctor will determine the most appropriate dose and schedule for your child.

Inhalation Solution—0.5%

- Children 2 to 11 years: Dosing is based on body weight, 0.045 to 0.048 mg per lb of body weight per dose, not to exceed 1.13 mg per dose taken 3 or 4 times daily.
- Children 12 years and older: 2.5 mg 3 or 4 times daily by nebulizer. More frequent or higher dosing is not recommended.

Inhalation Aerosol

- Children 4 years and older: Ventolin, 2 inhalations every 4 to 6 hours for severe bronchial spasm or to prevent asthmatic symptoms.
- Children 12 years and older: Proventil and Proventil HFA, 2 inhalations every 4 to 6 hours for severe bronchial spasm or to prevent asthmatic symptoms.

Tablets

- Children 6 to 11 years: Starting dose is 2 mg 3 or 4 times daily. Your doctor may increase the dose as needed, with the maximum daily dose not exceeding 32 mg.
- Children 12 years and older: Starting dose is 2 or 4 mg, 3 to 4 times daily. Your doctor may increase the dose as needed, with the maximum daily dose not exceeding 32 mg.

Proventil Repetabs and Volmax Extended-Release Tablets

- Children 6 to 11 years: For Proventil Repetabs, starting dose is 4 mg every 4 hours. Your doctor may increase the dose, with the maximum daily dosage not exceeding 24 mg.
- Children 12 years and older: 8 mg every 12 hours.

Syrup

- Children 2 to 6 years: Starting dose is 0.041 mg per lb of body weight 3 times a day.
- Children 7 to 14 years: Starting dose is 1 teaspoon, 3 or 4 times daily.
- Children 15 years and older: Starting dose is 1 or 2 teaspoons, 3 or 4 times daily.

If your child misses a dose, give it as soon as you remember. However, if it is nearly time for the next dose, do not give the missed dose. Continue with the regular dosing schedule. Do not give a double dose.

If your child is using an inhaler, make sure he or she inhales during the second half of the intake breath. If your doctor wants your child to take 2 inhalations, he or she should wait 5 minutes between puffs. If your child takes the extended-release tablet, you may notice the tablet coating in the stool, as the medicine does not dissolve in the stomach.

TIME UNTIL IT TAKES EFFECT

5 to 15 minutes for oral inhalation; up to 30 minutes for tablets.

POSSIBLE DRUG, FOOD, AND/OR SUPPLEMENT INTERACTIONS

Tell your doctor if your child is taking any prescription or over-the-counter medications or any vitamins, herbs, or other supplements. Possible interactions with albuterol may include the following:

- Amphetamines, dopamine, ephedrine, isoproterenol, and phenylephrine may worsen adverse effects on the heart.

- Theophylline may cause albuterol to leave the body rapidly and thus your child will lose the drug's benefits.
- Thiazide and loop diuretics (e.g., furosemide) may cause additional reductions in potassium levels.
- Tricyclic antidepressants may cause a significant rise in blood pressure.

SYMPTOMS OF OVERDOSE

An overdose of inhaled albuterol can cause chest pain, high blood pressure, and, rarely, death. If your child overdoses on the tablets, symptoms may include palpitations, unusual heart rhythm, chest pain, high blood pressure, fever, chills, cold sweats, nausea, vomiting, convulsions, tremors, or collapse. If overdose occurs, seek medical attention immediately and bring the prescription container with you.

THINGS TO TELL YOUR DOCTOR

- Tell your doctor if your child has had allergic reactions to any medications in the past or if he or she is taking any medications now.
- Tell your doctor if your child has a heart condition, seizure disorder, high blood pressure, hyperthyroidism, or diabetes.
- Seek immediate medical attention if your child experiences a serious allergic reaction (symptoms include hives, swelling of the mouth, lips, tongue, and throat) or if your child has skin reddening or peeling (the latter two signs are associated with use of the syrup).
- If your child is pregnant or becomes pregnant while taking albuterol, consult your doctor. Albuterol may cause high blood pressure, rapid heartbeat, and other reactions.

IMPORTANT PRECAUTIONS

- Store the syrup and solution for inhalation in the refrigerator or at room temperature. The aerosol can be stored at temperatures as low as 60° F, but should be at room temperature before use. Nebules must be used within 2 weeks of removing them from the refrigerator.

- If your child is using an inhaler, the device should be cleaned at least once a week. Remove the medication container from the plastic mouthpiece, wash the mouthpiece with warm water, and dry thoroughly. Make sure that your child uses the inhaler properly by observation.
- If your child is using albuterol inhalation aerosol, he or she should not be using any other inhaled medications without the consent of your doctor.

ALCLOMETASONE—
see *Corticosteroids, Topical*

AMANTADINE

BRAND NAME
Symmetrel
Generic Available

ABOUT THIS DRUG
Amantadine is an antiviral agent that is used to prevent or treat type A influenza (flu) infections. It is not effective against other types of flu or other viral infections, or against the common cold. This drug has been tested in children older than 1 year of age.

SIDE EFFECTS
Contact your physician if your child experiences any side effects that are persistent or troubling, including any that are not listed here.

- *More common:* agitation, anxiety, blurry vision, difficulty concentrating, dizziness, headache, irritability, loss of appetite, nausea, nightmares, red blotchy spots on the skin, difficulty sleeping
- *Less common or rare:* constipation; diarrhea; dry mouth, nose, and throat; headache, vomiting, unusual weakness or tiredness

HOW TO USE THIS DRUG

Amantadine is available in capsules and tablets, and as a syrup. The dosages given here are ones that are usually recommended for children. However, your doctor will determine the most appropriate dose and schedule for your child.

- Children 1 to 9 years: dose is based on body weight and must be determined by your doctor. The usual dose is 2 to 4 mg per lb of body weight given in two divided doses, not to exceed 70 mg per day.
- Children 10 to 12 years: 100 mg 2 times a day.
- Children 13 years and older: 200 mg once daily or 100 mg twice daily

Your child can take amantadine with food or milk to help prevent stomach irritation. If your child misses a dose, give it as soon as you remember. However, if it is nearly time for the next dose, do not give the forgotten dose and return to the regular dosing schedule. Do not give a double dose.

If you are using the syrup, use the measuring spoon that comes with the prescription, as using a kitchen spoon will likely dispense an incorrect dose.

TIME UNTIL IT TAKES EFFECT

For treatment of flu, this drug works best if started within 24 to 48 hours after the onset of signs or symptoms and should continue to be taken for 24 to 48 hours after signs and symptoms disappear. To prevent flu, amantadine should be started as soon as possible after exposure to the flu virus and continued for at least 10 days.

POSSIBLE DRUG, FOOD, AND/OR SUPPLEMENT INTERACTIONS

Tell your doctor if your child is taking any prescription or over-the-counter medications or any vitamins, herbs, or other supplements. Possible interactions with amantadine may include the following:

- Amphetamines; appetite suppressants; medications for asthma or other respiratory problems; medications for colds, sinus problems, or allergies (including sprays and nose drops); methylphenidate, or nabilone may cause irregular heartbeat, seizures, irritability, nervousness, or sleep problems.
- Use of anticholinergics (medications to treat stomach spasms or cramps) may increase the risk of blurry vision, dry mouth, hallucinations, nightmares, and confusion.
- Use of quinidine, trimethoprim and sulfamethoxazole may increase the level of amantadine in the blood and thus the chance for side effects.

SYMPTOMS OF OVERDOSE

Symptoms may include confusion, hallucinations, urinary retention; death is possible. If overdose occurs, seek medical attention immediately and bring the prescription container with you to the hospital.

THINGS TO TELL YOUR DOCTOR

- Tell your physician if your child has had allergic reactions to any medications in the past or if he or she is taking any medications now.
- Let your doctor know if your child has a history of epilepsy or seizures, heart disease, recurrent eczema, kidney disease, or emotional illness.
- Consult your doctor if your child is pregnant or becomes pregnant while taking amantadine.

IMPORTANT PRECAUTIONS

- This medication can cause blurry vision and dizziness, so be sure you know how your child reacts to the drug before he or she participates in potentially hazardous activities, such as riding a bike, driving a car, or operating machinery.
- Keep the capsules in a tightly closed container away from excess heat and moisture (e.g., in a bathroom, near a stove or sink).

- Amantadine can exacerbate mental problems in individuals who have a history of substance abuse or psychiatric disorders.

AMCINONIDE—see *Corticosteroids, Topical*

AMINOPHYLLINE— see *Xanthine Bronchodilators*

AMITRIPTYLINE— see *Tricyclic Antidepressants*

AMOXICILLIN—see *Penicillin Antibiotics*

AMPICILLIN—see *Pencillin Antibiotics*

CLASS: ANALGESIC-DECONGESTANT-ANTITUSSIVE-(ANTIHISTAMINE) COMBINATION

GENERICS
(1) acetaminophen + pseudoephedrine + dextromethorphan;
(2) acetaminophen + pseudoephedrine + dextromethorphan + (chlorpheniramine)

BRAND NAMES
(1) Comtrex Daytime Maximum Strength Cold, Cough, and Flu Relief, Contac Cold/Flu Day Caplets, TheraFlu Maximum Strength Non-Drowsy Formula Flu, Cold, and Cough, Triaminic Sore Throat Formula, Tylenol Cold & Flu No Drowsiness Powder, Tylenol Cold Non-Drowsy, Tylenol Multi-Symptom Cough, Vicks DayQuil Multi-Symptom

Cold/Flu LiquiCaps; (2) Alka-Seltzer Plus Cold & Cough
Liqui-Gels, Children's Tylenol Cold Plus Cough Multi-
Symptom, TheraFlu Flu, Cold & Cough, Tylenol Cold,
Tylenol Cold Multi-Symptom

ABOUT THESE DRUGS
Drug combinations that consist of an analgesic (acetaminophen), a decongestant (pseudoephedrine), an antitussive
(dextromethorphan), and an antihistamine (chlorpheniramine) are used to treat symptoms of cold and flu. Because
of the great variety of combination medications available,
we recommend that you consult your doctor about dosing
instructions for your child or carefully follow the instructions on the package. For additional information about these
drugs, see individual entries for *Acetaminophen*, *Dextromethorphan*, *Pseudoephedrine*, and *Chlorpheniramine*.
Also refer to the section in the introductory material on
"Combination Cold/Flu Medications for Children."

CLASS: ANTIEMETICS

GENERICS
(1) dolasetron; (2) granisetron; (3) ondansetron; (4)
palonosetron

BRAND NAMES
(1) Anzemet; (2) Kytril; (3) Zofran; (4) Aloxi
Generic Available for ondansetron only

ABOUT THESE DRUGS
Antiemetics, or antinausea drugs, are used to prevent and
treat the nausea and vomiting that frequently occur postsurgery or after treatment with chemotherapy. They work
by interfering with the nerve transmissions and the serotonin chemical receptor sites that stimulate nausea and
vomiting.

SIDE EFFECTS
Contact your physician if your child experiences any side effects that are persistent or troubling, including any that are not listed here.

Dolasetron
- *Most common:* chills, diarrhea, dizziness, fatigue, fever, headache, hypertension, indigestion, rapid or slow heartbeat
- *Less common or rare:* abnormal vision, flushing, hypotension, rash, taste changes, vertigo

Granisetron
- *Most common:* abdominal pain, constipation, diarrhea, headache, nausea, vomiting
- *Less common:* anxiety, dizziness, fever, hair loss, insomnia, loss of appetite

Ondansetron
- *More common:* constipation, diarrhea, fever, headache
- *Less common:* abdominal pain or cramps, dizziness, drowsiness, dry mouth, feeling cold, itching, unusual weakness
- *Rare:* chest pain, hives, shortness of breath, tight chest, wheezing

HOW TO USE THESE DRUGS
Dolasetron is available in tablets and solution and via injection. Granisetron comes in tablets, and ondansetron is available in tablets, oral disintegrating tablets, and oral solution and via injection. Palonosetron is available by injection only; therefore, dosage information is not provided here. The dosages given here are ones that are usually recommended for children. However, your doctor will determine the most appropriate dose and schedule for your child.

Dolasetron
- Children younger than 2 years: not recommended
- Children 2 to 16 years of age, for prevention of nausea

and vomiting after chemotherapy: 0.82 mg per lb of
body weight given within 1 hour before chemotherapy
is given. The injectable form may be given orally, diluted in apple or apple-grape juice.
- Children 2 to 16 years of age, to prevent nausea and
vomiting postsurgery: 0.54 mg per lb of body weight
given within 2 hours before surgery. The injectable
form may be given orally, diluted in apple or apple-
grape juice.

Granisetron
- Children younger than 12 years: dose to be determined
by your doctor
- Children 12 years and older, to prevent nausea and
vomiting caused by anticancer medication: 1 mg tablet
taken up to 1 hour before anticancer medication, then
1 mg 12 hours after the first dose. Alternatively, 2 mg
may be taken as one dose up to 1 hour before anticancer medication.
- Children 12 years and older, to prevent nausea and
vomiting caused by radiation treatment: two 1-mg
tablets taken within 1 hour of radiation

Ondansetron
- Children 4 to 11 years: one 4-mg tablet or 1 teaspoon
oral solution taken 3 times daily, the first dose taken 30
minutes before start of chemotherapy and the other two
doses 4 and 8 hours after the first dose. One 4-mg
tablet or 1 teaspoon oral solution should be taken 3
times daily (every 8 hours) for 1 to 2 days after completion of chemotherapy.
- Children 12 years and older: one 8-mg tablet or 2 teaspoons oral solution taken twice daily, the first dose
taken 30 minutes before start of chemotherapy and the
other dose taken 8 hours after the first dose. One 8-mg
tablet or 2 teaspoons oral solution should be taken
twice daily for 1 to 2 days after completion of
chemotherapy.
- Note: In early 2005, ondansetron was approved for

prevention of nausea and vomiting associated with general anesthesia in children as young as 1 month and for nausea and vomiting associated with chemotherapy in children as young as 6 months. Dose is by injection and determined by your doctor.

If your child is taking the orally disintegrating tablet form of ondansetron, the drug can be swallowed with saliva alone. The tablet should not be removed from the blister pack until your child is ready to take it. Peel off the foil backing from the blister pack and gently remove the tablet with dry hands. Do not try to push the tablets through the foil.

If your child misses a dose of dolasetron or granisetron, give it as soon as you remember. However, if it is nearly time for the next dose, skip the missed dose and resume the regular dosing schedule. Do not give a double dose.

If your child misses a dose of ondansetron and he or she does not feel nauseated, do not give the missed dose and continue with the regular dosing schedule. However, if your child does feel nauseated or has vomited, give him or her the missed dose as soon as possible. If vomiting continues, contact your doctor as soon as possible. Do not give a double dose.

These antiemetics can be taken with or without food; however, taking them with food can help prevent stomach upset.

TIME UNTIL THEY TAKE EFFECT
30 to 60 minutes

POSSIBLE DRUG, FOOD, AND/OR SUPPLEMENT INTERACTIONS
Granisetron and ondansetron have not been reported to interact with other medications, food, or supplements.

- If your child is taking dolasetron, your doctor may need to change your child's doses of the following medications or monitor your child for side effects. Note, however, that the following drugs usually are not

administered to children: amiodarone, cimetidine, cisapride, disopyramide, diuretics, erythromycin, moxi-
floxacin, pimozide, procainamide, quinidine, rifampin,
sotalol, sparfloxacin, and thioridazine.
- If your child is taking granisetron, ketoconazole may
interact with this drug.

SYMPTOMS OF OVERDOSE
- For dolasetron: dizziness, fainting
- For granisetron: headache
- For ondansetron: fainting, low blood pressure, sudden
blindness, and severe constipation

If an overdose occurs, seek immediate medical attention
and bring the drug container(s) with you.

THINGS TO TELL YOUR DOCTOR
- Tell your physician if your child has had allergic reactions to any medications in the past, if he or she is taking any medications now, or if your child has any
disease or medical condition.

IMPORTANT PRECAUTIONS
- Ondansetron oral disintegrating tablets contain phenylalanine, which should be avoided by anyone who has
phenylketonuria, a rare genetic disorder.
- These drugs can cause dizziness, so be sure you know
how your child reacts to them before he or she participates in potentially dangerous activities, such as riding
a bike, driving a car, or operating machinery.
- Store these medications in tightly closed containers at
room temperature and away from excess heat and
moisture (e.g., in the bathroom, near a stove or sink).

CLASS: ANTIHISTAMINE-DECONGESTANT-(ANTITUSSIVE) COMBINATION

GENERICS
(1) acrivastine + pseudoephedrine; (2) azatadine + pseudoephedrine; (3) brompheniramine + pseudoephedrine; (4) dexbrompheniramine + pseudoephedrine; (5) chlorpheniramine + pseudoephedrine; (6) fexofenadine + pseudoephedrine; (7) loratadine + pseudoephedrine; (8) chlorpheniramine + phenylephrine + (dextromethorphan); (9) chlorpheniramine + pseudoephedrine + (dextromethorphan)

BRAND NAMES
(1) Semprex-D; (2) Trinalin Repetabs; (3) Allent, Bromfed, Dallergy-JR, Endafed, Lodrane LD, Respahist, Rondec, Touro A&H, UltraBrom; (4) Disobrom; (5) Anamine, Chlordrine SR, Codimal-LA, Fedahist Gyrocaps, Histalet, Novafed A, Rescon-ED, and others; (6) Allegra-D; (7) Claritin-D 12-Hour, Claritin-D 24-Hour; (8) Alka-Seltzer Plus Cold & Cough; Tussar DM; (9) PediaCare Cough-Cold, PediaCare NightRest Cough & Cold Liquid, Triaminic Night Time Cough & Cold, Vicks Children's NyQuil Cold/Cough Relief
Generics Available/Over-the-Counter Available

ABOUT THESE DRUGS
The antihistamine and decongestant (pseudoephedrine) combinations listed here are used to treat symptoms of upper respiratory conditions, seasonal allergies such as hay fever, and the common cold. The antihistamine component relieves allergy symptoms (sneezing, watery eyes, swelling, hives, itching) while the decongestant portion constricts the blood vessels, which reduces the flow of blood to the nasal passages. Some also have an antitussive (anticough) component.

SIDE EFFECTS
Contact your doctor if your child experiences any side effects that are persistent or troubling, including any that are not listed here.

- *Most common:* dizziness, drowsiness, dry mouth, excitation, nervousness, poor coordination, restlessness, sedation, sleeplessness, upset stomach
- *Less common/rare:* abnormal heartbeat, agitation, anxiety, back pain, difficulty breathing, change in taste, chest pain, conjunctivitis, constipation, convulsions, depression, diarrhea, earache, eye pain, facial swelling, fatigue, flushing, gas, high blood pressure, indigestion, itching, leg cramps, migraine, mood disorders, muscle pain, nasal congestion, nosebleed, pneumonia, ringing in the ears, thirst, toothache, tremor, upper respiratory infection, urinary difficulties, viral infections, vision problems, vomiting, weakness, weight loss, wheezing

HOW TO USE THESE DRUGS

These drugs are available in many different formulations, including capsules, tablets, extended-release formulas, syrup, oral solutions, and oral suspensions. The dosages vary considerably, as do the ages for which each drug is appropriate; therefore, you should carefully follow the dosing instructions provided on the packaging or those given to you by your doctor or pharmacist.

In many cases, these drugs should be taken at least 1 hour before or 2 hours after a meal. However, if your child experiences stomach irritation, they can be taken with food.

If your child misses a dose, give it as soon as you remember. If, however, it is nearly time for the next dose, skip the missed dose and follow the regular dosing schedule. Never give a double dose.

TIME UNTIL THEY TAKE EFFECT

1 to 2 hours

POSSIBLE DRUG, FOOD, AND/OR SUPPLEMENT INTERACTIONS

Tell your doctor if your child is taking any prescription or over-the-counter medications or any vitamins, herbs, or other supplements. Possible interactions with these antihistamine-decongestant combinations may include the following:

- Use of any of these antihistamine-decongestant combination drugs along with any other antihistamines, decongestants, or antihistamine-decongestant combinations, whether prescription or over-the-counter medicine, may cause sedation.
- Monoamine oxidase (MAO) inhibitors (e.g., phenelzine) may make the side effects of antihistamines much more severe. MAO inhibitors should not be taken within 2 weeks of taking any antihistamine-decongestant combination medications.
- Blood pressure medications (e.g., metoprolol, propranolol) may cause unusually slow heart beat or raise blood pressure.
- Cimetidine, if taken with the loratadine-pseudoephedrine combination, may significantly increase blood levels of loratadine and may cause toxicity.
- Tricyclic antidepressants (e.g., amitriptyline, clomipramine) may make the side effects of antihistamines more severe.
- Grapefruit and grapefruit juice should be avoided if your child is taking the loratadine-pseudoephedrine combination.

SYMPTOMS OF OVERDOSE

Symptoms include anxiety, chest pain, chills, convulsions, drowsiness, dry mouth, fever, irregular or rapid heartbeat, loss of consciousness, nausea, nervousness, trembling, and urinary difficulties. If overdose occurs, seek immediate medical attention and bring the drug container(s) with you.

THINGS TO TELL YOUR DOCTOR

- Tell your doctor if your child has had allergic reactions to any medications in the past or if he or she is taking any medications, herbal remedies, or supplements now.
- Let your doctor know if your child has any of the following medical conditions: asthma, high blood pressure, diabetes, heart disease, peptic ulcer or other stomach problems, increased eye pressure, hyperthyroidism, or kidney disease.

- If your child is pregnant or becomes pregnant while taking any of these medications, consult your doctor.

IMPORTANT PRECAUTIONS
- These drugs can cause drowsiness and dizziness. Therefore, make sure you know how your child reacts before allowing him or her to participate in potentially dangerous activities, such as riding a bike, driving a car, or operating machinery.
- Store antihistamine-decongestant medications in a tightly closed container and keep away from excess heat and moisture (e.g., the bathroom, near a stove or sink). Liquid forms of these medications can be refrigerated, but do not allow them to freeze.
- Because of an increased sensitivity to sunlight when taking these drugs, your child should be protected against the sun by sunscreen and/or wearing long sleeves and pants when outdoors.

ASPIRIN

BRAND NAMES
Anacin, Ascriptin, Bayer, Bufferin, Easprin, Ecotrin, Empirin, Measurin, ZORprin
Generic Available/Over-the-Counter Available

ABOUT THIS DRUG
Aspirin is an analgesic (painkiller), anti-inflammatory drug given to treat mild to moderate pain and inflammation. It also may be used to prevent blood clots. Do not use it to treat fever in children unless specifically instructed to do so by your doctor.

SIDE EFFECTS
Contact your physician if your child experiences any side effects that are persistent or troubling, including any that are not listed here.

- *Common:* drowsiness, heartburn, nasal discharge, nausea, rash, ringing in the ears, stomach irritation, vomiting
- *Less common or rare:* abnormal bleeding, bruising, fever, insomnia, sore throat, weakness; Symptoms of Reye's syndrome, a rare but serious disorder that affects children 16 years of age and younger in response to aspirin intake include: agitation, confusion, difficulty breathing, extreme fatigue, itching, redness of the face, vomiting. Seek immediate medical attention.

HOW TO USE THIS DRUG

Aspirin is available in short-acting tablets, chewable tablets, delayed-release (enteric-coated) tablets, and suppositories. The dosages given here are ones that are usually recommended for children. However, your doctor will determine the most appropriate dose and schedule for your child.

All Tablet Forms and Suppositories, for Pain or Fever

- Children younger than 2 years: to be determined by your doctor
- Children 2 to 4 years: 160 mg every 4 hours as needed
- Children 4 to 6 years: 240 mg every 4 hours as needed
- Children 6 to 9 years: 320 to 325 mg every 4 hours as needed
- Children 9 to 11 years: 320 to 400 mg every 4 hours as needed
- Children 11 to 12 years: 320 to 480 mg every 4 hours as needed
- Children older than 12 years: 325 to 500 mg every 3 or 4 hours; 650 mg every 4 to 6 hours, or 1,000 mg every 6 hours as needed

All Tablet Forms and Suppositories, for Arthritis

- Children younger than 12 years: Based on body weight and determined by your doctor. Typically, 32 to 40 mg per lb of body weight daily, divided into several doses
- Children 12 years and older: 3,600 to 5,400 mg daily, divided into smaller doses

Do not give your child aspirin for more than 5 consecutive days without first consulting with your doctor. Aspirin should be taken with food or a full glass of water to help prevent stomach irritation.

If your child misses a dose, give it to him or her as soon as you remember. However, if it is nearly time for the next dose, do not give the missed dose. Continue with the regular dosing schedule. Do not give a double dose.

TIME UNTIL IT TAKES EFFECT
Mild pain and fever usually respond within 30 to 60 minutes. Full effect for other uses may take 2 to 3 weeks.

POSSIBLE DRUG, FOOD, AND/OR SUPPLEMENT INTERACTIONS
Tell your doctor if your child is taking any prescription or over-the-counter medications or any vitamins, herbs, or other supplements. The following medications should not be taken along with aspirin for more than a day or two unless under supervision by a doctor. (Note: Most of these medications are not recommended for use in children.)

- Acetaminophen, diclofenac, diflunisal, etodolac, fenoprofen, flurbiprofen, ibuprofen, indomethacin, ketoprofen, ketorolac, meclofenamate, mefenamic, nabumetone, naproxen, phenylbutazone, piroxicam, sulindac, tenoxicam, tiaprofenic acid, and tolmetin.
- Insulin may require dosage adjustments.
- Zafirlukast levels may rise and increase adverse effects.
- The herbs dong quai, feverfew, garlic, ginkgo, ginger, horse chestnut, and red clover may cause an increased risk of bleeding or stomach irritation if taken with aspirin.
- Supplements of fish oil or vitamin E may cause a significantly increased risk of bleeding.

SYMPTOMS OF OVERDOSE
Symptoms include delirium, disorientation, dizziness, fever, impaired hearing, nausea, rapid breathing, ringing in the ears,

seizures, and vomiting. If overdose occurs, seek immediate medical attention and bring the drug container with you.

THINGS TO TELL YOUR DOCTOR
- Tell your physician if your child has had allergic reactions to aspirin or to any medications in the past or if he or she is taking any medications now.
- Tell your physician if your child has a history of peptic ulcer disease or kidney or liver disease, or if he or she has asthma, nasal polyps, or lupus erythematosus.
- Consult your doctor if your child is pregnant or becomes pregnant while taking aspirin. Use of aspirin during pregnancy has been associated with an increased risk of stillbirth and newborn death.

IMPORTANT PRECAUTIONS
- Consult your doctor before giving aspirin to your child. Children 16 years and younger should not take aspirin if they have flu, chicken pox, or similar infections, because aspirin use can cause an often-fatal condition called Reye's syndrome.
- Keep the suppositories in a cool place, such as the refrigerator, but do not allow them to freeze.
- Store other forms of aspirin in a tightly closed container and away from excess heat or moisture (e.g., in a bathroom or near a stove or sink).
- Do not use aspirin tablets that have a strong odor of vinegar.

ATOMOXETINE

BRAND NAME
Strattera
Generic Not Available

ABOUT THIS DRUG
Atomoxetine is a selective norepinephrine reuptake inhibitor that is used as part of an overall program to treat attention

deficit/hyperactivity disorder (ADHD) in children and adults. It is believed to work by enhancing levels of norepinephrine, a chemical in the brain that regulates activity.

SIDE EFFECTS
Contact your doctor if your child experiences any side effects that are persistent or troubling, including any that are not listed here.

- *Most common:* constipation, cough, crying, diarrhea, dizziness, drowsiness, dry mouth, ear infection, fatigue, headache, indigestion, influenza, irritability, loss of appetite, mood swings, nausea, runny nose, skin inflammation, stomach pain, vomiting, weight loss
- *Less common/rare:* allergic reactions (edema, hives, rash)

HOW TO USE THIS DRUG
Atomoxetine is available in 10-, 18-, 25-, 40-, and 60-mg capsules. The dosages given here are ones that are usually recommended for children. However, your doctor will determine the most appropriate dose and schedule for your child.

- Children younger than 6 years: atomoxetine has not been tested in this age group.
- Children and adolescents who weigh up to 154 lbs: Typical starting dose is 0.23 mg per lb of body weight daily. After at least 3 days, your doctor may increase the daily total to 0.54 mg per lb of body weight. Daily doses should not exceed 0.63 mg per lb or a total of 100 mg, whichever is less.
- Children and adolescents who weigh more than 154 lbs: Usual starting dose is 40 mg per day. After at least 3 days, your doctor may increase the daily total to 80 mg. After 2 to 4 weeks, dosage may be increased to a maximum of 100 mg per day.

Atomoxetine may be taken with or without food. If your child misses a dose, give it as soon as you remember. If it is nearly time for the next dose, skip the missed dose and return to the regular dosing schedule. Do not give a double dose.

TIME UNTIL IT TAKES EFFECT
Unknown

POSSIBLE DRUG, FOOD, AND/OR SUPPLEMENT INTERACTIONS
Tell your doctor if your child is taking any prescription or over-the-counter medications or any vitamins, herbs, or other supplements. Possible interactions with atomoxetine may include the following:

- Albuterol and related asthma medications, as well as any drug that causes a rise in blood pressure (e.g., phenylephrine, which is found in some over-the-counter cold medications), may increase the effects of atomoxetine.
- If your child is also taking fluoxetine, paroxetine, or quinidine, your doctor may reduce the dose of atomoxetine.

SYMPTOMS OF OVERDOSE
Symptoms of overdose are not known. If you believe an overdose has occurred, seek immediate medical attention and bring the drug container(s) with you.

THINGS TO TELL YOUR DOCTOR
- Tell your doctor if your child has had allergic reactions to any medications in the past or if he or she is taking any medications now.
- Let your doctor know if your child has any of the following medical conditions: liver disorder, high blood pressure, urinary retention, narrow-angle glaucoma, or abnormally rapid heartbeat.
- Consult your doctor if your child is pregnant or becomes pregnant while taking atomoxetine.
- Monitor your child closely and contact your physician if he or she displays any unusual behavior during early treatment.

IMPORTANT PRECAUTIONS

- Atomoxetine can slow children's average rate of growth, but it is not yet known whether an individual's final adult height and weight are affected. Your doctor may interrupt use of atomoxetine if your child does not grow or gain weight at an appropriate rate.
- Atomoxetine can cause dizziness, so make sure you know how your child reacts to it before you allow him or her to ride a bike, drive a car, or participate in other activities that require alertness.
- The efficacy of atomoxetine past 9 weeks and its safety beyond 1 year have not been evaluated systematically.
- Store atomoxetine in a tightly closed container and keep at room temperature away from excess heat and moisture (e.g., the bathroom, near sinks).

ATTAPULGITE

BRAND NAMES

Diar-Aid, Diarrest, Diasorb, Diatrol, Donnagel, Kaopek, K-Pek, Parepectolin, Rheaban (Note: In the United States, Kaopectate no longer contains attapulgite.)
Generic Available/Over-the-Counter Available

ABOUT THIS DRUG

Attapulgite is an antidiarrheal drug. Experts believe it works by binding to bacteria and toxins in the digestive tract that cause diarrhea and facilitating their removal from the body. It may also reduce the amount of fluid in stool.

SIDE EFFECTS

Contact your doctor if your child experiences any side effects that are persistent or troubling, including any that are not listed here.

- *Most common:* constipation
- *Less common/rare:* none

HOW TO USE THIS DRUG

Attapulgite is available in tablets, chewable tablets, and as an oral suspension. The dosages given here are ones that are usually recommended for children. However, your doctor will determine the most appropriate dose and schedule for your child.

- Children younger than 3 years: not recommended
- Children 3 to 6 years: 300 mg (chewable tablet or oral suspension) after each loose bowel movement, but no more than 2,100 mg within a 24-hour period
- Children 7 to 12 years: 1,200 mg (chewable tablet or oral suspension) after each loose bowel movement, but no more than 8,400 mg within a 24-hour period. If taking tablets, 750 mg after each loose bowel movement, but no more than 4,500 mg within a 24-hour period
- Children 13 years and older: 1,200 to 1,500 mg (tablets or oral suspension) after each loose bowel movement, but no more than 9,000 mg within a 24-hour period. If taking chewable tablets, 1,200 mg after each loose bowel movement, but no more than 8,400 mg within a 24-hour period

If your child misses a dose, give it as soon as you remember. However, if it is nearly time for the next dose, skip the missed dose and continue with the regular dosing schedule. Do not give a double dose.

TIME UNTIL IT TAKES EFFECT

1 to 2 days. If the diarrhea has not improved or if it has gotten worse in 2 days, call your doctor.

POSSIBLE DRUG, FOOD, AND/OR SUPPLEMENT INTERACTIONS

Tell your doctor if your child is taking any prescription or over-the-counter medications or any vitamins, herbs, or other supplements. Generally, if your child is taking any other medications, he or she should not take them within 2 to 3 hours of attapulgite, because taking the medications at the same time as attapulgite may prevent the other drugs from being absorbed by the body.

SYMPTOMS OF OVERDOSE

No cases of overdose have been reported. However, if you believe your child has taken an excessive amount of atta-pulgite, seek immediate medical attention and bring the drug container(s) with you.

THINGS TO TELL YOUR DOCTOR

- Tell your doctor if your child has had allergic reactions to any medications in the past or if he or she is taking any medications now.
- Let your doctor know if your child has any medical conditions.
- If your child's diarrhea does not improve after 2 days of treatment, if it gets worse, if he or she develops a fever, or if there is blood or mucus in the stool, contact your doctor as soon as possible and discontinue use of attapulgite.

IMPORTANT PRECAUTIONS

- Store attapulgite in a tightly closed container and keep at room temperature away from excess heat and mois-ture (e.g., the bathroom, near sinks).
- Make sure your child drinks lots of liquids, as the loss of body water due to diarrhea can cause dizziness, lightheadedness, decreased urination, dry mouth, and wrinkling of the skin. Contact your doctor immediately if your child develops any of these symptoms.
- A nonirritating diet and plenty of fluids are recom-mended as your child recovers from diarrhea. In addi-tion to encouraging intake of fluids, mild foods such as applesauce, bananas, rice, cooked cereals, and plain breads are recommended.

AZELASTINE

BRAND NAMES
Astelin (nasal); Optivar (ophthalmic)
Generic Not Available

ABOUT THIS DRUG
Azelastine is an antihistamine that is used to treat or relieve symptoms of allergies and chronic nasal inflammation and obstruction (vasomotor rhinitis) (nasal form) or itchy eyes (ophthalmic form). It works by blocking the effects of histamine, a naturally occurring substance in the body that causes sneezing, watery eyes, hives, itching, and other symptoms of allergies.

SIDE EFFECTS
Contact your doctor if your child experiences any side effects that are persistent or troubling, including any that are not listed here.

- *Most common:* nasal form—bitter taste in the mouth, drowsiness, headache, unexpected weight gain; ophthalmic form—bitter taste in the mouth, eye burning/stinging, headache
- *Less common/rare:* nasal form—dizziness, dry mouth, fatigue, nasal burning, nosebleeds, sneezing, sore throat; ophthalmic form—asthma, conjunctivitis, eye pain, fatigue, flulike symptoms, inflamed pharynx, runny nose, temporary blurry vision

HOW TO USE THIS DRUG
Azelastine is available as a nasal spray and eye drops. The dosages given here are ones that are usually recommended for children. However, your doctor will determine the most appropriate dose and schedule for your child.

Nasal Form
- Children younger than 5 years: not recommended
- Children 5 to 11 years: one spray per nostril twice daily; for allergies only

- Children 12 years and older: 2 sprays per nostril, not to exceed twice daily

Ophthalmic Form
- Children younger than 3 years: not recommended
- Children 3 years and older: one drop in each affected eye twice daily

If your child misses a dose, give it as soon as you remember. If it is nearly time for the next dose, skip the missed dose and continue with the regular dosing schedule. Never give a double dose.

TIME UNTIL IT TAKES EFFECT
1 to 3 hours

POSSIBLE DRUG, FOOD, AND/OR SUPPLEMENT INTERACTIONS
Tell your doctor if your child is taking any prescription or over-the-counter medications or any vitamins, herbs, or other supplements. Possible interactions with azelastine may include the following:

- Azelastine may increase the sedative effects of alcohol, barbiturates, other antihistamines, painkillers, sedatives, and tranquilizers.

SYMPTOMS OF OVERDOSE
No cases of overdose have been reported. However, if you believe an overdose has occurred or your child has accidentally ingested the medication, seek immediate medical attention and bring the drug container(s) with you.

THINGS TO TELL YOUR DOCTOR
- Tell your doctor if your child has had allergic reactions to any medications in the past or if he or she is taking any medications, herbal remedies, or supplements now.

IMPORTANT PRECAUTIONS

- Your doctor will prescribe azelastine for a specific amount of time. Your child should take azelastine for the entire prescribed time, even if he or she feels better before the end of scheduled treatment.
- Because azelastine can cause drowsiness, make sure you know how your child reacts before he or she participates in potentially hazardous activities, such as riding a bike, driving a car, or operating machinery.
- Store azelastine in a tightly closed container and away from excess heat and moisture (e.g., the bathroom, near a stove or sink). It can be refrigerated, but do not allow it to freeze.

AZITHROMYCIN

BRAND NAME
Zithromax
Generic Not Available

ABOUT THIS DRUG
Azithromycin is a type of antibiotic that is used to treat various bacterial infections. In children it is used to treat middle ear infections, strep throat, tonsillitis, and pneumonia. It works by preventing the bacteria from manufacturing the special proteins they need to survive.

SIDE EFFECTS
Contact your doctor if your child experiences any side effects that are persistent or troubling, including any that are not listed here.

- *More common:* abdominal discomfort, diarrhea, dizziness, headache, nausea, vomiting
- *Less common/rare (seen more often in children than in adults):* agitation, constipation, cough, fever, fungal infection, insomnia, loss of appetite, nervousness, pink-

eye, runny nose, shortness of breath, sore throat, stomach inflammation, sweating

Very rarely, azithromycin can cause a serious reaction, characterized by swelling of the lips, face, and neck, that hinders swallowing, breathing, and speaking; it can also cause serious skin disease. Seek medical attention immediately if any of these symptoms occurs.

HOW TO USE THIS DRUG
Azithromycin is available in capsules, tablets, and powder (to be mixed with water) and via injection. (Information on the injectable form is not provided here.) The dosages given here are ones that are usually recommended for children. However, your doctor will determine the most appropriate dose and schedule for your child.

Middle Ear Infection
- Children 6 months and older: There are three options: a single dose of 13.6 mg per lb of body weight; 4.5 mg per lb once daily for 3 days; or 4.5 mg per lb once on day 1 followed by 2.3 mg per lb once daily for 4 days

Pneumonia
- Children 6 months and older: 4.5 mg suspension per lb of body weight once on day 1, followed by 2.3 mg per lb of body weight daily for 4 days

Strep Throat, Tonsillitis
- Children 2 years and older: 5.4 mg per lb of body weight once daily for 5 days

If your child misses a dose, give it as soon as you remember. If you miss a day completely, skip the missed dose and resume the regular dosing schedule. Do not give a double dose.

The capsules should be taken at least 1 hour before or 2 hours after a meal. If your child cannot swallow the capsule, you can open it and mix the contents with a little bit of water. The tablets can be taken with or without food.

TIME UNTIL IT TAKES EFFECT

The speed at which azithromycin takes effect depends partly on the severity of your child's infection. Usually an improvement is seen within 3 to 5 days.

POSSIBLE DRUG, FOOD, AND/OR SUPPLEMENT INTERACTIONS

Tell your doctor if your child is taking any prescription or over-the-counter medications or any vitamins, herbs, or other supplements. Possible interactions with azithromycin may include the following:

- Do not take azithromycin at the same time as an aluminum- or magnesium-based antacid (e.g., Mylanta, Maalox), because the antacids can prevent the azithromycin from being absorbed by the body.
- Cyclosporine, digoxin, hexobarbital, nelfinavir, phenytoin, theophylline, and warfarin may interact with azithromycin.

SYMPTOMS OF OVERDOSE

No cases of overdose have been reported. If you believe an overdose has occurred, seek immediate medical attention and bring the drug container(s) with you.

THINGS TO TELL YOUR DOCTOR

- Tell your doctor if your child has had allergic reactions to any medications in the past or if he or she is taking any medications now.
- Let your doctor know if your child has any type of liver disease.
- Consult your doctor if your child is pregnant or becomes pregnant while taking azithromycin.

IMPORTANT PRECAUTIONS

- Store azithromycin in a tightly closed container and keep at room temperature away from excess heat and moisture (e.g., the bathroom, near sinks).
- Make sure your child takes azithromycin for the entire

course prescribed by the doctor, even if he or she has
no more symptoms, because the infection may return if
the medication is stopped too soon.
- Azithromycin may cause dizziness, so make sure you
know how your child reacts before he or she participates in potentially hazardous activities, such as riding
a bike, driving a car, or operating machinery.
- Azithromycin may make your child more sensitive to
sunlight, so be sure he or she wears sunscreen and/or
long pants and long sleeves when outside.

BACITRACIN

BRAND NAMES
AK-Tracin, Bacticin (ophthalmic forms); Baciguent (derma-
tologic)
Generic Available

ABOUT THIS DRUG
Bacitracin is an antibiotic that is available for two primary
purposes: as an ointment to treat cuts and abrasions; and as
an ophthalmic preparation to treat minor bacterial infections
of the eyelids. It works by preventing the bacteria from manufacturing cells walls, which then leads to the death of the
bacteria.

SIDE EFFECTS
Contact your doctor if your child experiences any side effects that are persistent or troubling, including any that are
not listed here.

- *Most common:* ophthalmic form—temporary minor
stinging of the eyes
- *Less common/rare:* dermatologic form—minor irritation of the skin

In very rare cases, both the dermatologic and ophthalmic
formulations can cause a severe allergic reaction, character-

ized by hives, difficulty breathing, or total closure of the airways. Similarly, in very rare cases the ophthalmic preparations can cause severe eye pain, headache, pain on exposure to light, double vision, itching, burning, inflammation, and a rapid change in vision. Seek immediate medical attention if any of these symptoms occurs.

HOW TO USE THIS DRUG
Bacitracin is available as an ointment and solution for ophthalmic purposes and as an ointment for skin conditions. The dosages given here are ones that are usually recommended for children. However, your doctor will determine the most appropriate dose and schedule for your child.

- For skin conditions: apply to the affected area 2 to 5 times daily, or as directed by your doctor
- For ophthalmic conditions: apply to the eye 1 or more times daily, or as directed by your doctor

If your child misses a dose, apply it as soon as you remember, then resume your regular dosing schedule.

TIME UNTIL IT TAKES EFFECT
4 to 7 days

POSSIBLE DRUG, FOOD, AND/OR SUPPLEMENT INTERACTIONS
Tell your doctor if your child is taking any prescription or over-the-counter medications or any vitamins, herbs, or other supplements. Possible interactions with bacitracin may include the following:

- When using the ophthalmic ointment or solution, avoid use of other ophthalmic products unless allowed by your doctor.
- No other topically applied medications should be used if your child is using the dermatologic form of bacitracin.

SYMPTOMS OF OVERDOSE

Symptoms of an overdose with the ophthalmic form include appearance of floating spots, double vision, headache, inflammation, itching, rapid change in vision, and severe eye pain. If you think an overdose has occurred, rinse the eye with water and call the Poison Control Center or your local emergency department.

THINGS TO TELL YOUR DOCTOR

- Tell your doctor if your child has had allergic reactions to any medications in the past or if he or she is taking any medications now.
- Let your doctor know if your child has any medical conditions.
- Consult your doctor if your child is pregnant or becomes pregnant while using bacitracin.

IMPORTANT PRECAUTIONS

- Store bacitracin in a tightly closed container and keep at room temperature away from excess heat and moisture (e.g., the bathroom, near sinks).
- For the ophthalmic ointment, do not touch the tube opening to any surface, including the eye. The tube opening is sterile, and if it becomes contaminated it could cause an eye infection. Keep the ointment properly capped when it is not in use.
- Because ophthalmic bacitracin may cause blurry vision, make sure you know how your child reacts to the medication before he or she rides a bike, drives a car, or participants in other activities that require alertness.
- If your child wears contact lenses, ask your doctor if they can be worn while your child is being treated with ophthalmic bacitracin.

BACLOFEN

BRAND NAME
Lioresal
Generic Available

ABOUT THIS DRUG
Baclofen is a muscle relaxant used to relieve muscle pain
from spasms and cramping that are related to medical conditions such as multiple sclerosis and spinal injuries. The
drug helps reduce the transmission of nerve signals from the
spinal cord to certain muscles.

SIDE EFFECTS
Contact your doctor if your child experiences any side effects that are persistent or troubling, including any that are
not listed here.

- *Most common:* dizziness, drowsiness, fatigue, headache,
  insomnia, muscle weakness, nausea
- *Less common/rare:* clumsiness, constipation, diarrhea,
  loss of appetite, muscle or joint pain, numbness or tingling in the hands or feet, painful urination, stomach
  pain, unsteadiness, unusual excitability

HOW TO USE THIS DRUG
Baclofen is available in tablets. The dosages given here are
ones that are usually recommended for children. However,
your doctor will determine the most appropriate dose and
schedule for your child.

- Children younger than 12 years: to be determined by
  your doctor
- Children 12 years and older: starting dose is 5 mg 3
  times daily. Your doctor may increase the dose as
  needed. The maximum dose is 80 mg daily.

To reduce stomach irritation, baclofen can be taken with
food or milk. If your child misses a dose, give it as soon as

you remember if it is within 1 hour of the scheduled dose. If more than 1 hour has passed since the scheduled dose, do not give the missed dose and give the next scheduled dose at the proper time. Do not give a double dose.

TIME UNTIL IT TAKES EFFECT
Some benefit may occur within 3 to 4 days, but it may take 1 week to reach full effect.

POSSIBLE DRUG, FOOD, AND/OR SUPPLEMENT INTERACTIONS
Tell your doctor if your child is taking any prescription or over-the-counter medications or any vitamins, herbs, or other supplements. Possible interactions with baclofen may include the following:

- Antidepressants, including doxepin, imipramine, nortriptyline, fluoxetine, paroxetine, sertraline, phenelzine, and tranylcypromine
- Antihistamines, including brompheniramine, chlorpheniramine, azatadine, and clemastine
- Narcotics, including meperidine, morphine, propoxyphene, oxycodone, and codeine
- Sedatives, including phenobarbital, amobarbital, and secobarbital
- Alcohol (should be avoided)

SYMPTOMS OF OVERDOSE
Symptoms include blurry vision, drowsiness, loss of consciousness, muscle weakness, seizures, slowed breathing, twitching, vision loss, and vomiting. If overdose occurs, seek immediate medical attention and bring the drug container(s) with you.

THINGS TO TELL YOUR DOCTOR
- Tell your doctor if your child has had allergic reactions to any medications in the past or if he or she is taking any medications now.
- Let your doctor know if your child has any medical

conditions, especially diabetes, emotional disorder, kidney disease, or epilepsy.

- Consult your doctor if your child is pregnant or becomes pregnant while taking baclofen.

IMPORTANT PRECAUTIONS

- Store baclofen in a tightly closed container and keep away from excess heat and moisture (e.g., the bathroom, near a stove or sink).
- Because baclofen can causes dizziness and faintness when rising from a seated or reclined position, make sure you know how your child reacts to the drug before he or she rides a bike, drives a car, or participates in other activities that require alertness.
- It is dangerous to stop taking baclofen suddenly. Your doctor must help your child slowly reduce his or her dosing, because abrupt withdrawal can cause hallucinations and seizures.

BECLOMETHASONE—
see *Corticosteroids, Oral Inhalants* and *Corticosteroids, Nasal Inhalants*

BETAMETHASONE—
see *Corticosteroids, Oral* and *Corticosteroids, Topical*

BISMUTH SUBSALICYLATE

BRAND NAMES
Bismatrol, Pepto-Bismol, Pink Bismuth
Generic Available/Over-the-Counter Available

ABOUT THIS DRUG
Bismuth is an antidiarrheal medication used to treat diarrhea, acid indigestion, heartburn, and duodenal ulcers. It can also help prevent traveler's diarrhea. Bismuth works by stimulat-

ing the movement of fluids across the intestinal tract wall, neutralizing some bacterial toxins, promoting the activity of the intestinal muscles, and reducing intestinal inflammation.

SIDE EFFECTS
Contact your doctor if your child experiences any side effects that are persistent or troubling, including any that are not listed here.

- *Most common:* black stools, dark tongue
- *Less common/rare:* abdominal pain, confusion, dizziness, hearing loss, increased sweating, muscle weakness, nausea, thirst, difficulty breathing, and vomiting. If these symptoms occur, call your doctor immediately.

HOW TO USE THIS DRUG
Bismuth is available in tablets and as an oral suspension. The dosages given here are ones that are usually recommended for children. However, your doctor will determine the most appropriate dose and schedule for your child.

- Children younger than 12 years: As of spring 2004, the FDA required the maker of Pepto-Bismol to remove dosing instructions for children younger than 12 years and to advise parents to ask their doctor about giving this product to children.
- Children 12 years and older: 2 tablets or 2 tablespoons of liquid every 30 to 60 minutes, not to exceed 16 doses daily for no more than 2 days

TIME UNTIL IT TAKES EFFECT
Within 30 to 60 minutes

POSSIBLE DRUG, FOOD, AND/OR SUPPLEMENT INTERACTIONS
Tell your doctor if your child is taking any prescription or over-the-counter medications or any vitamins, herbs, or other supplements. Possible interactions with bismuth may include the following:

- Bismuth may interact with other salicylates, anticoagulants, oral diabetes medications, heparin, probenecid, thrombolytic agents, oral tetracycline, or sulfinpyrazone.

SYMPTOMS OF OVERDOSE
Symptoms include confusion, drowsiness (severe), hearing loss or ringing in the ears, loss of consciousness, rapid or deep breathing, seizures, and severe excitability. If overdose occurs, seek immediate medical attention and bring the drug container(s) with you.

THINGS TO TELL YOUR DOCTOR
- Tell your doctor if your child has had allergic reactions to any medications in the past or if he or she is taking any medications, herbal remedies, or supplements now.
- Let your doctor know if your child has mucus in stool, black or bloody stool, fever, diabetes, kidney disease, dehydration, stomach ulcers, dysentery or a bleeding problem, or is taking medication for arthritis.
- Consult your doctor before giving bismuth to your child if he or she is recovering from flu or chicken pox.

IMPORTANT PRECAUTIONS
- Use of bismuth for longer than 2 days may result in constipation. Consult your doctor if your child does not get relief within 2 days.
- Do not use bismuth to treat diarrhea if your child has a fever or if there is blood or mucus in the stool.
- Store bismuth in a tightly closed container and keep at room temperature away from excess heat and moisture (e.g., the bathroom, near a stove or sink). The oral form may be kept in the refrigerator, but do not allow it to freeze.

BROMPHENIRAMINE

BRAND NAMES
Bromarest, Bromfed, Bromphen, Dimetane, Dimetapp Allergy, Nasahist B, ND-Stat, Oraminic II, Rondec, Veltane
Generic Available

ABOUT THIS DRUG
Brompheniramine is an antihistamine that is used to prevent or relieve symptoms associated with hay fever, allergies, and the common cold. The drug blocks the effects of histamine, a naturally occurring substance in the body that causes itching, sneezing, watery eyes, hives, swelling, and other symptoms characteristic of an allergic reaction. It also can be used to relieve itching associated with insect bites, poison ivy, and poison oak.

SIDE EFFECTS
Contact your doctor if your child experiences any side effects that are persistent or troubling, including any that are not listed here.

- *Most common:* drowsiness; dry mouth, nose, or throat; unusual excitability. Drowsiness usually subsides within a few days.
- *Less common/rare:* dizziness, difficult or painful urination, loss of appetite, vision changes

HOW TO USE THIS DRUG
Brompheniramine is available as capsules, tablets, extended-release tablets, and elixir and via injection. (Information on the injectable form is not provided here.) The dosages given here are ones that are usually recommended for children. However, your doctor will determine the most appropriate dose and schedule for your child.

Capsules, Tablets, Elixir
- Children 2 to 6 years: 1 mg every 4 to 6 hours
- Children 7 to 12 years: 2 mg every 4 to 6 hours
- Children 13 years and older: 4 mg every 4 to 6 hours

Extended-Release Tablets
- Children 6 years and older: 8 to 12 mg every 12 hours

If your child misses a dose, give it as soon as you remember. If it is nearly time for the next dose, skip the missed dose and resume the regular dosing schedule. Do not double the next dose.

Brompheniramine can be taken with food to help reduce stomach upset.

TIME UNTIL IT TAKES EFFECT
15 to 60 minutes

POSSIBLE DRUG, FOOD, AND/OR SUPPLEMENT INTERACTIONS
Tell your doctor if your child is taking any prescription or over-the-counter medications or any vitamins, herbs, or other supplements. Possible interactions with brompheniramine may include the following:

- Antidepressants, anticonvulsants, medications for colds or allergies, muscle relaxants, narcotics, sedatives, and tranquilizers may interact with brompheniramine.
- Brompheniramine should not be taken within 2 weeks of taking a monoamine oxidase (MAO) inhibitor (e.g., phenelzine or tranylcypromine).

SYMPTOMS OF OVERDOSE
Symptoms include loss of consciousness, hallucinations, severe drowsiness, and seizures. If overdose occurs, seek immediate medical attention and bring the drug container(s) with you.

THINGS TO TELL YOUR DOCTOR
- Tell your doctor if your child has had allergic reactions to any medications in the past or if he or she is taking any medications now.
- Let your doctor know if your child has any of the following medical conditions: asthma, diabetes, glau-

coma, ulcers, high blood pressure, seizures, an overactive thyroid gland, heart disease.
- If your child is scheduled to undergo surgery (including dental surgery), tell the doctor or dentist that your child is taking brompheniramine.
- If your child becomes pregnant while using this drug, consult your doctor.

IMPORTANT PRECAUTIONS
- Store brompheniramine in a tightly closed container and keep at room temperature away from excess heat and moisture (e.g., the bathroom, near sinks).
- Brompheniramine can cause drowsiness and dizziness; therefore, make sure you know how your child reacts before he or she rides a bike, drives a car, or participates in other activities that require alertness.

BUDESONIDE

BRAND NAMES
Pulmicort Turbuhaler, Rhinocort Aqua, Rhinocort Turbuhaler
Generic Not Available

ABOUT THIS DRUG
Budesonide is a respiratory corticosteroid that is used to treat the symptoms of allergic rhinitis (seasonal allergies, hay fever). Its primary effect is to reduce or prevent inflammation of the lining of the airways and reduce the symptoms associated with allergic rhinitis, such as sneezing, watery eyes, itching, and swelling.

SIDE EFFECTS
Contact your doctor if your child experiences any side effects that are persistent or troubling, including any that are not listed here.

- *Most common:* nasal inhalant—burning or irritation of the nasal passages, nosebleed, sore throat; oral in-

halant—hoarseness, sore throat, white patches in the mouth or throat
- *Less common/rare:* digestive discomfort, eye pain, gradually reduced vision, stomach pain, watery eyes

HOW TO USE THIS DRUG
Budesonide is available as a nasal inhalant, an oral inhalant, in nebulized form (jet nebulizer), and as capsules. The dosages given here are ones that are usually recommended for children. However, your doctor will determine the most appropriate dose and schedule for your child.

- Infants and children 1 to 8 years: As maintenance treatment of asthma and preventive therapy, the inhalation suspension is a nebulized formulation, with a recommended dose range of 0.5 to 1 mg daily in 1 or 2 doses.
- Children 6 years and older: For seasonal rhinitis, use the nasal inhaler: 2 inhalations in each nostril twice daily or 4 inhalations in each nostril in the morning (256 µg is the maximum daily dose).

Budesonide can be used with or without food. After each use, your child should rinse his or her mouth with water. If your child misses a dose, give it as soon as you remember. If it is nearly time for the next dose, however, do not give the missed dose. Continue with the regular dosing schedule. Do not give a double dose.

TIME UNTIL IT TAKES EFFECT
Some relief can be expected within 24 hours, but it can take 3 to 7 days to reach full benefit.

POSSIBLE DRUG, FOOD, AND/OR SUPPLEMENT INTERACTIONS
Tell your doctor if your child is taking any prescription or over-the-counter medications or any vitamins, herbs, or other supplements. Possible interactions with budesonide may include the following:

- Use of some anticonvulsive drugs can increase the risk of osteoporosis.
- Oral bronchodilators (e.g., aminophylline, ephedrine) and inhalant bronchodilators (e.g., methylphenidate) may increase the effects of budesonide.
- Use of methylphenidate and budesonide together can cause increased suppression of growth in children.

SYMPTOMS OF OVERDOSE
Symptoms include fluid retention, stomach irritation, nervousness, and facial flushing. If overdose occurs, seek immediate medical attention and bring the drug container(s) with you.

THINGS TO TELL YOUR DOCTOR
- Tell your doctor if your child has had allergic reactions to any medications in the past or if he or she is taking any medications now.
- Let your doctor know if your child has any of the following medical conditions: any type of respiratory infection, herpes of the eye, liver damage, chronic bronchitis, or nose ulcers.
- Consult your doctor if your child is pregnant or becomes pregnant while using budesonide.

IMPORTANT PRECAUTIONS
- Store budesonide in a tightly closed container and keep away from excess heat and moisture (e.g., the bathroom, near a stove or sink).
- Budesonide should not be used if your child has severe acute asthma or status asthmaticus that requires more intense treatment, if the asthma can be controlled with other antiasthmatic drugs that are not related to cortisone, or if your child needs cortisone-like drugs infrequently to control his or her asthma.
- Because corticosteroids can have a negative effect on growth, it is important to have your child's growth rate monitored regularly by your doctor.
- Use of budesonide can suppress the immune system

and thus may increase your child's risk of infection. As a precaution, while your child is taking budesonide he or she should avoid contact with people who have an infection, such as measles or chicken pox. Tell your doctor if your child is exposed to anyone with these or other infections or if he or she develops blisters or sores that do not heal properly.

BUPROPION

BRAND NAME
Wellbutrin
Generic Not Available

ABOUT THIS DRUG
Bupropion is an antidepressant that is used in the treatment of major depression as well as attention deficit/hyperactivity disorder (ADHD) and bipolar disorder. It appears to help balance the levels of neurotransmitters, chemicals in the brain that are associated with emotions, mental state, and mood.

SIDE EFFECTS
Contact your doctor if your child experiences any side effects that are persistent or troubling, including any that are not listed here.

- *Most common:* constipation, dizziness, dry mouth, increased sweating, loss of appetite, nausea, trembling, unusual weight loss, vomiting
- *Less common/rare:* acne, blisters in the mouth and eyes, blurry vision, chills, difficulty concentrating, drowsiness, fatigue, fever, hallucinations, hostility, impotence, indigestion, insomnia, irregular heartbeat, rash, seizures, severe headache

HOW TO USE THIS DRUG
Bupropion is available in tablets and extended-release tablets. The dosages given here are ones that are usually

recommended for children. However, your doctor will determine the most appropriate dose and schedule for your child.

- Bupropion is usually given in 2 to 4 doses daily in evenly spaced intervals (at least 6 hours in between). Your doctor will determine the most appropriate dose and schedule for your child.

Bupropion can be taken with food to help reduce stomach irritation. If your child misses a dose, give it as soon as you remember. If it is nearly time for the next dose, skip the missed dose and continue with the regular dosing schedule. Do not give a double dose.

TIME UNTIL IT TAKES EFFECT
If you give this drug to your child for ADHD, you should see an effect within 2 weeks. For treatment of depression, an effect may take 3 to 4 weeks or longer.

POSSIBLE DRUG, FOOD, AND/OR SUPPLEMENT INTERACTIONS
Tell your doctor if your child is taking any prescription or over-the-counter medications or any vitamins, herbs, or other supplements. Possible interactions with bupropion may include the following:

- Carbamazepine may reduce the blood levels of bupropion.
- Haloperidol, lithium, loxapine, molindone, phenothiazine tranquilizers, thioxanthene tranquilizers, and tricyclic antidepressants increase the risk of seizures.

SYMPTOMS OF OVERDOSE
Symptoms include hallucinations, seizures, chest pain, difficulty breathing, rapid heartbeat, and loss of consciousness. If overdose occurs, seek immediate medical attention and bring the drug container(s) with you.

THINGS TO TELL YOUR DOCTOR

- Tell your doctor if your child has had allergic reactions to any medications in the past or if he or she is taking any medications now.
- Let your doctor know if your child has any of the following medical conditions: history of seizures; Tourette's syndrome; anorexia nervosa; bulimia; addiction to narcotics, cocaine, or alcohol; heart disease; kidney or liver disease; head injury; or brain or spinal cord tumor.
- Tell your doctor if there is a history of depression, bipolar disorder, or any other mental health condition in your child's family.
- Consult your doctor if your child is pregnant or becomes pregnant while taking bupropion.

IMPORTANT PRECAUTIONS

- Bupropion is one of the antidepressants for which the U.S. Food and Drug Administration (FDA) ordered manufacturers to place a "black box warning" on the label, alerting patients to the possibility of clinical worsening of depression or the emergence of suicidality when using this drug (see "Psychiatric Drugs" in the introductory material of this book). These risks are especially relevant when beginning the drug or when the dose changes (either increases or decreases).
- Your child should not stop taking this drug suddenly, because withdrawal symptoms may occur. Withdrawal from bupropion should be supervised by your child's doctor.
- Store bupropion in a tightly closed container and keep away from excess heat and moisture (e.g., the bathroom, near a stove or sink).
- Bupropion can cause dizziness or shaking; therefore, you should make sure you know how your child reacts before he or she participates in potentially hazardous activities, such as riding a bike, driving a car, or operating machinery.

CALCITRIOL

BRAND NAME
Rocaltrol
Generic Not Available

ABOUT THIS DRUG
Calcitriol is a vitamin D analog used to treat abnormally low
blood levels of calcium, which can be associated with
chronic kidney failure or other conditions, such as hypoparathyroidism. This drug promotes the absorption and
use of calcium and phosphorus in the body, which are necessary to support the constant turnover of bone.

SIDE EFFECTS
Contact your doctor if your child experiences any side effects that are persistent or troubling, including any that are
not listed here.

- *Most common:* none
- *Rare:* abdominal cramps, dizziness, dry mouth, fatigue, headache, loss of appetite, metallic taste in
  mouth, muscle and/or joint pain, nausea, vomiting. If
  any of these occurs, call your doctor immediately.

HOW TO USE THIS DRUG
Calcitriol is available in capsules and oral solution. The
dosages given here are ones that are usually recommended
for children. However, your doctor will determine the most
appropriate dose and schedule for your child.

Dialysis Patients
- Children 1 to 5 years: 0.25 to 2 µg once daily.
- Children 6 years and older: Starting dose is 0.25 µg
  once daily. Your doctor may increase the dose every 4
  to 8 weeks to no more than 1 µg daily. Maintenance
  dose is typically 0.25 µg every other day up to 1.25 µg
  daily.

Hypoparathyroidism

- Children 1 to 5 years: 0.25 to 0.75 µg once daily
- Children 6 years and older: Starting dose is 0.25 µg once daily. Your doctor may gradually increase the dose every 2 to 4 weeks to no more than 0.5 to 2 µg daily.

If your child misses a dose, give it as soon as you remember. However, if it is nearly time for the next dose, skip the missed dose and resume the regular dosing schedule. Do not give a double dose.

TIME UNTIL IT TAKES EFFECT

An effect begins in about 2 to 6 hours, but it can take up to 4 weeks to reach full benefit.

POSSIBLE DRUG, FOOD, AND/OR SUPPLEMENT INTERACTIONS

Tell your doctor if your child is taking any prescription or over-the-counter medications or any vitamins, herbs, or other supplements. Possible interactions with calcitriol may include the following:

- Many over-the-counter (OTC) drugs interact with calcitriol. Talk to your doctor before you give any OTC drugs to your child while he or she is using calcitriol.
- Antacids, calcium supplements, cholestyramine, colestipol, digoxin, diuretics, ketoconazole, laxatives, oral steroids (e.g., dexamethasone, methylprednisolone, prednisone), other forms of vitamin D, phenobarbital, and phenytoin

SYMPTOMS OF OVERDOSE

Early symptoms include constipation, diarrhea, dry mouth, increased thirst, loss of appetite, headache, metallic taste, nausea, and vomiting. Advanced symptoms include bone pain, irregular heartbeat, itching, extreme drowsiness, and mental changes. If overdose occurs, seek immediate medical attention and bring the drug container(s) with you.

THINGS TO TELL YOUR DOCTOR

- Tell your doctor if your child has had allergic reactions to any medications in the past, especially other forms of vitamin D (e.g., calcifediol, dihydrotachysterol, doxercalciferol, ergocalciferol, paricalcitol), or if he or she is taking any medications now.
- Let your doctor know if your child has any of the following medical conditions: heart disease, blood vessel disease, hypoparathyroidism, hypercalcemia, hypervitaminosis D, or kidney disease.
- Consult your doctor if your child is pregnant or becomes pregnant while taking calcitriol.

IMPORTANT PRECAUTIONS

- Store calcitriol in a tightly closed container and keep away from excess heat and moisture (e.g., the bathroom, near a stove or sink).

CARBAMAZEPINE

BRAND NAMES
Carbatrol, Epitol, Equetro, Tegretol
Generic Available

ABOUT THIS DRUG
Carbamazepine is an anticonvulsant and analgesic medication used to control certain types of seizures associated with epilepsy. It is also effective in the treatment of facial pain related to trigeminal neuralgia (tic douloureux). One form—Equetro—is approved for treatment of bipolar disorder. Carbamazepine inhibits the repeated and uncontrolled firing of neurons in the brain that causes seizures.

SIDE EFFECTS
Contact your doctor if your child experiences any side effects that are persistent or troubling, including any that are not listed here.

- *Most common:* blurry vision, constipation, diarrhea, dizziness, drowsiness, increased sensitivity of the skin to sunlight, incoordination, itching, nausea, stomach pain, vomiting
- *Less common/rare:* abnormal eye movements, agitation, depression, heart rhythm abnormalities, impaired speech, impotence, involuntary movements (limbs, tongue, or face), ringing in the ears, tingling or numbness in the extremities, yellow skin discoloration, and others.

In extremely rare cases, potentially deadly side effects occur with use of carbamazepine. If your child experiences fever, rash, mouth ulcers, easy bruising, reddish or purplish spots on the skin, or sore throat, contact your doctor immediately.

HOW TO USE THIS DRUG
Carbamazepine is available in tablets, chewable tablets, extended-release tablets, and capsules and as oral suspension. The dosages given here are ones that are usually recommended for children. However, your doctor will determine the most appropriate dose and schedule for your child.

Anticonvulsant
- Children 6 to 12 years: Starting dose is 100 mg in divided doses on day 1, increased by 100 mg per day until the best response is achieved; maximum daily dosage is 1,000 mg.
- Children 13 years and older: Starting dose is 100 to 200 mg once or twice daily, increased in divided doses until the best response is obtained; optimal daily dosage is 800 to 1,200 mg. Once seizures are under control, your doctor will likely reduce the dosage gradually to an effective minimum dose.

Bipolar Disorders
- Starting dose is 200 to 400 mg per day in divided doses, increased gradually until symptoms are under control. If given along with lithium and neuroleptics,

the starting dosage should be 100 to 200 mg daily and
then increased gradually.

Trigeminal Neuralgia

- Children 13 years and older: Starting dose is 100 mg tablet
  twice daily (50 mg 4 times daily when using the suspension), increased by 200 mg per day until the pain is eliminated. Doses should not exceed 1,200 mg daily. Once pain
  relief is maintained, progressive reduction in dosage
  should be attempted until a minimum effective dosage is
  reached. Because trigeminal neuralgia periodically goes
  into remission, your doctor will attempt to reduce or discontinue the drug at intervals of not more than 3 months.

If your child misses a dose, give it as soon as you remember. If it is nearly time for the next dose, skip the missed
dose and resume the regular dosing schedule. Do not give a
double dose. If you miss an entire day or more of dosing,
call your doctor as soon as possible for instructions.

Carbamazepine suspension and tablets should be taken
with food to reduce the chance of stomach distress. The
extended-release capsules, however, do not need to be
taken with food unless they cause stomach distress. If your
child cannot swallow the capsule, its contents can be sprinkled over a teaspoon of applesauce or a similar food. The
capsule or its contents should not be chewed or crushed.

TIME UNTIL IT TAKES EFFECT
Several hours or longer

POSSIBLE DRUG, FOOD, AND/OR SUPPLEMENT
INTERACTIONS
Tell your doctor if your child is taking any prescription or
over-the-counter medications or any vitamins, herbs, or
other supplements. Possible interactions with carbamazepine may include the following:

- Cimetidine, clarithromycin, danazol, diltiazem, isoniazid, propoxyphene, erythromycin-type antibiotics,

fluoxetine, fluvoxamine, mexiletine, nicotinamide, terfenadine, valproate, and verapamil may increase blood levels of carbamazepine and could result in carbamazepine toxicity.

- Cisplatin, doxorubicin, felbamate, rifampin, and theophylline may reduce the effectiveness of carbamazepine.
- Lithium may increase nervous system side effects.
- Carbamazepine counteracts the effects of acetaminophen, warfarin, theophylline, cyclosporine, digitalis drugs, disopyramide, doxycycline, haloperidol, levothyroxine, and quinidine.
- Use of other antiseizure drugs along with carbamazepine may cause unpredictable side effects.
- Grapefruit and grapefruit juice may increase the effects of carbamazepine. Your child should not consume these foods while taking this drug.

SYMPTOMS OF OVERDOSE
Symptoms include abnormal heartbeat, confusion, double vision, extreme drowsiness, irregular breathing, loss of consciousness, seizures, spasms, and tremors. If overdose occurs, seek immediate medical attention and bring the drug container(s) with you.

THINGS TO TELL YOUR DOCTOR
- Tell your doctor if your child has had allergic reactions to any medications in the past or if he or she is taking any medications now.
- Let your doctor know if your child has any of the following medical conditions: history of heart, liver, or kidney damage; glaucoma; bone marrow depression.
- Tell your doctor if your child is pregnant or becomes pregnant while taking carbamazepine. Use of this drug during pregnancy increases the risk of birth defects.

IMPORTANT PRECAUTIONS
- Store carbamazepine in a tightly closed container and keep away from excess heat and moisture (e.g., the bathroom, near a stove or sink).

- If your child is taking carbamazepine to control seizures, do not stop treatment suddenly, as this can cause serious consequences. Only your doctor can determine how to gradually withdraw your child from this drug.
- Because carbamazepine can cause dizziness, blurry vision, and drowsiness, make sure you know how your child reacts to the drug before allowing him or her to ride a bike, drive a car, or engage in other potentially dangerous activities that require alertness.
- Some people who take carbamazepine become more sensitive to sunlight and experience itching, rash, or severe sunburn. Make sure your child's skin is protected from sunlight (sunscreen, long sleeves, long pants) while he or she is taking this drug.

CEFACLOR—see *Cephalosporins*

CEFADROXIL—see *Cephalosporins*

CEFDINIR—see *Cephalosporins*

CEFIXIME—see *Cephalosporins*

CEFPODOXIME—see *Cephalosporins*

CEFPROZIL—see *Cephalosporins*

CEFTIBUTEN—see *Cephalosporins*

CEFUROXIME—see *Cephalosporins*

CEPHALEXIN—see *Cephalosporins*

CLASS: CEPHALOSPORINS

GENERICS
(1) cefaclor; (2) cefadroxil; (3) cefdinir; (4) cefixime; (5) cefpodoxime; (6) cefprozil; (7) ceftibuten; (8) cefuroxime; (9) cephalexin; (10) cephradine

BRAND NAMES
(1) Ceclor; (2) Cefadroxil, Duricef, Ultracef; (3) Omnicef; (4) Suprax; (5) Vantin; (6) Cefzil; (7) Cedax; (8) Ceftin; (9) Keflex, Keftab; (10) Velosef
Generics Available

ABOUT THESE DRUGS
The cephalosporin antibiotics are related to cephalosporin C, an antibiotic that is similar to penicillin. The drugs in this class are used to treat a variety of common bacterial infections, and experts have identified certain infections that typically respond to each of the antibiotics. Overall, all of the cephalosporin antibiotics prevent bacteria from manufacturing cell walls, which they need to survive.

SIDE EFFECTS
Contact your doctor if your child experiences any side effects that are persistent or troubling, including any that are not listed here.

- *Most common:* abdominal pain, diarrhea, gas, itching, nausea, rash, vomiting
- *Less common/rare:* changes in taste, colitis (severe abdominal cramps and perhaps severe, bloody diarrhea), confusion, dizziness, headache, loss of appetite, muscle ache and swelling, seizures, tingling in the hands or feet, tiredness. Serum sickness (fever, joint pain, rash) is associated with cefaclor.

HOW TO USE THESE DRUGS

Cephalosporins are available in tablets, granules or powder for oral suspension (flavored), drops, and capsules and via injection. (Information on the injectable form is not provided here.) The dosages given here are ones that are usually recommended for children. However, your doctor will determine the most appropriate dose and schedule for your child.

Cefaclor

- Children up to 12 years: 9 mg per lb of body weight daily in 2 to 3 equal doses
- Children 13 years and older: 250 mg every 9 hours, or 375 to 500 mg every 12 hours

Cefadroxil

- Children up to 12 years: 13 mg per lb of body weight daily in 1 to 2 doses
- Children 13 years and older: 1 to 2 g daily in 1 to 2 doses

Cefdinir

- Children up to 12 years: 3 to 6.5 mg per lb of body weight daily in 1 to 2 doses for 5 to 10 days
- Children 13 years and older: 300 to 600 mg daily for 5 to 10 days

Cefixime

- Children up to 12 years: 3.5 mg per lb of body weight daily in 1 to 2 doses
- Children 13 years and older: 400 mg daily in 1 to 2 doses

Cefpodoxime Proxetil

- Children 5 months to 12 years: 2.5 to 5 mg per lb of body weight daily. Maximum when treating middle ear infections: 400 mg daily; when treating sore throat or tonsillitis, 200 mg daily
- Children 13 years and older: 400 mg daily in 1 to 2 doses

Cefprozil
- Children 6 months to 12 years: 13 mg per lb of body weight every 12 hours
- Children 13 years and older: 250 to 1,000 mg daily

Ceftibuten
- Children up to 12 years: 4 mg per lb of body weight once daily for 10 days
- Children 13 years and older: 400 mg once daily for 10 days

Cefuroxime
- Children up to 12 years: oral suspension, 9 to 13.6 mg per lb of body weight per day given in 2 divided doses for 10 days
- Children 13 years and older: tablets, 125 to 500 mg every 12 hours for up to 10 days, depending on the condition being treated

Cephalexin
- Children up to 12 years: 11 to 23 mg per lb of body weight daily. If treating middle ear infections, your doctor may increase the dose to 46 mg per lb of body weight
- For children 13 years and older: 250 to 1,000 mg every 6 hours. If treating urinary infections, your doctor may prescribe up to 500 mg every 12 hours

Cephradine
- Children 9 months and older: 11 to 45 mg per lb of body weight daily in 2 to 4 doses

Your child can take any of the cephalosporin antibiotics with food or milk to reduce the possibility of stomach upset. Food increases the absorption of cefpodoxime and cefuroxime.

If your child misses a dose of a medication he or she takes once daily, give it as soon as you remember. If it is nearly time for the next dose, give the missed dose immedi-

ately and give the next dose 10 to 12 hours later, then return
to the regular dosing schedule. If the medication is one your
child takes twice daily, give the missed dose as soon as you
remember and the next dose 5 to 6 hours later, then return to
the regular schedule. If the medication is one your child
takes three or more times daily, give the missed dose immediately and the next 2 to 4 hours later, then return to the regular schedule. Never give a double dose.

TIME UNTIL THEY TAKE EFFECT
Your child should begin to feel better within a few days, but
the exact length of time until you notice benefits will vary
depending on the type and severity of the infection. If your
child fails to improve or gets worse after taking any of these
antibiotics for a few days, call your doctor.

POSSIBLE DRUG, FOOD, AND/OR SUPPLEMENT
INTERACTIONS
Tell your doctor if your child is taking any prescription or
over-the-counter medications or any vitamins, herbs, or
other supplements. Possible interactions with cephalosporin
antibiotics may include the following:

- Antacids can reduce the amount of cefaclor, cefdinir,
  and cefpodoxime in the bloodstream. To prevent this
  from occurring, antacids should be taken at least 2
  hours before or after taking these antibiotics.
- Cimetidine, famotidine, nizatidine, and ranitidine can
  reduce the effectiveness of cefuroxime and cefpodoxime and so should not be taken with these drugs.
- Iron supplements and iron-fortified foods may hinder
  the absorption of cefdinir. Your child should consume
  these items at least 2 hours before or after taking this
  cephalosporin.

SYMPTOMS OF OVERDOSE
Symptoms include seizures, severe abdominal pain, vomiting, and bloody diarrhea. If overdose occurs, seek immediate
medical attention and bring the drug container(s) with you.

THINGS TO TELL YOUR DOCTOR
- Tell your doctor if your child has had allergic reactions to any medications in the past or if he or she is taking any medications, herbal remedies, or supplements now. About 15 percent of people who are allergic to penicillin are also allergic to cephalosporins. Symptoms of an allergic reaction include rash, fever, hives, and joint pain.
- Let your doctor know if your child shows signs of anemia (paleness, tiredness, difficulty breathing, weakness, abnormal heart rhythms).
- Consult your doctor if your child is pregnant or becomes pregnant while taking any of the cephalosporins.

IMPORTANT PRECAUTIONS
- Store cephalosporin antibiotics in a tightly closed container and keep at room temperature away from excess heat and moisture (e.g., the bathroom, near a stove or sink). Do not allow the liquid forms of these medications to freeze.
- Long-term or frequent use of cephalosporins can cause a secondary infection that will not respond to the antibiotic being given.

CEPHRADINE—see *Cephalosporins*

CETIRIZINE

BRAND NAME
Zyrtec
Generic Not Available

ABOUT THIS DRUG
Cetirizine is a histamine blocker that is used to treat symptoms of perennial and seasonal allergies. This drug helps relieve sneezing, itchy skin, watery eyes, and other symptoms of allergic reactions by blocking the effects of a naturally occurring substance called histamine.

SIDE EFFECTS

Contact your doctor if your child experiences any side effects that are persistent or troubling, including any that are not listed here.

- *Most common (in children 6 to 11 years):* abdominal pain, cough, diarrhea, drowsiness, headache, nosebleed, sore throat, wheezing
- *Less common/rare (in children 6 to 11 years):* nausea, vomiting

HOW TO USE THIS DRUG

Cetirizine is available in syrup, regular tablets, and chewable tablets. The dosages given here are ones that are usually recommended for children. However, your doctor will determine the most appropriate dose and schedule for your child.

- Children 2 to 5 years: Usual starting dose is ½ teaspoon syrup (2.5 mg) once daily. Your doctor may increase the dosage to a maximum of 1 teaspoon once daily or ½ teaspoon every 12 hours.
- Children 6 to 11 years: Usual starting dose is 1 to 2 teaspoons syrup (5 to 10 mg) once daily
- Children 12 years and older: 5 to 10 mg once daily

If your child misses a dose, give it as soon as you remember. If it is nearly time for the next dose, do not give the missed dose. Continue with the regular dosing schedule. Never give a double dose.

TIME UNTIL IT TAKES EFFECT

20 to 40 minutes

POSSIBLE DRUG, FOOD, AND/OR SUPPLEMENT INTERACTIONS

Tell your doctor if your child is taking any prescription or over-the-counter medications or any vitamins, herbs, or other supplements. Cetirizine may interact with the following:

- Barbiturates such as phenobarbital
- Some antidepressants, such as amitriptyline, desipramine, doxepin, and nortriptyline
- Certain narcotics, such as codeine, hydrocodone, morphine, and oxycodone
- Certain antianxiety or sleep-inducing drugs, such as alprazolam, diazepam, lorazepam
- Certain antihistamines found in cold medications, such as diphenhydramine or chlorpheniramine

SYMPTOMS OF OVERDOSE
Symptoms in children include irritability and restlessness followed by severe drowsiness. If overdose occurs, seek immediate medical attention and bring the drug container(s) with you.

THINGS TO TELL YOUR DOCTOR
- Tell your doctor if your child has had allergic reactions to any medications in the past or if he or she is taking any medications now.
- Let your doctor know if your child has kidney or liver disease.
- Consult your doctor if your child is pregnant or becomes pregnant while taking cetirizine.

IMPORTANT PRECAUTIONS
- Store cetirizine in a tightly closed container and keep at room temperature away from excess heat and moisture (e.g., the bathroom, near a stove or sink). Do not allow the syrup to freeze.
- Because cetirizine can cause drowsiness, be sure you know how your child reacts to the drug before he or she participates in potentially hazardous activities, such as riding a bike, driving a car, or operating machinery.

CHLORDIAZEPOXIDE

BRAND NAMES
Libritabs, Lithobid
Generic Available

ABOUT THIS DRUG
Chlordiazepoxide is a benzodiazepine tranquilizer and an antianxiety agent that is prescribed to treat anxiety and muscle spasms. It produces mild sedation by enhancing the effect of GABA (gamma-aminobutyric acid), a natural chemical in the brain that inhibits the firing of neurons and depresses the transmission of nerve messages.

SIDE EFFECTS
Contact your doctor if your child experiences any side effects that are persistent or troubling, including any that are not listed here.

- *Most common:* dizziness, drowsiness, lightheadedness, loss of coordination, slurred speech, unsteady gait
- *Less common/rare:* constipation, false sense of well-being, nausea, unusual fatigue, urinary problems, vomiting

HOW TO USE THIS DRUG
Chlordiazepoxide is available in capsules and tablets and via injection. (Information on injections is not provided here.) The dosages given here are ones that are usually recommended for children. However, your doctor will determine the most appropriate dose and schedule for your child.

- Children younger than 6 years: not recommended
- Children 6 years and older: 5 mg 2 to 4 times daily. Some children may need 10 mg 2 or 3 times daily.

If your child misses a dose, give it as soon as you remember. If it is nearly time for the next dose, skip the missed dose and continue with the regular dosing schedule. Never give a double dose.

TIME UNTIL IT TAKES EFFECT
Within 1 to 2 hours

POSSIBLE DRUG, FOOD, AND/OR SUPPLEMENT INTERACTIONS
Tell your doctor if your child is taking any prescription or over-the-counter medications or any vitamins, herbs, or other supplements. Possible interactions with chlordiazepoxide may include the following:

- The effects of antacids, antidepressants, barbiturates, blood thinners, cimetidine, cough medicines, decongestants, disulfiram, levodopa, major tranquilizers, narcotics, and oral contraceptives may be altered or they may change the effects of chlordiazepoxide.
- Alcohol should be avoided.

SYMPTOMS OF OVERDOSE
Symptoms include confusion, extreme drowsiness, loss of consciousness, slowed breathing, slow reflexes, slurred speech, staggering gait, and tremor. If overdose occurs, seek immediate medical attention and bring the drug container(s) with you.

THINGS TO TELL YOUR DOCTOR
- Tell your doctor if your child has had allergic reactions to any medications in the past or if he or she is taking any medications, herbal remedies, or supplements now.
- Let your doctor know if your child has any of the following medical conditions: brain disease, any chronic lung disease, hyperactivity, depression or other mental illness, sleep apnea, epilepsy, porphyria, kidney disease, or liver disease.
- If your child is hyperactive and/or aggressive, contact your doctor if your child reacts to chlordiazepoxide with acute rage, excitement, or stimulation.
- Tell your doctor if your child is pregnant or becomes pregnant during treatment with chlordiazepoxide. This drug can cause birth defects if taken during the first trimester.

IMPORTANT PRECAUTIONS

- Your child can experience withdrawal symptoms, including seizures, if he or she stops taking this drug abruptly. Talk to your doctor about withdrawing slowly from chlordiazepoxide.
- Because this drug causes dizziness and drowsiness, make sure you know how your child responds before he or she participates in potentially hazardous activities, such as riding a bike, driving a car, or operating machinery.
- Store chlordiazepoxide in a tightly closed container and keep away from excess heat and moisture (e.g., the bathroom, near a stove or sink).

CHLORPHENIRAMINE (ORAL)

BRAND NAMES

Aller-Chlor, Chlo-Amine, Chlophen, Chlor-Trimeton, Phenetron Oral, Telachlor, Teldrin
Generic Available

ABOUT THIS DRUG

Chlorpheniramine is an antihistamine used to relieve the symptoms of hay fever and other allergies, and for hives and itchy skin. This drug works by blocking the effects of histamine, a naturally occurring substance that causes itching, sneezing, watery eyes, hives, and swelling.

SIDE EFFECTS

Contact your doctor if your child experiences any side effects that are persistent or troubling, including any that are not listed here.

- *Most common:* drowsiness; dry mouth, nose, and throat; excitability,
- *Less common/rare:* difficult urination, dizziness, loss of appetite, vision changes

HOW TO USE THIS DRUG

Chlorpheniramine is available as regular tablets and capsules, sustained-release tablets and capsules, liquid, and syrup. The dosages given here are ones that are usually recommended for children. However, your doctor will determine the most appropriate dose and schedule for your child.

- Children 2 to 6 years: 1 mg syrup every 6 hours
- Children 7 to 12 years: 2 mg syrup, liquid, or regular tablets or capsules 3 to 4 times daily, not to exceed 12 mg daily
- Children 13 years and older: 4 mg tablets 3 to 4 times daily as needed for a maximum dose of 24 mg. Sustained-release capsules, 8 mg every 8 hours or 12 mg every 12 hours as needed

Do not give sustained-release tablets or capsules to a child who is younger than 12 years of age or give regular or chewable tablets or liquid to a child who is younger than 6 years of age unless directed to do so by your doctor.

Chlorpheniramine may be taken with food or milk to reduce the chance of stomach upset. If your child misses a dose, give it as soon as you remember if you are up to 2 hours late. If it is more than 2 hours late, skip the missed dose and continue with your regular dosing schedule. Never give a double dose.

TIME UNTIL IT TAKES EFFECT

15 to 60 minutes

POSSIBLE DRUG, FOOD, AND/OR SUPPLEMENT INTERACTIONS

Tell your doctor if your child is taking any prescription or over-the-counter medications or any vitamins, herbs, or other supplements. Possible interactions with chlorpheniramine may include the following:

- Maprotiline and tricyclic antidepressants (e.g., amitriptyline, clomipramine) may make the side effects of chlorpheniramine more severe.

- Excessive drowsiness may occur if chlorpheniramine is taken along with 5-HTP (5-hydroxytryptophan), GABA (gamma-aminobutyric acid), kava, melatonin, melissa, or valerian.

SYMPTOMS OF OVERDOSE

Symptoms include severe drowsiness, combativeness, confusion, dilated and sluggish pupils, excessive excitability, loss of coordination, weak pulse, seizures, loss of consciousness. If overdose occurs, seek immediate medical attention and bring the drug container(s) with you.

THINGS TO TELL YOUR DOCTOR

- Tell your doctor if your child has had allergic reactions to any medications in the past or if he or she is taking any medications now.
- Let your doctor know if your child has any of the following medical conditions: glaucoma, ulcers, asthma, diabetes, difficulty urinating, heart disease, high blood pressure, seizures, or hyperthyroidism.

IMPORTANT PRECAUTIONS

- Store chlorpheniramine in a tightly closed container and keep at room temperature away from excess heat and moisture (e.g., the bathroom, near a stove or sink). Do not allow the liquid or syrup to freeze.
- Chlorpheniramine can cause drowsiness; therefore, you should know how it affects your child before he or she participates in potentially hazardous activities, such as riding a bike, driving a car, or operating machinery.

CLARITHROMYCIN

BRAND NAME
Biaxin
Generic Not Available

ABOUT THIS DRUG
Clarithromycin is an antibacterial agent (a macrolide antibiotic) used to treat various bacterial infections, such as those that affect the tonsils, respiratory tract (e.g., bronchitis, pneumonia), ears, sinuses, and skin. It prevents bacterial cells from producing the proteins that are necessary for their survival.

SIDE EFFECTS
Contact your doctor if your child experiences any side effects that are persistent or troubling, including any that are not listed here.

- *Less common:* fungal infection of the mouth or throat, gas, headache, nausea, taste changes, upset stomach, vomiting
- *Rare:* colitis (severe abdominal cramps and severe, possibly bloody diarrhea), allergic reactions (swelling of the lips, tongue, face, and throat; breathing problems, rash, hives). Seek immediate medical attention if these symptoms occur.

HOW TO USE THIS DRUG
Clarithromycin is available in tablets and as an oral suspension. The dosages given here are ones that are usually recommended for children. However, your doctor will determine the most appropriate dose and schedule for your child.

- Children 6 months to 12 years: 3.4 mg per lb of body weight, up to 500 mg every 12 hours for 10 days
- Children 13 years and older: 250 to 500 mg every 12 hours for 1 to 2 weeks

The suspension form should be shaken well before each use. Clarithromycin may be taken with or without food, but it should be taken at the same time each day. If your child misses a dose, give it as soon as you remember. If it is within 4 hours of the next dose, do not give the missed dose, and return to the regular dosing schedule. Never give a double dose.

TIME UNTIL IT TAKES EFFECT
There is some benefit within 2 hours, but the full impact normally takes 2 to 5 days.

POSSIBLE DRUG, FOOD, AND/OR SUPPLEMENT INTERACTIONS
Tell your doctor if your child is taking any prescription or over-the-counter medications or any vitamins, herbs, or other supplements. Possible interactions with clarithromycin may include the following:

- Use of clarithromycin with omeprazole, carbamazepine, or ranitidine can increase the blood levels of both drugs.
- Clarithromycin may prolong the effects of alprazolam, diazepam, midazolam, and triazolam and result in serious nervous system depression.
- Clarithromycin may raise theophylline levels and cause an overdose.
- Fluconazole increases the blood levels of clarithromycin.
- Clarithromycin increases the effects of buspirone and causes adverse reactions.
- Cyclosporine, digoxin, ergot drugs (e.g., ergotamine, methysergide), tacrolimus, and triazolam may cause drug side effects.
- Clarithromycin may increase the blood-thinning effects of warfarin.

SYMPTOMS OF OVERDOSE
Symptoms include diarrhea, stomach cramps, severe nausea, and vomiting. If overdose occurs, seek immediate medical attention and bring the drug container(s) with you.

THINGS TO TELL YOUR DOCTOR
- Tell your doctor if your child has had allergic reactions to any medications in the past, especially other macrolide antibiotics, or if he or she is taking any medications now.
- Let your doctor know if your child has kidney or liver disease.
- Consult your doctor if your child is pregnant or becomes pregnant while taking clarithromycin.

IMPORTANT PRECAUTIONS
- Store clarithromycin in a tightly closed container and keep away from excess heat and moisture (e.g., the bathroom, near a stove or sink). Do not refrigerate the suspension.
- Clarithromycin may increase your child's sensitivity to sunlight. Make sure your child wears sunscreen and long sleeves/long pants when exposed to sunlight.

CLINDAMYCIN

BRAND NAMES
Systemic: Cleocin, Cleocin Pediatric; Topical: Cleocin T, Clinda-Derm
Generic Available

ABOUT THIS DRUG
Clindamycin is an antibacterial agent used to treat serious bacterial infections as well as acne. This drug is unusual in that it is one of the few oral antibiotics that is effective against anaerobic bacteria, which thrive in the absence of oxygen, such as in wounds, the abdomen, and the lung. It works by inhibiting the synthesis of certain proteins needed by the bacteria for their survival.

SIDE EFFECTS
Contact your doctor if your child experiences any side effects that are persistent or troubling, including any that are not listed here.

- *Most common:* for oral doses—diarrhea, nausea, painful swallowing, stomach pain, vomiting; for topical doses—dry skin, itching, and red, burning, or peeling skin
- *Less common/rare:* for oral doses—difficulty breathing, colitis (severe abdominal cramps and severe, possibly bloody diarrhea), itching, joint pain, rash, yellowing of the skin or eyes; for topical doses—abdominal pain, colitis, diarrhea, gastrointestinal upset

HOW TO USE THIS DRUG
Clindamycin is available as capsules, oral solution, gel, topical solution, suspension, cream, and vaginal suppository and via injection. (Information on the injectable form is not provided here.) The dosages given here are ones that are usually recommended for children. However, your doctor will determine the most appropriate dose and schedule for your child.

Oral Forms
- Children 1 month to 12 years: 0.9 to 2.3 mg per lb of body weight daily every 6 hours or as instructed by your doctor
- Children 13 years and older: 150 to 300 mg every 6 hours

Topical Forms
- Children up to 12 years: determined by your doctor
- Children 13 years and older: apply a thin layer to the affected areas twice daily

The oral forms should be taken with a full glass of water or with food to help prevent stomach upset. If your child misses a dose, give it as soon as you remember. However, if it is nearly time for the next dose, do not give the missed dose. Continue with the regular dosing schedule, and never give a double dose.

TIME UNTIL IT TAKES EFFECT
Oral clindamycin begins to work within 1 hour, but noticeable effects won't be evident for about 3 to 5 days. Call your

doctor if you don't see some improvement within that time. Improvement from use of the topical form (for acne) takes several weeks. If you don't notice any improvement after 6 weeks, talk to your doctor.

POSSIBLE DRUG, FOOD, AND/OR SUPPLEMENT INTERACTIONS
Tell your doctor if your child is taking any prescription or over-the-counter medications or any vitamins, herbs, or other supplements. Possible interactions with clindamycin may include the following:

- Erythromycins, chloramphenicol, or any diarrhea medication that contains kaolin or attapulgite should not be used along with clindamycin, as they may decrease the effects of clindamycin.
- Alcohol should be avoided.

SYMPTOMS OF OVERDOSE
Symptoms include severe diarrhea or other drug side effects in a severe form. If overdose occurs, seek immediate medical attention and bring the drug container(s) with you.

THINGS TO TELL YOUR DOCTOR
- Tell your doctor if your child has had allergic reactions to any medications in the past or if he or she is taking any medications now.
- Let your doctor know if your child has any of the following medical conditions: severe liver or kidney disease, history of stomach or intestinal disease, especially enteritis or colitis caused by antibiotics.
- Contact your doctor if your child develops severe or worsening diarrhea.
- Consult your doctor if your child is pregnant or becomes pregnant while taking clindamycin.

IMPORTANT PRECAUTIONS
- Store clindamycin in a tightly closed container and keep away from excess heat and moisture (e.g., the

bathroom, near a stove or sink). Do not refrigerate the oral liquid form.
- Because diarrhea is a common side effect of clindamycin, your physician may recommend giving your child probiotics (e.g., *Lactobacillus acidophilus, Bifidobacterium longum*)—"friendly" bacteria supplements—during and for a week or two after your child takes this drug.

CLOBETASOL—see *Corticosteroids, Topical*

CLOCORTOLONE—
see *Corticosteroids, Topical*

CLOMIPRAMINE—
see *Tricyclic Antidepressants*

CLOTRIMAZOLE (TOPICAL)

BRAND NAMES
Lotrimin, Lotrimin AF, Mycelex, Mycelex OTC
Generic Available

ABOUT THIS DRUG
Clotrimazole is an antifungal medication used to treat fungal infections that affect the skin (e.g., ringworm, athlete's foot, jock itch), mouth, and vaginal tract. It works by preventing fungi from producing the substances they need to reproduce.

SIDE EFFECTS
Contact your doctor if your child experiences any side effects that are persistent or troubling, including any that are not listed here.

- *Most common:* lozenges—if swallowed, may cause diarrhea, nausea, stomach cramps, vomiting; vaginal cream—may cause discharge, itching, vaginal burning or other irritation; topical form—not associated with common side effects
- *Less common/rare:* topical form or lozenges—may cause burning, hives, itching, peeling, stinging or other skin irritation; vaginal cream—may cause headache or stomach cramps

HOW TO USE THIS DRUG

Clotrimazole is available as topical cream, lotion, and solution, oral lozenge, and vaginal cream and vaginal tablets. The dosages given here are ones that are usually recommended for children. However, your doctor will determine the most appropriate dose and schedule for your child.

Skin Infections
- Apply a thin layer to the affected areas twice daily, morning and evening

Mouth Infections
- Children younger than 3 years: lozenges should not be given to children younger than 3 years
- Children 3 years and older: dissolve one 10-mg lozenge completely in the mouth 5 times daily for at least 14 days

Vaginal Infections
- Children 12 years and older: Vaginal cream—insert with an applicator, 50 mg of 1% cream for 6 to 14 nights, or 100 mg of 2% cream for 3 nights, or 500 mg of 10% for 1 night
- Children 12 years and older (nonpregnant): Vaginal tablets—insert one 100-mg tablet for 6 to 14 nights, or one 200-mg tablet for 3 nights, or one 500-mg tablet for 1 night

The lozenges work best when taken on an empty stomach. However, they can be taken with food if stomach irritation results and if your child allows the lozenge to dissolve completely in the mouth.

If your child misses a dose, give it as soon as you remember. If it is nearly time for the next dose, do not give the missed dose. Continue with the regular dosing schedule. Do not give double doses.

TIME UNTIL IT TAKES EFFECT

It depends on the severity of the infection, but significant improvement should occur within 1 week. In cases involving use of the 2% or 10% vaginal cream or 200-mg or 500-mg vaginal tablet, improvement should be evident within 3 to 4 days using the lower doses and 1 to 2 days using the higher ones.

POSSIBLE DRUG, FOOD, AND/OR SUPPLEMENT INTERACTIONS

Tell your doctor if your child is taking any prescription or over-the-counter medications or any vitamins, herbs, or other supplements. No drug-drug interactions have been reported for clotrimazole, nor any food, vitamin, or herbal interactions.

SYMPTOMS OF OVERDOSE

Overdose with clotrimazole is unlikely. However, if you believe an overdose has occurred or if the vaginal tablets are accidentally ingested, seek immediate medical attention and bring the drug container(s) with you.

THINGS TO TELL YOUR DOCTOR

- Tell your doctor if your child has had allergic reactions to any medications in the past or if he or she is taking any medications now.
- If you are using the topical form of clotrimazole, talk to your physician before using any other topical medication in the same areas.
- Consult your doctor if your child is pregnant or becomes pregnant while using clotrimazole.

IMPORTANT PRECAUTIONS

- Store clotrimazole in a tightly closed container and keep at room temperature away from excess heat and moisture (e.g., the bathroom, near a stove or sink).
- Your child should take the entire course of clotrimazole as prescribed by your doctor, even if the symptoms disappear before treatment is done. Stopping the medication too soon may allow the infection to return.

CLOXACILLIN—see *Penicillin Antibiotics*

CLOZAPINE

BRAND NAME
Clozaril
Generic Not Available

ABOUT THIS DRUG
Clozapine is an atypical antipsychotic that has been approved for treatment of severe schizophrenia in individuals who have not responded to other treatments. It is also increasingly being prescribed for children and adolescents who have bipolar disorder, attention deficit/hyperactivity disorder (ADHD), and other behavioral disorders.

This drug inhibits the activity of dopamine, a chemical in the brain. It is believed that overstimulation of specific areas in the brain by dopamine is associated with some psychiatric conditions.

SIDE EFFECTS
Contact your doctor if your child experiences any side effects that are persistent or troubling, including any that are not listed here.

- *Most common:* abdominal upset, abnormal muscle movements, agitation, confusion, constipation, dizziness, drowsiness, dry mouth, fainting, fever, headache, heartburn, high blood pressure, low blood pressure, nausea, rapid heartbeat and other heart-related conditions, salivation, sedation, sleep problems, sweating, vertigo, vision problems, vomiting, weight gain. About 5 percent of patients experience seizures.

- *Less common:* agranulocytosis (severe decline in white blood cell count; see "Important Precautions"), anemia, angina, anxiety, blood clots, bluish tinge in the skin, breast pain, difficulty breathing, bronchitis, chills, constant involuntary eye movements, cough, depression, diarrhea, dilated pupils, disorientation, dry throat, fatigue, fever, hallucinations, heart problems, hives, impotence, irritability, itching, jerky movements, joint pain, lethargy, loss of appetite, muscle spasm, painful menstruation, paranoia, poor coordination, skin inflammation, slurred speech, stuttering, swollen salivary glands, urinary difficulties, vaginal itch, weakness, wheezing, yellow skin and eyes.

Use of this drug may also cause a rare but life-threatening syndrome called neuroleptic malignant syndrome (NMS). Symptoms include fever, difficulty breathing, rapid heartbeat, rigid muscles, mental changes, increased sweating, irregular blood pressure, and convulsions. If your child displays these symptoms, seek immediate medical attention.

Very rarely in young people, a disorder known as tardive dyskinesia may occur. Characteristics include wormlike movements of the tongue, lip smacking, and slow, rhythmical, involuntary movements, which may become permanent. If your child experiences these side effects, contact your doctor immediately, and he or she will likely advise you to stop giving your child the medication.

HOW TO USE THIS DRUG

Clozapine is available in tablets. The dosages given here are ones that are often recommended for children. However, your doctor will determine the most appropriate dose and schedule for your child.

- Children younger than 6 years: not recommended
- Children 6 years and older: Starting dose often is 6.25 mg given twice per day. Your doctor may increase the dose as needed.

Clozapine can be taken with or without food. If your child misses a dose, give it as soon as you remember. If it is nearly time for the next dose, do not give the missed dose. Continue with the regular dosing schedule. Never give a double dose.

TIME UNTIL IT TAKES EFFECT
It can take several weeks for the full effect of this drug to occur.

POSSIBLE DRUG, FOOD, AND/OR SUPPLEMENT INTERACTIONS
Tell your doctor if your child is taking any prescription or over-the-counter medications or any vitamins, herbs, or other supplements. Possible interactions with clozapine may include the following:

- Use of lithium and clozapine together may cause neuroleptic malignant syndrome (see "Side Effects"), which is potentially fatal.
- Clozapine may increase the blood levels of digoxin, heparin, phenytoin, and warfarin.
- Isoniazid, phenothiazines, theophylline, and tricyclic antidepressants, among others, may increase the risk of seizure when combined with clozapine.
- Anticholinergic drugs such as tricyclic antidepressants (e.g., amitriptyline, imipramine) can increase anticholinergic effects, including confusion, blurry vision, and dry mouth.
- Central nervous system depressants (e.g., alcohol, benzodiazepines, antipsychotics) may increase the sedative effects of clozapine. These drugs should not be used when taking clozapine.
- Drugs that help reduce blood pressure (e.g., antihyper-

tensives, beta-blockers, diuretics) may increase the blood pressure–lowering effects of clozapine.
- Cigarette smoking may alter dosage needs.
- Herbs that produce a sedative effect may cause significant depressant interactions if used with clozapine. Such herbs include calendula, capsicum, catnip, goldenseal, gotu kola, hops, kava, lady's slipper, sage, Siberian ginseng, skullcap, St. John's wort, and valerian, among others.

SYMPTOMS OF OVERDOSE
Symptoms of overdose include difficulty breathing, delirium, drowsiness, excessive salivation, low blood pressure, fainting, pneumonia, rapid heartbeat, seizures, and coma. If overdose occurs, seek immediate medical attention and bring the drug container(s) with you.

THINGS TO TELL YOUR DOCTOR
- Tell your doctor if your child has had allergic reactions to any medications in the past or if he or she is taking any medications now.
- Tell your doctor if your child has a history of blood disorders, serious bowel problems, seizures not controlled by medication, breathing problems, diabetes or a family history of diabetes, glaucoma, heart problems, kidney problems, liver problems, obesity or a family history of obesity, or difficulty urinating.
- Because clozapine may make your child dizzy, drowsy, and/or sedated, make sure you know how your child reacts to the drug before he or she participates in potentially hazardous activities, such as riding a bike, driving a car, or operating machinery.
- If your child is scheduled for surgery (including dental surgery), tell your doctor or dentist that your child is taking clozapine.
- The rapidly dissolving form of clozapine may contain phenylalanine or aspartame. Consult your doctor or pharmacist about your child taking clozapine if he or she has phenylketonuria or any other condition

that requires the restriction of aspartame or phenyl-lalanine.

IMPORTANT PRECAUTIONS
- Clozapine can cause significant weight gain. Your doctor should carefully monitor your child's growth and development while he or she is taking this drug.
- This drug can cause blood sugar levels to rise, which can cause serious or even fatal conditions if your child has diabetes. Blood sugar levels should be monitored carefully.
- Store clozapine in a tightly closed container and keep at room temperature away from excess heat and moisture (e.g., the bathroom, near a stove or sink).

CODEINE/CODEINE PLUS GUAIFENESIN

BRAND NAMES
Codeine combined with guaifenesin in Brontex, Gani-Tuss NR, Mytussin AC Cough Syrup, Robitussin A-C Syrup, Tussi-Organidin NR, and others
Generic Available

ABOUT THIS DRUG
Codeine is an opioid (narcotic) painkiller used to treat moderate to severe pain and to control severe cough. It acts on specific areas of the spinal cord and brain where pain messages are processed. In the treatment of cough, it blocks the cough reflex center in the brain. (See also *Acetaminophen plus Codeine; Guaifenesin.*)

SIDE EFFECTS
Contact your doctor if your child experiences any side effects that are persistent or troubling, including any that are not listed here.

- *Most common:* constipation, drowsiness, dizziness, loss of appetite, nausea, sweating, vomiting
- *Less common/rare:* agitation, anemia, headache, rash

HOW TO USE THIS DRUG

Codeine is available in tablets, oral solution, and syrup. The dosages given here are ones that are usually recommended for children. However, your doctor will determine the most appropriate dose and schedule for your child.

For Pain
- Children up to 12 years: 0.23 mg of oral solution per lb of body weight every 4 to 6 hours as needed
- Children 13 years and older: 15 to 60 mg every 3 to 6 hours as needed

For Cough—Codeine Alone
- Age 2 years: 3 mg every 4 to 6 hours, not to exceed 12 mg daily
- Age 3 years: 3.5 mg every 4 to 6 hours, not to exceed 14 mg daily
- Age 4 years: 4 mg every 4 to 6 hours, not to exceed 16 mg daily
- Age 5 years: 4.5 mg every 4 to 6 hours, not to exceed 18 mg daily
- Ages 6 to 12 years: 5 to 10 mg every 4 to 6 hours, not to exceed 60 mg daily

For Cough—Combination Formulas
- See individual product instructions

If your child misses a dose, give it as soon as you remember. If it is nearly time for the next dose, skip the missed dose and continue with the regular dosing schedule. Never give a double dose.

TIME UNTIL IT TAKES EFFECT

Your child should experience pain relief 30 to 60 minutes after taking a dose. When taken for cough, relief takes about 1 to 2 hours.

POSSIBLE DRUG, FOOD, AND/OR SUPPLEMENT INTERACTIONS

Tell your doctor if your child is taking any prescription or over-the-counter medications or any vitamins, herbs, or other supplements. Possible interactions with codeine may include the following:

- Tranquilizers, sleeping pills, and other drugs that affect the central nervous system should not be taken along with codeine.
- Drugs that lower blood pressure (e.g., beta-blockers, antihypertensives) may result in abnormally low blood pressure, in which case the codeine should be stopped.
- Herbs that produce a sedative effect (e.g., capsicum, catnip, goldenseal, gotu kola, hops, kava, passionflower, sage, Siberian ginseng, St. John's wort, and valerian, among others) should be avoided, as they may cause potentially serious depressant interactions.

SYMPTOMS OF OVERDOSE

Symptoms include pinpoint pupils, seizures, confusion, dizziness, severe drowsiness, troubled breathing, stupor, and coma. If overdose occurs, seek immediate medical attention and bring the drug container(s) with you.

THINGS TO TELL YOUR DOCTOR

- Tell your doctor if your child has had allergic reactions to any medications in the past or if he or she is taking any medications now.
- Let your doctor know if your child has any of the following medical conditions: kidney, liver, heart, or thyroid disease; asthma, seizures, urinary difficulties, or colitis.
- Tell your doctor if your child has had a head injury.
- Consult your doctor if your child is pregnant or becomes pregnant while taking codeine. This drug may cause breathing problems in infants during delivery, and excessive use during pregnancy may cause infants to be drug dependent.

- Before your child has any type of surgery, including dental surgery, tell your doctor that your child is taking this drug.

IMPORTANT PRECAUTIONS
- Store codeine in a tightly closed container and keep at room temperature away from excess heat and moisture (e.g., the bathroom, near a stove or sink). Do not allow the liquid forms to freeze.
- Because this drug can cause drowsiness, dizziness, light-headedness, and/or sedation, monitor your child carefully when he or she takes it and do not let your child participate in potentially dangerous activities, such as riding a bike, driving a car, or operating machinery.
- If your child takes codeine regularly for several weeks, talk to your doctor, as physical dependence can develop and side effects may occur if the codeine is stopped abruptly.

CLASS: CORTICOSTEROIDS, NASAL INHALANTS

GENERICS
(1) beclomethasone; (2) budesonide (see *Budesonide*); (3) dexamethasone; (4) flunisolide; (5) fluticasone; (6) mometasone; (7) triamcinolone

BRAND NAMES
(1) Beconase, Beconase AQ, Vancenase, Vancenase AQ; (2) see *Budesonide*; (3) Dexacort Turbinaire; (4) Nasalide, Nasarel, Rhinalar; (5) Flonase; (6) Nasonex; (7) Nasacort, Nasacort AQ, Tri-Nasal
Generics Available

ABOUT THESE DRUGS
Nasal inhalation corticosteroids are used to treat severe symptoms of chronic and seasonal allergic hay fever (rhinitis) that have not responded to other medications. These

drugs reduce inflammation of the mucous membranes in the nasal passages.

SIDE EFFECTS

Contact your doctor if your child experiences any side effects that are persistent or troubling, including any that are not listed here.

- *Most common:* burning or dry nasal passages, headache, irritated nasal passages and throat
- *Less common:* bronchial asthma, lightheadedness, loss of sense of taste, nasal congestion, nausea, nosebleed, sneezing attacks
- *Rare:* hypersensitivity reaction (e.g., breathing problems, itching, rash, swelling), increased eye pressure, sore throat, ulcers in the nasal passages, watery eyes, wheezing, vomiting. Seek immediate medical attention if your child experiences breathing problems.

HOW TO USE THESE DRUGS

Nasal inhalation corticosteroids are available in nasal inhalers. The dosages given here are ones that are usually recommended for children. However, your doctor will determine the most appropriate dose and schedule for your child.

Beclomethasone

- Children 6 to 12 years: 1 spray in each nostril 3 times daily
- Children 13 years and older: 1 spray in each nostril 2 to 4 times daily

Budesonide—see *Budesonide*

Dexamethasone

- Children younger than 6 years: to be determined by your doctor
- Children 6 to 12 years: 1 to 2 sprays in each nostril 2 times daily for up to 2 weeks

- Children 13 years and older: 2 sprays in each nostril 2 to 3 times daily for up to 2 weeks

Flunisolide
- Children 6 to 14 years: 1 spray in each nostril 3 times daily, or 2 sprays in each nostril 2 times daily
- Children 15 years and older: starting dose, 2 sprays in each nostril 2 times daily, which your doctor may increase to up to 8 sprays daily in each nostril

Fluticasone
- Children 4 years and older: 1 spray in each nostril once daily, which your doctor may increase to 2 sprays per day in each nostril

Mometasone
- Children 12 years and older: 1 or 2 sprays in each nostril once daily, which your doctor may increase to 4 sprays daily in each nostril

Triamcinolone
- Children 6 to 12 years: 1 (Nasacort AQ) or 2 (Nasacort) sprays in each nostril once daily, which your doctor may increase to 2 sprays daily in each nostril
- Children 13 years and older: 2 sprays in each nostril once daily, which your doctor may increase to 4 sprays daily in each nostril

If your child misses a dose, give it as soon as you remember. However, if it is nearly time for the next dose, skip the missed dose and continue with the regular dosing schedule. Never give a double dose.

TIME UNTIL THEY TAKE EFFECT
Beclomethasone, dexamethasone, flunisolide, fluticasone, and triamcinolone, usually within 1 week but up to 3 weeks for a full effect; mometasone, 11 hours to 2 days

•

POSSIBLE DRUG, FOOD, AND/OR SUPPLEMENT INTERACTIONS

Tell your doctor if your child is taking any prescription or over-the-counter medications or any vitamins, herbs, or other supplements. No interactions with other medications, foods, or supplements have been noted. However, you should consult your physician before your child uses any of these drugs if he or she is also using any oral corticosteroids, other inhaled corticosteroids, or any drugs that suppress the immune system.

SYMPTOMS OF OVERDOSE

No specific symptoms of overdose have been reported. If, however, you believe an overdose has occurred, or if your child accidentally takes one of these drugs orally, seek immediate medical attention and bring the drug container(s) with you.

THINGS TO TELL YOUR DOCTOR

- Tell your doctor if your child has had allergic reactions to any medications in the past or if he or she is taking any medications, herbal remedies, or supplements now. Also tell your doctor if your child is sensitive or allergic to any of the propellants in the nasal spray, which include benzalkonium chloride, disodium edetate, phenylethanol, fluorocarbons, and propylene glycol.
- Let your doctor know if your child has undergone recent nasal surgery or has any of the following medical conditions: tuberculosis; ocular herpes simplex; any untreated fungal, bacterial, or viral infection; nasal polyps
- Use of corticosteroids increases the risk of infection. While your child is taking these drugs, he or she should avoid contact with people who have an infection. If your child is exposed to chicken pox or measles while using any of these corticosteroids or if he or she develops blisters or sores, contact your physician immediately.
- If your child is scheduled to undergo any type of surgery (including dental surgery), tell your doctor or dentist that your child is taking corticosteroids.

- Consult your doctor if your child is pregnant or becomes pregnant while taking corticosteroids. Use of large amounts of corticosteroids during pregnancy may suppress fetal development.

IMPORTANT PRECAUTIONS
- In rare cases, use of nasal inhalation corticosteroids can cause *Candida* yeast infections in the nose and throat.
- Store nasal inhalation corticosteroids in a tightly closed container and keep away from excess heat and moisture (e.g., the bathroom, near a stove or sink).

CLASS: CORTICOSTEROIDS, ORAL

GENERICS
(1) betamethasone; (2) cortisone; (3) dexamethasone; (4) hydrocortisone (systemic); (5) methylprednisolone (systemic); (6) prednisolone (systemic); (7) prednisone; (8) triamcinolone

BRAND NAMES
(1) Celestone; (2) Cortone Acetate; (3) Decadron, Dexone, Hexadrol; (4) Cortef, Hydrocortone; (5) Medrol; (6) Cortolone, Delta-Cortef, Pediapred, Prelone; (7) Deltasone, Liquid Pred, Meticorten, Orasone, Panasol-S, Prednicen-M; (8) Aristocort A, Kenacort
Generics Available

ABOUT THESE DRUGS
Oral corticosteroids are used to treat various inflammatory conditions in children, including asthma and other severe respiratory diseases, gastrointestinal diseases, skin disorders, and inflammation of the heart, nerves, and other organs.

Synthetic corticosteroids have been designed to mimic the ones produced naturally by the adrenal glands. They are given to provide relief from swelling, itching, redness, and other allergic reactions.

SIDE EFFECTS

Contact your doctor if your child experiences any side effects that are persistent or troubling, including any that are not listed here.

- *Most common:* acne, dizziness, gas, headache, insomnia, increased appetite, indigestion, poor wound healing, swollen legs or feet
- *Less common:* bloody or tarry stool, blurry vision, euphoria, fatigue, fever, frequent urination, mood changes, muscle cramps, restlessness, stomach or hip pain, thirst
- *Rare:* confusion, convulsions, hallucinations, irregular heartbeat, joint pain, leg or thigh pain, skin color changes, unusual hair growth on the body or face

HOW TO USE THESE DRUGS

These drugs are available in tablets, elixir, and oral solution. The dosages given here are ones that are usually recommended for children. Doses for children up to age 12 are highly individualized and must be determined by your physician. However, your doctor will determine the most appropriate dose and schedule for your child.

Betamethasone
- Children up to age 12 years: dose depends on body weight and will be determined by your physician
- Children 13 years and older: 0.25 to 7.2 mg daily in 1 or 2 divided doses

Cortisone
- Children up to age 12 years: dose depends on body weight and will be determined by your physician
- Children 13 years and older: 25 to 300 mg daily in 1 or 2 divided doses

Dexamethasone
- Children up to age 12 years: dose depends on body weight and will be determined by your physician

- Children 13 years and older: 0.5 to 10 mg as determined by your doctor

Hydrocortisone
- Children up to age 12 years: dose depends on body weight and will be determined by your physician
- Children 13 years and older: 20 to 800 mg every 1 or 2 days as a single or divided dose

Methylprednisolone
- Children up to age 12 years: dose depends on body weight and will be determined by your physician
- Children 13 years and older: 4 to 160 mg every 1 or 2 days as a single or divided dose

Prednisolone
- Children up to age 12 years: dose depends on body weight and will be determined by your physician
- Children 13 years and older: 5 to 200 mg as needed and prescribed by your doctor

Prednisone
- Children up to age 12 years: dose depends on body weight and will be determined by your physician
- Children 13 years and older: 5 to 200 mg every 1 to 2 days as a single or divided dose

Triamcinolone
- Children up to age 12 years: dose depends on body weight and will be determined by your physician
- Children 13 years and older: 2 to 60 mg in 1 or 2 divided doses

Oral corticosteroids should be taken with food to help prevent stomach upset. If your child experiences stomach burning or pain, consult your doctor.

If your child misses a dose, give it as soon as you remember. If it is nearly time for the next dose, do not give the missed dose. Continue with your regular dosing schedule. Never give a double dose.

TIME UNTIL THEY TAKE EFFECT
Varies, depending on the condition and its severity and the medication used

POSSIBLE DRUG, FOOD, AND/OR SUPPLEMENT INTERACTIONS
Tell your doctor if your child is taking any prescription or over-the-counter medications or any vitamins, herbs, or other supplements. Possible interactions with oral corticosteroids may include the following:

- Oral corticosteroids may reduce the effects of anticoagulants (e.g., warfarin), antidiabetic drugs (e.g., glipizide), and salicylates (e.g., aspirin).
- Use of antacids may reduce the effects of prednisone and dexamethasone.
- Antihistamines (e.g., clemastine, cetirizine), carbamazepine, cholestyramine, colestipol, cyclosporine, ephedrine, glutethimide, rifampin, primidone, phenytoin, and phenobarbital may reduce the effects of oral corticosteroids.
- Tricyclic antidepressants (e.g., clomipramine, imipramine) may increase the risk of mental side effects.
- Nonsteroidal anti-inflammatory drugs (NSAIDs) may increase the risk of ulcers and increase the effects of oral corticosteroids.
- Corticosteroids can cause severe potassium depletion, which can increase the risk of digoxin toxicity.

SYMPTOMS OF OVERDOSE
Symptoms include convulsions, fluid retention, heart failure, and severe headache. If overdose occurs, seek immediate medical attention and bring the drug container(s) with you.

THINGS TO TELL YOUR DOCTOR

- Tell your doctor if your child has had allergic reactions to any medications in the past, including other corticosteroids, or if he or she is taking any medications now.
- Let your doctor know if your child has any of the following medical conditions: severe kidney disease, ulcerative colitis, high blood pressure, Cushing's disease, diabetes, hypothyroidism, stomach ulcers, seizure disorder, chicken pox or measles (or recent exposure to either), a fungal infection, or an antibiotic-resistant infection.
- Use of corticosteroids increases the risk of infection. While your child is taking these drugs, he or she should avoid contact with people who have an infection. If your child is exposed to chicken pox or measles while using any of these corticosteroids or if he or she develops blisters or sores, contact your physician immediately.
- If you want your child to stop taking these drugs, do not stop treatment yourself. Talk to your doctor, as only he or she can safely withdraw your child from the drug.
- If your child is scheduled to undergo any type of surgery (including dental surgery), tell your doctor or dentist that your child is taking corticosteroids.
- Consult your doctor if your child is pregnant or becomes pregnant while taking oral corticosteroids. Long-term use of high doses of these drugs may cause birth defects.

IMPORTANT PRECAUTIONS

- Corticosteroids compromise the immune system, which can make your child more susceptible to infections.
- Oral corticosteroids may contain sulfite preservatives and tartrazine dyes that can cause allergic reactions in some people.
- Oral corticosteroids may hinder the normal growth of your child. Talk to your doctor about this issue and make sure he or she regularly monitors your child's development.

- Store corticosteroids in a tightly closed container and keep away from excess heat and moisture (e.g., the bathroom, near a stove or sink). Do not allow the liquid forms to freeze.

CLASS: CORTICOSTEROIDS, ORAL INHALANTS

GENERICS
(1) beclomethasone; (2) budesonide (see *Budesonide*); (3) dexamethasone; (4) flunisolide; (5) fluticasone; (6) triamcinolone

BRAND NAMES
(1) Beclodisk, Becloforte, Beclovent, Beclovent Rotacaps, Qvar, Vanceril; (2) see *Budesonide*; (3) Decadron Respihaler; (4) AeroBid, AeroBid-M, Bronalide; (5) Flovent Oral Inhaler, Rotadisk; (6) Azmacort
Generics Available

ABOUT THESE DRUGS
Oral inhalation corticosteroids are used to prevent symptoms of chronic bronchial asthma. They are not effective in the treatment of acute asthma attacks. These drugs help prevent inflammation in the lungs and breathing passages.

SIDE EFFECTS
Contact your doctor if your child experiences any side effects that are persistent or troubling, including any that are not listed here.

- *Most common:* cough, dry mouth, hoarseness, throat irritation
- *Less common:* bruising, dry throat, headache, nausea, painful swallowing, thrush (yeast infection of the throat or mouth)
- *Rare:* breathing problems, tight or painful chest

HOW TO USE THESE DRUGS

Oral inhalation corticosteroids are available in oral inhalers.
The dosages given here are ones that are usually recommended for children. However, your doctor will determine
the most appropriate dose and schedule for your child.

Beclomethasone

- Children 6 to 12 years: 1 to 2 inhalations 3 to 4 times
  daily
- Children 13 years and older: 2 inhalations 3 to 4 times
  daily, or 4 inhalations twice daily; if your child has severe asthma, up to 16 inhalations daily can be taken.

Budesonide—see *Budesonide*

Flunisolide

- Children 6 to 15 years: 1 inhalation in the morning and
  1 inhalation in the evening; do not exceed 4 inhalations
  daily
- Children 16 years and older: 2 inhalations in the morning and 2 inhalations in the evening; do not exceed 8
  inhalations daily.

Fluticasone

- Children 12 years and older: 88 to 880 µg twice daily
- Children 12 years and older: Rotadisk—100 to 1,000
  µg twice daily

Triamcinolone

- Children 6 to 12 years: 1 to 2 inhalations 3 to 4 times
  daily; maximum of 12 inhalations daily
- Children 12 years and older: 2 inhalations 3 to 4 times
  daily; maximum of 16 inhalations daily

Before using the inhaler, your child should drink water to
moisten his or her throat. He or she should wait at least 1
minute between inhalations and rinse the mouth after com-
pleting dosing.

If your child misses a dose, give it as soon as you remem-

ber. However, if it is nearly time for the next dose, skip the missed dose and continue with the regular dosing schedule. Never give a double dose.

TIME UNTIL THEY TAKE EFFECT
Usually within 1 week but up to 3 weeks for a full effect

POSSIBLE DRUG, FOOD, AND/OR SUPPLEMENT INTERACTIONS
Tell your doctor if your child is taking any prescription or over-the-counter medications or any vitamins, herbs, or other supplements. No interactions with other medications, foods, or supplements have been noted. However, you should consult your physician before your child uses any of these drugs if he or she is also using any oral corticosteroids, other inhaled corticosteroids, or any drugs that suppress the immune system.

SYMPTOMS OF OVERDOSE
No specific symptoms of overdose have been reported. If, however, you believe an overdose has occurred, or if your child accidentally ingests the drug, seek immediate medical attention and bring the drug container(s) with you.

THINGS TO TELL YOUR DOCTOR
- Tell your doctor if your child has had allergic reactions to any medications in the past or if he or she is taking any medications, herbal remedies, or supplements now.
- Let your doctor know if your child has tuberculosis, herpes simplex virus of the eye, chronic bronchitis or bronchiectasis, hypothyroidism, liver disease, glaucoma, or any active infection.
- Use of corticosteroids increases the risk of infection. While your child is taking these drugs, he or she should avoid contact with people who have an infection. If your child is exposed to chicken pox or measles while using any of these corticosteroids or if he or she develops blisters or sores, contact your physician immediately.

- If your child is scheduled to undergo any type of surgery (including dental surgery), tell your doctor or dentist that your child is taking corticosteroids.
- Consult your doctor if your child is pregnant or becomes pregnant while using oral inhalant corticosteroids. Use of large amounts of these medications during pregnancy may suppress fetal development.

IMPORTANT PRECAUTIONS
- In rare cases, use of oral inhalation corticosteroids can cause *Candida* yeast infections in the mouth and throat. To help prevent this, after each use of the inhaler your child should rinse his or her mouth with water and spit out the water.
- These medications must be used regularly to prevent the shortness of breath and wheezing associated with asthma, bronchitis, and emphysema.
- There is a slight chance oral inhalation corticosteroids may cause a slowing of growth in children. Monitor your child's growth regularly while he or she is using these drugs.
- Store oral inhalation corticosteroids in a tightly closed container and keep away from excess heat and moisture (e.g., the bathroom, near a stove or sink).

CLASS: CORTICOSTEROIDS, TOPICAL

GENERICS
(1) alclometasone; (2) amcinonide; (3) betamethasone; (4) clobetasol; (5) clocortolone; (6) desonide; (7) desoximetasone; (8) dexamethasone; (9) diflorasone; (10) fluocinolone; (11) fluocinonide; (12) flurandrenolide; (13) fluticasone; (14) halcinonide; (15) halobetasol; (16) hydrocortisone; (17) mometasone; (18) prednicarbate; (19) triamcinolone

BRAND NAMES
(1) Aclovate; (2) Cyclocort; (3) Alphatrex, Diprosone, Luxiq, Teladar, Valisone; (4) Cormax, Embeline, Temovate;

(5) Cloderm; (6) Desonate, DesOwen, Verdeso; (7) Topicort; (8) Aeroseb-Dex, Decadron; (9) Florone, Maxiflor, Psorcon; (10) Fluonid, Flurosyn, Synalar; (11) Fluonex, Lidex; (12) Cordran, Cordran SP; (13) Cutivate; (14) Halog; (15) Ultravate; (16) Acticort 100, Bactine Hydrocortisone, Cortaid Intensive Therapy, Delcort, Lanacort-5, Penecort, Tegrin-HC, and others; (17) Elocon; (18) Dermatop; (19) Aristocort, Flutex, Kenalog, Kenonel, Triderm
Generics Available

ABOUT THESE DRUGS
Topical corticosteroids are prescribed to treat itching, inflammation, and other types of skin irritation. Many brands and strengths are available, and each one has conditions for which it is better suited than others. Your doctor will identify the best product for your child's condition.

These medications interfere with the production of various substances that cause inflammation, redness, swelling, and pain associated with skin conditions.

SIDE EFFECTS
Contact your doctor if your child experiences any side effects that are persistent or troubling, including any that are not listed here.

- *Most common:* acne, burning, dryness, itching, irritation, redness, stinging and cracking, tingling or numbness in the extremities
- *Less common:* blistering and pus near hair follicles (with prolonged use), increased susceptibility to infection, unusual bleeding or bruising

HOW TO USE THESE DRUGS
Topical corticosteroids are available in gel, cream, lotion, tape, aerosol, and ointment. Dosages and dosing schedules differ for each medication. Your doctor will determine the best product, dose, and dosing schedule for your child's needs.

Generally, if your child misses a dose, give it as soon as

you remember. If it is nearly time for the next dose, skip the missed dose and continue with the regular dosing schedule. Do not give a double dose.

TIME UNTIL THEY TAKE EFFECT
Varies

POSSIBLE DRUG, FOOD, AND/OR SUPPLEMENT INTERACTIONS
Tell your doctor if your child is taking any prescription or over-the-counter medications or any vitamins, herbs, or other supplements. No interactions with other medications, foods, or supplements have been noted. However, you should consult your doctor before your child uses any of these drugs if he or she is also using any other topical medications.

SYMPTOMS OF OVERDOSE
No specific symptoms of overdose have been reported. If, however, you believe an overdose has occurred or if your child accidentally ingests the drug, seek immediate medical attention and bring the drug container(s) with you.

THINGS TO TELL YOUR DOCTOR
- Tell your doctor if your child has had allergic reactions to any medications in the past or if he or she is taking any medications, herbal remedies, or supplements now.
- Contact your doctor if symptoms worsen or do not improve within 1 week of use.
- Do not use these drugs more often or longer than your doctor prescribes.
- Let your doctor know if your child has cataracts, diabetes, glaucoma, any type of infection or sores, or tuberculosis.
- Consult your doctor if your child is pregnant or becomes pregnant while using topical corticosteroids. Use of large amounts of these medications during pregnancy may cause birth defects.

IMPORTANT PRECAUTIONS

- Store topical corticosteroids in a tightly closed container and keep away from excess heat or cold.
- Use of corticosteroids increases the risk of infection. While your child is taking these drugs, he or she should avoid contact with people who have an infection. If your child is exposed to chicken pox or measles while using any of these corticosteroids or if he or she develops blisters or sores, contact your physician immediately.

CORTISONE—see *Corticosteroids, Oral*

CROMOLYN SODIUM

BRAND NAMES

Children's Nasalcrom, Crolom, Intal, Intal Aerosol Spray, Intal Nebulizer Solution, Nasalcrom, Opticrom
Generic Available

ABOUT THIS DRUG

Cromolyn is an antiallergy and antiasthmatic medication used to help control symptoms of seasonal allergies, chronic bronchial asthma, and conjunctivitis (inflammation of the mucous membranes of the eyelids and whites of the eyes), which often accompanies allergies.

This drug inhibits the release of histamine, a naturally occurring chemical that is released by the body during allergic reactions. Histamine causes sneezing, hives, itchy and watery eyes, swelling, and other allergic reactions.

SIDE EFFECTS

Contact your doctor if your child experiences any side effects that are persistent or troubling, including any that are not listed here.

- *Most common:* nasal and inhalant forms—burning or irritated nose, dry or irritated throat, sneezing; ophthalmic form—burning or stinging of the eyes

- *Less common/rare:* nasal and inhalant forms—cough, headache, postnasal drip, unpleasant taste; ophthalmic form—dry or puffy around the eyes, increased itching or watering of the eyes

HOW TO USE THIS DRUG

Cromolyn is available as an aerosol, inhalation solution (20-mg capsule), ampoule (20 mg), nasal solution, and ophthalmic drops. The dosages given here are ones that are usually recommended for children. However, your doctor will determine the most appropriate dose and schedule for your child.

Inhalation Aerosol

- Children 4 years and younger: this form of cromolyn should not be used in this age group
- Children 5 years and older: to prevent asthma symptoms, 2 inhalations 4 times daily
- Children 5 years and older: to prevent bronchospasm, 2 inhalations at least 10 to 15 minutes but not more than 60 minutes before exercise or exposure to allergens

Inhalation Solution

- Children younger than 2 years: this form of cromolyn should not be used in this age group
- Children 2 years and older: to prevent asthma symptoms, 20 mg (contents of 1 capsule, used in an inhaler, or 1 ampoule used in a nebulizer) 4 times daily, 4 to 6 hours apart
- Children 2 years and older: for prevention of bronchospasm, 20 mg (contents of 1 capsule, used in an inhaler, or 1 ampoule used in a nebulizer), taken at least 10 to 15 minutes but not more than 60 minutes before exercise or exposure to allergens

Nasal Solution

- Children 5 years and younger: use and dosage to be determined by your doctor

- Children 6 years and older: 1 spray in each nostril 3 to 6 times daily

Ophthalmic Drops
- Children up to 4 years: dose and schedule to be determined by your doctor
- Children 4 years and older: 1 drop 4 to 6 times daily in evenly spaced intervals

The inhalation solution form is a capsule that is placed in an inhaler for use; the ampoule is used in a nebulizer. You should regularly clean your child's inhaler or nebulizer; follow the instructions provided with the unit or ask your health-care professional.

If your child misses a dose, give it if it is within 2 hours of the scheduled dose. If it is more than 2 hours past the scheduled dose, skip the missed dose and continue with the regular dosing schedule. Never give a double dose.

TIME UNTIL IT TAKES EFFECT
Response time varies. For the ophthalmic form, relief may occur within a few days or it may take weeks. For the nasal and inhalant forms, cromolyn must be taken for about 6 weeks before it reaches full effect.

POSSIBLE DRUG, FOOD, AND/OR SUPPLEMENT INTERACTIONS
Tell your doctor if your child is taking any prescription or over-the-counter medications or any vitamins, herbs, or other supplements. No significant drug, food, or supplement interactions have been reported for cromolyn.

SYMPTOMS OF OVERDOSE
No specific symptoms of overdose have been reported. However, if you believe your child has taken an excessive amount of this drug, or if the ophthalmic form is accidentally ingested, seek immediate medical attention and bring the drug container(s) with you.

THINGS TO TELL YOUR DOCTOR
- Tell your doctor if your child has had allergic reactions to any medications in the past or if he or she is taking any medications now.
- Let your doctor know if your child has any of the following medical conditions: kidney or liver disease, polyps or growths inside the nose, abnormal heart rhythm, or diseased coronary blood vessels.
- Consult your doctor if your child is pregnant or becomes pregnant during treatment.

IMPORTANT PRECAUTIONS
- Store cromolyn in a tightly closed container and keep away from excess heat, direct light, and moisture (e.g., the bathroom, near a stove or sink). Do not allow the ophthalmic form to freeze.
- Your child should use this drug for the full treatment period, even if he or she feels better before the scheduled end of therapy.

CYPROHEPTADINE

BRAND NAME
Periactin
Generic Available

ABOUT THIS DRUG
Cyproheptadine is an antihistamine used to prevent or relieve symptoms of hay fever and other seasonal allergies. This drug blocks the effects of histamine, a naturally occurring substance in the body that causes symptoms such as sneezing, itching, watery eyes, and other symptoms of allergic reactions. Cyproheptadine is sometimes used as an appetite stimulant.

SIDE EFFECTS
Contact your physician if your child experiences any side effects that are persistent or troubling, including any that are not listed here.

- *Most common:* dry mouth, dry nose, drowsiness
- *Less common/rare:* difficult urination, dizziness, excitement, increased sensitivity to sunlight, irritability, rash, restlessness, weight gain

HOW TO USE THIS DRUG
Cyproheptadine is available as tablets and a syrup. The dosages given here are ones that are usually recommended for children. However, your doctor will determine the most appropriate dose and schedule for your child.

- Children 2 to 6 years: 2 mg (one-half tablet) every 8 to 12 hours
- Children 7 to 14 years: 4 mg every 8 to 12 hours
- Children 15 years and older: 4 mg every 8 hours, which your doctor may gradually increase

Cyproheptadine may be taken with or without food. If your child misses a dose, give it as soon as you remember. However, if it is nearly time for the next dose, skip the missed dose and resume the regular dosing schedule. Do not give a double dose.

TIME UNTIL IT TAKES EFFECT
15 to 60 minutes

POSSIBLE DRUG, FOOD, AND/OR SUPPLEMENT INTERACTIONS
Tell your doctor if your child is taking any prescription or over-the-counter medications or any vitamins, herbs, or other supplements. Possible interactions with cyproheptadine may include the following:

- Use of cyproheptadine along with monoamine oxidase (MAO) inhibitors, sedatives, other antihistamines, cough medicines, or tranquilizers may alter the effects of these drugs in your child's system.
- Alcohol should be avoided.

SYMPTOMS OF OVERDOSE

Symptoms include hallucinations, convulsions, blurry vision, flushing, very dry warm skin, dilated pupils, and severe sedation. If overdose occurs, seek immediate medical attention and bring the drug container(s) with you.

THINGS TO TELL YOUR DOCTOR

- Tell your doctor if your child has had allergic reactions to any medications in the past or if he or she is taking any medications, herbal remedies, or supplements now.
- Let your doctor know if your child has any difficulties with urination or has glaucoma or other vision disorders.
- Consult your doctor if your child is pregnant or becomes pregnant during treatment.

IMPORTANT PRECAUTIONS

- Store cyproheptadine in a tightly closed container and keep away from excess heat and moisture (e.g., the bathroom, near a stove or sink). Keep the liquid form refrigerated, but do not allow it to freeze.
- Cyproheptadine may make your child drowsy, so be sure you know how he or she reacts before you allow him or her to participate in potentially hazardous activities, such as riding a bike, driving a car, or operating machinery.

DANTROLENE

BRAND NAME
Dantrium
Generic Not Available

ABOUT THIS DRUG
Dantrolene is a muscle relaxant that is used to control recurring muscle spasms and cramps that accompany conditions such as cerebral palsy, multiple sclerosis, spinal cord injuries, and others. This drug blocks the release of calcium, a

substance necessary for muscle contraction, in skeletal muscle, which results in control of muscle spasms and cramping.

SIDE EFFECTS
Contact your doctor if your child experiences any side effects that are persistent or troubling, including any that are not listed here.

Most common: dizziness, drowsiness, headache, muscle weakness

Less common/rare: blood pressure changes, chills, confusion, cramps, difficulty swallowing, double vision, frequent urination, hallucinations, irregular or rapid heartbeat, muscle pain, nervousness, watery eyes, weight loss

HOW TO USE THIS DRUG
Dantrolene is available in capsules and via injection. (Injection dosage is not provided here.) The dosages given here are ones that are usually recommended for children. However, your doctor will determine the most appropriate dose and schedule for your child.

• Dose is based on body weight and will be determined by your doctor. Beginning dose is typically 0.23 mg per lb of body weight twice daily. Your doctor may increase the dose as needed. The dose is usually not more than 100 mg 4 times daily.

Dantrolene can be taken with food or milk to prevent stomach irritation. If your child misses a dose, give it as soon as you remember. If it is nearly time for the next dose, skip the missed dose and continue with the dosing schedule. Never give a double dose.

If your child has difficulty taking the capsules, you can open them and add the contents to a small amount of juice or other liquid. Shake well and make sure your child drinks the entire amount of liquid.

TIME UNTIL IT TAKES EFFECT
1 to 2 weeks

POSSIBLE DRUG, FOOD, AND/OR SUPPLEMENT INTERACTIONS
Tell your doctor if your child is taking any prescription or over-the-counter medications or any vitamins, herbs, or other supplements. Possible interactions with dantrolene may include the following:

- Talk to your doctor before giving any of the following drugs to your child along with dantrolene: acetaminophen, amiodarone, antiviral medications, antithyroid medications, carbamazepine, central nervous system depressants, chloroquine, disulfiram, divalproex, mercaptopurine, methotrexate, methyldopa, naltrexone, phenothiazines, phenytoin, tricyclic antidepressants, or valproic acid.
- Warfarin and clofibrate can reduce the effects of dantrolene.
- Tolbutamide can increase the effects of dantrolene.

SYMPTOMS OF OVERDOSE
Symptoms include bloody urine, chest pains, convulsions, loss of consciousness, and shortness of breath. If overdose occurs, seek immediate medical attention and bring the drug container(s) with you.

THINGS TO TELL YOUR DOCTOR
- Tell your doctor if your child has had allergic reactions to any medications in the past or if he or she is taking any medications now.
- Let your doctor know if your child has any of the following medical conditions: asthma, bronchitis, emphysema, other chronic lung disease, heart disease, or liver disease
- Consult your doctor if your child is pregnant or becomes pregnant during treatment.

IMPORTANT PRECAUTIONS

- If your child needs to take dantrolene for a prolonged time, your doctor may conduct periodic blood tests.
- Store dantrolene in a tightly closed container and keep at room temperature away from excess heat and moisture (e.g., the bathroom, near stoves or sinks).

DEMECLOCYCLINE–
see *Tetracycline Antibiotics*

DESIPRAMINE–
see *Tricyclic Antidepressants*

DESLORATADINE/DESLORATADINE PLUS PSEUDOEPHEDRINE

BRAND NAMES
Clarinex, Clarinex Syrup; Clarinex-D 24 Hour (with pseudoephedrine)
Generic Not Available

ABOUT THIS DRUG
Desloratadine is a tricyclic antihistamine antagonist that is used to treat the symptoms of seasonal and perennial allergic rhinitis, which include sneezing, itchy and watery eyes, runny nose, swelling, and scratchy throat; it is also used to treat hives or itching of unknown cause. It works by inhibiting the release of histamine, a chemical produced by the body and released in response to allergens. The combination of desloratadine and pseudoephedrine adds a decongestant benefit.

SIDE EFFECTS
Contact your doctor if your child experiences any side effects that are persistent or troubling, including any that are not listed here.

- *Most common:* dry mouth (more common in the combination product), fatigue, headache, insomnia, inflamed pharynx, menstrual problems, muscle pain
- *Rare:* drowsiness (in most other antihistamines, this side effect is common)

HOW TO USE THIS DRUG

Desloratadine is available in tablets, syrup, and oral disintegrating tablets. The combination product is available in extended-release tablets. The dosages given here are ones that are usually recommended for children. However, your doctor will determine the most appropriate dose and schedule for your child.

Regular and Oral Disintegrating Tablets
- Children younger than 12 years: to be determined by your doctor
- Children 12 years and older: 5 mg once daily

Syrup
- Children 6 to 11 months: 2 mL (1 mg) once daily
- Children 12 months to 5 years: ½ teaspoon (1.25 mg in 2.5 mL) once daily
- Children 6 to 11 years: 1 teaspoon (2.5 mg in 5 mL) once daily
- Children 12 years and older: 2 teaspoons (5 mg in 10 mL) once daily

Extended-Release Tablets (Combination Product)
- Children younger than 12 years: not recommended
- Children 12 years and older: 1 tablet once daily

Desloratadine can be taken with or without food. If using the syrup, use the measuring spoon or dropper that comes with the medication, not a kitchen teaspoon. If using the oral disintegrating tablets, remove the tablets from the package by peeling away the backing on the blister pack; do not push the tablets through the bubble.

If your child misses a dose, give it as soon as you remem-

ber. If it is nearly time for the next dose, do not give the missed dose. Continue with the regular dosing schedule. Do not give a double dose.

TIME UNTIL IT TAKES EFFECT
1 week or more until the full effect occurs

POSSIBLE DRUG, FOOD, AND/OR SUPPLEMENT INTERACTIONS
Tell your doctor if your child is taking any prescription or over-the-counter medications or any vitamins, herbs, or other supplements. No significant interactions have been reported for this drug; however, the following precautions are noted:

- Use of Clarinex-D 24 Hour along with other antihistamines and decongestants may have an adverse effect on the cardiovascular system.
- Talk to your doctor if your child is taking clarithromycin, erythromycin, itraconazole, or ketoconazole.

SYMPTOMS OF OVERDOSE
Symptoms may include rapid heartbeat and sleepiness. If overdose occurs, seek immediate medical attention and bring the drug container(s) with you.

THINGS TO TELL YOUR DOCTOR
- Tell your doctor if your child has had allergic reactions to any medications in the past or if he or she is taking any medications now, especially other antihistamines or decongestants.
- Let your doctor know if your child has liver or kidney disease. Due to its pseudoephedrine component, Clarinex-D 24 Hour extended-release tablets should be avoided if your child has narrow-angle glaucoma, high blood pressure, severe heart disease, or difficulty urinating.
- Consult your doctor if your child is pregnant or becomes pregnant during treatment.

IMPORTANT PRECAUTIONS

- Store desloratadine in a tightly closed container and keep away from excess heat and moisture (e.g., the bathroom, near a stove or sink). Do not allow the syrup to freeze.

DESMOPRESSIN

BRAND NAMES
DDAVP, Stimate
Generic Not Available

ABOUT THIS DRUG
Desmopressin is an antidiuretic used to control symptoms of diabetes insipidus (water diabetes) but is also useful in controlling bed-wetting in children. This drug works by increasing the amount of water that is reabsorbed by the kidneys, which results in reduced urine output.

SIDE EFFECTS
Contact your doctor if your child experiences any side effects that are persistent or troubling, including any that are not listed here.

- *Less common:* abdominal cramps, flushing, headache, nausea, slight increase in blood pressure
- *Rare:* a condition called water intoxication, characterized by confusion, drowsiness, decreased urination, headache, rapid weight gain, and seizures

HOW TO USE THIS DRUG
Desmopressin is available as nasal solution and tablets and via injection. (Information on the injectable form is not provided here.) The dosages given here are ones that are usually recommended for children. However, your doctor will determine the most appropriate dose and schedule for your child.

Bed-wetting
- Children younger than 6 years: to be determined by your doctor
- Children 6 years and older: starting dose of the nasal form is 10 µg inhaled into each nostril at bedtime. Your doctor may increase the dose. Starting dose of the tablets is 0.2 mg once at bedtime. Your doctor may increase the dose to as much as 0.6 mg daily

Diabetes Insipidus
- Children younger than 3 months: to be determined by your doctor
- Children 3 months to 12 years: Dose is based on body weight, usually 0.11 µg per lb when using the nasal solution. The dose is inhaled in a nostril 1 or 2 times daily.
- Children 13 years and older: Starting dose is 10 µg inhaled in a nostril at bedtime. Your doctor may increase the dose up to 40 µg daily, which may be divided into 2 or 3 doses a day. When using the tablets, starting dose is 0.05 mg twice daily. Your doctor may increase the dose to 0.1 to 0.8 mg and divide the dose into several per day.

Desmopressin can be taken with or without food. If your child misses a dose, give it as soon as you remember. If it is nearly time for the next dose, however, skip the missed dose. Continue with the regular dosing schedule. Do not give a double dose.

TIME UNTIL IT TAKES EFFECT
About 1 hour

POSSIBLE DRUG, FOOD, AND/OR SUPPLEMENT INTERACTIONS
Tell your doctor if your child is taking any prescription or over-the-counter medications or any vitamins, herbs, or other supplements. Possible interactions with desmopressin may include the following:

- Carbamazepine, chlorpropamide, and clofibrate may increase the effect of desmopressin.
- Demeclocycline, lithium, and norepinephrine may decrease the effect of desmopressin.

SYMPTOMS OF OVERDOSE

Symptoms include abdominal cramps, coma, confusion, headache, inability to urinate, nausea, seizures, and unusual weight gain. If overdose occurs, seek immediate medical attention and bring the drug container(s) with you.

THINGS TO TELL YOUR DOCTOR

- Tell your doctor if your child has had allergic reactions to any medications in the past or if he or she is taking any medications, herbal remedies, or supplements now.
- Let your doctor know if your child has any of the following medical conditions: asthma, allergic rhinitis, blood vessel disease, a cold or other upper respiratory infection, congestive heart failure, cystic fibrosis, kidney disease, migraine, or a seizure disorder.

IMPORTANT PRECAUTIONS

- Store desmopressin in a tightly closed container and keep at room temperature away from excess heat and moisture (e.g., the bathroom, near a stove or sink). Keep the nasal form refrigerated, but do not allow it to freeze.
- Desmopressin prevents the loss of water, so it is important that your child drink only enough water to satisfy thirst.

DESONIDE—see *Corticosteroids, Topical*

DESOXIMETASONE— see *Corticosteroids, Topical*

DEXAMETHASONE—see *Corticosteroids, Nasal Inhalants; Corticosteroids, Oral; Corticosteroids, Oral Inhalants;* and *Corticosteroids, Topical*

DEXMETHYLPHENIDATE

BRAND NAME
Focalin XR
Generic Not Available

ABOUT THIS DRUG
Dexmethylphenidate is an amphetamine-like drug that is used as a once-a-day treatment for attention deficit/hyperactivity disorder (ADHD) in children, adolescents, and adults. The drug works on the central nervous system by stimulating the brain stem and the release of various brain chemicals, including serotonin, dopamine, and norepinephrine, which results in improved alertness, concentration, and attention span. Dexmethylphenidate is available in a capsule, and when the beads are released, half of them act immediately. The other half provide a delayed reaction.

SIDE EFFECTS
Contact your doctor if your child experiences any side effects that are persistent or troubling, including any that are not listed here.

Most common: anorexia, anxiety, headache (25% of patients), increased appetite (30% of patients), insomnia, upset stomach
• *Less common:* blurry vision, dizziness, jitteriness

If your child experiences any of the following symptoms, contact your doctor immediately: severe nervousness, bruising, staring-type behavior, chest pain, irregular heartbeat, fever, hot dry skin, increased blood pressure, joint pain, rash, itching, or uncontrollable head, mouth, neck, or limb movements.

HOW TO USE THIS DRUG
Dexmethylphenidate is available as extended-release capsules. The dosages given here are ones that are usually recommended for children. However, your doctor will determine the most appropriate dose and schedule for your child.

- Children younger than 6 years old: not recommended
- Children 6 to 17 years: 5 mg capsule per day. Your doctor may adjust the dose in 5-mg increments per week up to a maximum of 20 mg daily

Your child should swallow the capsule whole; it should not be crushed or chewed. If this is difficult for your child, you can open the capsule and sprinkle the contents into one tablespoon of cool applesauce (using warm applesauce may result in improper dosing). Your child should take the applesauce immediately without chewing the sprinkles and then drink some fluids. This medication can be taken with or without food.

If your child misses a dose, give it as soon as you remember. However, if it is nearly time for the next dose, only give that dose; never give a double dose.

TIME UNTIL IT TAKES EFFECT
Within 1 hour

POSSIBLE DRUG, FOOD, AND/OR SUPPLEMENT INTERACTIONS
Tell your doctor if your child is taking any prescription or over-the-counter medications or any vitamins, herbs, or other supplements. Possible interactions with dexmethylphenidate may include the following:

- Dexmethylphenidate should not be used at the same time as monoamine oxidase (MAO) inhibitors or for at

least 2 weeks after use of MAO inhibitors has been discontinued.
- Dexmethylphenidate may decrease the effectiveness of drugs used to treat hypertension.
- Use of antacids or acid suppressants may change how dexmethylphenidate is released in the body.
- Doses of anticoagulants, anticonvulsants (e.g., phenobarbital, phenytoin, primidone), and tricyclic antidepressants (e.g., imipramine, desipramine) may need to be adjusted if these drugs are used along with dexmethylphenidate.
- Serious adverse effects have been reported when clonidine is used along with dexmethylphenidate. Use of clonidine and similar drugs along with dexmethylphenidate should be avoided.

SYMPTOMS OF OVERDOSE

Symptoms include cardiac arrhythmias, convulsions (may be followed by coma), confusion, delirium, euphoria, flushing, hallucinations, headache, high blood pressure, muscle twitching, palpitations, sweating, and tremors. If overdose occurs, seek immediate medical attention and bring the drug container(s) with you.

THINGS TO TELL YOUR DOCTOR

- Tell your doctor if your child has had allergic reactions to any medications in the past or if he or she is taking any medications, herbal remedies, or supplements now.
- Tell your doctor if your child has severe anxiety, tension, or agitation. Dexmethylphenidate can aggravate these symptoms and thus should not be given to your child.
- Let your doctor know if your child has any of the following medical conditions: glaucoma or other vision problems, high blood pressure, liver disease, heart problems, overactive thyroid, motor tics or spasms, a seizure disorder, or Tourette's syndrome.
- Before any type of surgical or dental procedure is performed, tell the doctor or dentist that your child is taking dexmethylphenidate.

- Consult your doctor if your child is pregnant or becomes pregnant during treatment.
- Loss of appetite (anorexia) is a common side effect and can result in significant weight loss. Contact your doctor if your child continues to have poor eating habits or is losing weight after being on dexmethylphenidate for more than a few weeks.

IMPORTANT PRECAUTIONS
- Long-term use of this drug can lead to dependence. Your physician should carefully monitor your child during treatment.
- To help prevent weight loss, encourage your child to eat small, frequent meals. Your physician should carefully monitor your child's growth during treatment.
- Store dexmethylphenidate in a tightly closed container and keep at room temperature away from excess heat and moisture (e.g., the bathroom, near a stove or sink).

DEXTROAMPHETAMINE/ DEXTROAMPHETAMINE PLUS AMPHETAMINE

GENERICS
(1) dextroamphetamine; (2) dextroamphetamine + amphetamine

BRAND NAMES
(1) Dexedrine, Dextrostat; (2) Adderall, Adderall XR
Generic Not Available

ABOUT THIS DRUG
Dextroamphetamine and the combination of dextroamphetamine and an amphetamine are central nervous system stimulants used to treat attention deficit/hyperactivity disorder (ADHD) and narcolepsy and to control weight.

These two drugs work by stimulating the nerve cells in the

spinal cord and brain, which enhances an individual's alertness and mental concentration and reduces drowsiness and fatigue.

SIDE EFFECTS

Contact your doctor if your child experiences any side effects that are persistent or troubling, including any that are not listed here.

- *Most common:* dizziness, high blood pressure, over-stimulation, palpitations, restlessness, sleeplessness
- *Less common:* constipation, diarrhea, diminished sex drive, dry mouth, euphoria, hallucinations, headache, itching, muscle spasms, taste changes
- *Rare:* psychotic reactions

HOW TO USE THIS DRUG

Dextroamphetamine is available in tablets and extended-release capsules; dextroamphetamine + amphetamine is available in tablets. The dosages given here are ones that are usually recommended for children. However, your doctor will determine the most appropriate dose and schedule for your child.

- Children 3 to 6 years: for ADHD—2.5 mg daily as a starting dose
- Children 7 years and older: for ADHD, 5 mg once or twice daily as a starting dose; for narcolepsy—5 mg once daily
- Children 12 to 18 years: for narcolepsy—10 mg once daily

Both of these drugs can be taken with food to help prevent stomach upset. If your child misses a dose, give it as soon as you remember unless it is within 6 hours of bedtime. If it is nearly time for the next dose, do not give the missed dose. Continue with the regular dosing schedule. Never give a double dose.

TIME UNTIL IT TAKES EFFECT

The tablets take effect usually within 30 to 45 minutes; the extended-release capsules may take longer.

POSSIBLE DRUG, FOOD, AND/OR SUPPLEMENT INTERACTIONS

Tell your doctor if your child is taking any prescription or over-the-counter medications or any vitamins, herbs, or other supplements. Possible interactions with dextroamphetamine or dextroamphetamine + amphetamine may include the following:

- Tricyclic antidepressants (e.g., amitriptyline, imipramine) chlorpromazine, guanethidine, haloperidol, lithium, methenamine, reserpine, and sodium acid phosphate may reduce the effects of dextroamphetamine.
- Acetazolamide, monoamine oxidase (MAO) inhibitors (e.g., phenelzine), propoxyphene, and thiazide diuretics (e.g., chlorothiazide) may increase the effects of dextroamphetamine.
- Dextroamphetamine may decrease the effects of antihistamines (e.g., loratadine), blood pressure medications (e.g., clonidine), ethosuximide, and veratrum alkaloids (present in some blood pressure medications).
- Citrus juices and vitamin C supplements can reduce the absorption of amphetamines. Your child should consume these items at least 1 hour before or 2 hours after taking his or her dose.

SYMPTOMS OF OVERDOSE

An overdose of these drugs can be fatal. Symptoms include confusion, coma, hallucinations, high fever, overaggressive behavior, rapid breathing, panic, restlessness, seizures, and tremors. If overdose occurs, seek immediate medical attention and bring the drug container(s) with you.

THINGS TO TELL YOUR DOCTOR

- Tell your doctor if your child has had allergic reactions

to any medications in the past or if he or she is taking any medications now.

- Let your doctor know if your child has glaucoma, heart disease, hypothyroidism, high blood pressure, or tics or Tourette's syndrome or is in an agitated state.
- Consult your doctor if your child is pregnant or becomes pregnant during treatment. These medications can cause birth defects when used during the early stages of pregnancy. There is also an increased risk of premature delivery, symptoms of drug withdrawal in newborns, and low-birth-weight infants.

IMPORTANT PRECAUTIONS

- Dextroamphetamine and dextroamphetamine + amphetamine can stunt your child's growth. Your doctor should conduct a comprehensive evaluation of your child before he or she prescribes these drugs.
- Because these drugs can interfere with sleep, make sure your child takes them at least 6 hours before bedtime.
- Use of these drugs can cause dizziness; therefore, make sure you know how your child reacts before you allow him or her to ride a bike, drive a car, or engage in activities that are potentially dangerous.
- These drugs contain FD&C Yellow No. 5 (tartrazine), which can cause allergic reactions (e.g., bronchial asthma) in certain hypersensitive individuals. This hypersensitivity is frequently seen in people who are hypersensitive to aspirin.
- Store dextroamphetamine and dextroamphetamine + amphetamine in a tightly closed container and keep at room temperature away from excess heat and moisture (e.g., the bathroom, near a stove or sink).

DEXTROMETHORPHAN

BRAND NAMES
Benylin Pediatric Cough Suppressant, Delsym, Hold DM, Pertussin DM Extra Strength, Robitussin Cough Gels, Robitussin

Honey Cough Suppressant, Robitussin Maximum Strength
Cough Suppressant, Robitussin Pediatric Cough Suppressant,
Simply Cough, St. Joseph Cough Suppressant, Sucrets 8 Hour
Cough Suppressant, Triaminic Cough Softchews, Vicks For-
mula 44 Pediatric Formula; there are also approximately 100
combination products that contain dextromethorphan. See also
Analgesic-Decongestant-Antitussive-(Antihistamine) and
Antihistamine-Decongestant-(Antitussive).
Generic Available/ Over-the-Counter Available

ABOUT THIS DRUG

Dextromethorphan is a cough suppressant that is used to relieve
a dry or minimally productive cough (e.g., one that produces a
small amount of mucus or phlegm). Such a cough is usually associated with allergies, colds, flu, and some lung conditions.
This drug suppresses cough by reducing the sensitivity of the
cough center in the brain. In recent years, abuse by adolescents
has become a concern (see "Important Precautions").

SIDE EFFECTS

Contact your doctor if your child experiences any side effects that are persistent or troubling, including any that are
not listed here.

- *Most common:* none
- *Less common/rare:* abdominal pain, dizziness, nausea,
  sedation, vomiting. These symptoms are more likely to
  occur at the start of treatment and diminish as the body
  becomes accustomed to the drug.

HOW TO USE THIS DRUG

Dextromethorphan is available in capsules, lozenges,
tablets, oral suspension, and syrup. The dosages given here
are ones that are usually recommended for children. However, your doctor will determine the most appropriate dose
and schedule for your child.

- Children younger than 2 years: to be determined by
  your doctor

- Children 2 to 6 years: 2.5 to 5 mg every 4 hours, or 7.5 mg every 6 to 8 hours, or 15 mg of the extended-release liquid twice daily
- Children 7 to 12 years: 5 to 10 mg every 4 hours or 30 mg of extended-release liquid twice daily
- Children 13 years and older: 10 to 20 mg every 4 hours or 30 mg every 6 to 8 hours, or 30 to 60 mg of extended-release liquid twice daily

If your child misses a dose, give it as soon as you remember. If it is nearly time for the next dose, however, skip the missed dose and resume the regular dosing schedule. Never give a double dose.

TIME UNTIL IT TAKES EFFECT
15 to 30 minutes

POSSIBLE DRUG, FOOD, AND/OR SUPPLEMENT INTERACTIONS
Tell your doctor if your child is taking any prescription or over-the-counter medications or any vitamins, herbs, or other supplements. Possible interactions with dextromethorphan may include the following:

- Doxepin increases the toxic effects of both drugs.
- Use of sedatives or other central nervous system depressants can increase the sedative effects of both drugs.
- Use of monoamine oxidase (MAO) inhibitors can cause disorientation, high fever, or loss of consciousness.
- Quinidine increases the risk of experiencing side effects.
- Cough, cold, or allergy products (prescription or over-the-counter medications) should not be used along with this drug unless recommended by your doctor.

SYMPTOMS OF OVERDOSE
Symptoms include agitation, blurry vision, confusion, coma, extreme drowsiness or dizziness, hallucinations, irritability, loss of consciousness, mood changes, nausea, nervousness,

uncontrollable eye movements, and vomiting. If overdose occurs, seek immediate medical attention and bring the drug container(s) with you.

THINGS TO TELL YOUR DOCTOR
- Tell your doctor if your child has had allergic reactions to any medications in the past or if he or she is taking any medications now.
- Let your doctor know if your child has any of the following medical conditions: asthma, emphysema, lung disease, liver disorder
- Consult your doctor if your child is pregnant or becomes pregnant during treatment.

IMPORTANT PRECAUTIONS
- In May 2005, the U.S. Food and Drug Administration issued a warning about dextromethorphan, noting a trend in abuse of this drug, especially among teenagers. The abuse involves the powdered form found in capsules. Parents should be aware that when dextromethorphan is taken as prescribed, it is considered to be a safe medication. In greater amounts, however, symptoms of overdose (see earlier) and death may occur. Because dextromethorphan is available without a prescription, availability and the potential for abuse are significant.
- Store dextromethorphan in a tightly closed container and keep away from excess heat and moisture (e.g., the bathroom, near a stove or sink). Do not allow the liquid forms of the drug to freeze.
- This drug should not be used to treat a cough that is caused by asthma or emphysema.

DIAZEPAM

BRAND NAMES
Diastat, Di-Tran, T-Quil, Valium, Valrelease, Vazepam, X-O'Spaz, Zetran
Generic Available

ABOUT THIS DRUG

Diazepam is a benzodiazepine tranquilizer, antianxiety medication, and muscle relaxant that is used mainly to treat anxiety, panic attacks, and muscle spasms. This drug produces mild sedation by enhancing the effect of GABA, a chemical that inhibits the firing of nerve cells and thus reduces nerve excitation.

SIDE EFFECTS

Contact your doctor if your child experiences any side effects that are persistent or troubling, including any that are not listed here.

- *Most common:* dizziness, drowsiness (most common during the first few days of treatment), lightheadedness, loss of coordination, slurred speech, unsteady gait
- *Less common/rare:* change in sexual desire or abilities, constipation, headache, hallucinations, jaundice, nausea, rage, rash, slow heartbeat, unusual fatigue, vertigo, vomiting

HOW TO USE THIS DRUG

Diazepam is available in tablets, capsules, and rectal gel and via injection. (Injection and gel information is not provided here.) The dosages given here are ones that are usually recommended for children. However, your doctor will determine the most appropriate dose and schedule for your child.

- Children 6 months and older: 1.0 to 2.5 mg 3 or 4 times daily. Your doctor may increase the dose if appropriate.

Diazepam can be taken with or without food. If your child misses a dose, give it as soon as you remember. If it is within 1 hour of the missed dose, give it. If not, skip the missed dose and continue with the regular dosing schedule. Never give a double dose.

TIME UNTIL IT TAKES EFFECT
30 minutes

POSSIBLE DRUG, FOOD, AND/OR SUPPLEMENT INTERACTIONS

Tell your doctor if your child is taking any prescription or over-the-counter medications or any vitamins, herbs, or other supplements. Possible interactions with diazepam may include the following:

- Cimetidine, oral contraceptives, disulfiram, fluoxetine, isoniazid, ketoconazole, rifampin, metoprolol, probenecid, propoxyphene, propranolol, and valproic acid may prolong the effects of diazepam.
- Diazepam may elevate the blood levels of digoxin and phenytoin and increase the risk of toxicity of both of these drugs.
- Narcotics (e.g., codeine, oxycodone), barbiturates (e.g., phenobarbital), monoamine oxidase (MAO) inhibitors (e.g., phenelzine), antihistamines (e.g., cetirizine), and antidepressants (e.g., amitriptyline) may lead to excessive drowsiness, breathing problems, and extreme depression.
- Alcohol should not be used while taking diazepam, because the drug can increase the effects of alcohol.
- Herbs that produce a sedative effect should be avoided, as they may cause significant depression. Some of these herbs include calendula, capsicum, catnip, goldenseal, gotu kola, hops, kava, passionflower, sage, Siberian ginseng, skullcap, St. John's wort, and valerian.
- Grapefruit and grapefruit juice can slow down the breakdown of diazepam, so have your child avoid these foods while using diazepam.

SYMPTOMS OF OVERDOSE

Symptoms include confusion, extreme drowsiness, loss of consciousness, poor coordination, slowed breathing, slurred speech, staggering, and tremor. If overdose occurs, seek immediate medical attention and bring the drug container(s) with you.

THINGS TO TELL YOUR DOCTOR
- Tell your doctor if your child has had allergic reactions to any medications in the past or if he or she is taking any medications now.
- Let your doctor know if your child has any of the following medical conditions: severe lung disease, severe depression, narrow-angle glaucoma, sleep apnea, psychotic disorder, hyperactivity, or kidney or liver disease, as diazepam can worsen them.
- Consult your doctor if your child is pregnant or becomes pregnant during treatment. Diazepam has the potential to cause birth defects if taken during the first trimester.

IMPORTANT PRECAUTIONS
- Diazepam can cause dizziness, drowsiness, and other symptoms of sedation. Make sure you know how your child responds to diazepam before you allow him or her to participate in potentially dangerous activities, such as riding a bike, driving a car, or operating machinery.
- Diazepam can cause physical and psychological dependence (addiction), even after only 4 weeks of use, and your child may experience withdrawal symptoms if he or she stops taking the drug suddenly. If you want your child to stop taking diazepam, talk to your doctor about how to taper treatment. Do **not** stop treatment on your own.
- Store diazepam in a tightly closed container and keep away from excess heat and moisture (e.g., the bathroom, near a stove or sink).

DICLOXACILLIN—see *Penicillin Antibiotics*

DIFLORASONE— see *Corticosteroids, Topical*

DIMENHYDRINATE

BRAND NAMES
Calm-X, Dimetabs, Dramamine, Marmine, Nico-Vert, Tega-Vert, Triptone, Vertab
Generic Available

ABOUT THIS DRUG
Dimenhydrinate is an antihistamine that is used to treat the symptoms of motion sickness, such as nausea, vomiting, dizziness, and vertigo. It accomplishes this by directly inhibiting the stimulation of certain nerves in the inner ear and brain that are associated with these symptoms.

SIDE EFFECTS
Contact your doctor if your child experiences any side effects that are persistent or troubling, including any that are not listed here.

- *Most common:* drowsiness
- *Less common/rare:* blurry vision, dry mouth, headache, low blood pressure (causing dizziness, weakness, ringing in the ears), loss of coordination

HOW TO USE THIS DRUG
Dimenhydrinate is available in tablets, capsules, syrup, elixir, and suppositories and via injection. (Information on the injectable form is not provided here.) The dosages given here are ones that are usually recommended for children. However, your doctor will determine the most appropriate dose and schedule for your child.

Oral Forms
- Children 2 to 6 years: 12.5 to 25 mg every 6 to 8 hours
- Children 7 to 12 years: 25 to 50 mg every 6 to 8 hours
- Children 13 years and older: 50 to 100 mg every 4 to 6 hours

Suppositories
- Children 6 to 8 years: 12.5 to 25 mg every 8 to 12 hours
- Children 9 to 12 years: 25 to 50 mg every 8 to 12 hours
- Children 13 years and older: 50 mg every 9 to 12 hours

If you give this drug to your child to prevent motion sickness, it should be taken at least 30 minutes but optimally 1 to 2 hours before traveling. Dimenhydrinate can be taken with food or milk to help prevent stomach upset.

If your child misses a dose, give it as soon as you remember. If it is nearly time for the next dose, however, do not give the missed dose and resume your regular dosing schedule. Never give a double dose.

TIME UNTIL IT TAKES EFFECT
Oral, within 20 to 30 minutes; injection, 2 to 20 minutes; suppositories, 30 to 45 minutes

POSSIBLE DRUG, FOOD, AND/OR SUPPLEMENT INTERACTIONS
Tell your doctor if your child is taking any prescription or over-the-counter medications or any vitamins, herbs, or other supplements. Possible interactions with dimenhydrinate may include the following:

- Excessive drowsiness may occur if dimenhydrinate is taken along with any of these natural supplements: 5-HTP, (5-hydroxytryptophan), valerian, melatonin, GABA (gamma-aminobutyric acid), kava, or melissa.
- Talk to your doctor before your child takes dimenhydrinate along with any of the following medications: narcotics, sedatives, tranquilizers, antidepressants, antibiotics, aspirin, barbiturates, cisplatin, diuretics, or theophylline.

SYMPTOMS OF OVERDOSE
Symptoms include difficulty breathing, drowsiness, hallucinations, loss of consciousness, and seizures. If overdose oc-

curs, seek immediate medical attention and bring the drug container(s) with you.

THINGS TO TELL YOUR DOCTOR
- Tell your doctor if your child has had allergic reactions to any medications in the past or if he or she is taking any medications now.
- Let your doctor know if your child has glaucoma.
- Consult your doctor if your child is pregnant or becomes pregnant during treatment.

IMPORTANT PRECAUTIONS
- Observe your child carefully for side effects, as children are more likely to develop serious complications.
- Store dimenhydrinate in a tightly closed container and keep away from excess heat and moisture (e.g., the bathroom, near a stove or sink). Do not allow the liquid forms to freeze.

DIPHENHYDRAMINE

BRAND NAMES
AllerMax, Banophen, Belix, Benadryl, Benadryl Topical, Benylin Cough Syrup, Bydramine Cough Syrup, Diphen Cough, Dormin, Genahist, Hydramyn Syrup, Nidryl, Nordryl, Nytol, Nytol Maximum Strength, Phendry, Silphen Cough, Sleep-Eze 3, Sleepinal, Sominex, Tusstat Syrup, Twilite, Uni-Bent Cough Syrup
Generic Available/Over-the-Counter Available

ABOUT THIS DRUG
Diphenhydramine is an antihistamine used to relieve symptoms of motion sickness, hay fever, sleep difficulties, and itchy skin and hives. This drug works by blocking the effects of histamine, a naturally occurring substance that causes sneezing, itching, swelling, and watery eyes.

SIDE EFFECTS
Contact your doctor if your child experiences any side effects that are persistent or troubling, including any that are not listed here.

- *Most common:* drowsiness, dry mouth, nausea, thickening of mucus
- *Less common/rare:* blurry vision, confusion, difficult urination

HOW TO USE THIS DRUG
Diphenhydramine is available in tablets, capsules, elixir, and syrup and via injection. (Information on the injectable form is not provided here.) The dosages given here are ones that are usually recommended for children. However, your doctor will determine the most appropriate dose and schedule for your child.

For Hay Fever
- Children younger than 6 years: 6.25 to 12.5 mg every 4 to 6 hours
- Children 6 to 12 years: 12.5 to 25 mg every 4 to 6 hours
- Children 13 years and older: 25 to 50 mg every 4 to 6 hours

For Nausea, Dizziness, and Vomiting
- Children: 0.45 to 0.7 mg per lb of body weight every 4 to 6 hours

For Cough
- Children 2 to 6 years: 6.25 mg (½ teaspoon) liquid forms every 4 to 6 hours
- Children 7 to 12 years: 12.5 mg (1 teaspoon) liquid forms every 4 to 6 hours
- Children 13 years and older: 25 mg every 4 to 6 hours

Diphenhydramine can be taken with food or milk to reduce stomach distress. If your child misses a dose, give it as soon as you remember. If it is nearly time for the next dose, skip the missed dose and resume the regular dosing schedule. Never give a double dose.

TIME UNTIL IT TAKES EFFECT
15 minutes

POSSIBLE DRUG, FOOD, AND/OR SUPPLEMENT INTERACTIONS
Tell your doctor if your child is taking any prescription or over-the-counter medications or any vitamins, herbs, or other supplements. Possible interactions with diphenhydramine may include the following:

- Do not use medications that may make your child feel drowsy or sleepy, including but not limited to alprazolam, diazepam, chlordiazepoxide, temazepam, or triazolam; or antidepressants, including amitriptyline, doxepin, nortriptyline, fluoxetine, sertraline, or paroxetine.
- Talk to your doctor before you give your child diphenhydramine along with over-the-counter cough, cold, allergy, or insomnia medications.
- Diphenhydramine should not be taken within 14 days of having taken a monoamine oxidase (MAO) inhibitor (e.g., phenelzine, isocarboxazid).

SYMPTOMS OF OVERDOSE
Symptoms include difficulty breathing, confusion, dilated pupils, excitability, fever, loss of consciousness, loss of coordination, seizures, and weak pulse. If overdose occurs, seek immediate medical attention and bring the drug container(s) with you.

THINGS TO TELL YOUR DOCTOR
- Tell your doctor if your child has had allergic reactions to any medications in the past or if he or she is taking any medications now.
- Let your doctor know if your child has any of the fol-

lowing medical conditions: asthma, heart problems, difficulty urinating, glaucoma or increased eye pressure, hyperthyroidism, hypertension, stomach ulcer
- Consult your doctor if your child is pregnant or becomes pregnant during treatment.

IMPORTANT PRECAUTIONS
- Observe your child carefully for side effects, as children are more likely to develop serious complications.
- Because this drug causes drowsiness, make sure you know how your child responds before he or she participates in potentially hazardous activities, such as riding a bike, driving a car, or operating machinery.
- Store diphenhydramine in a tightly closed container and keep away from excess heat and moisture (e.g., the bathroom, near a stove or sink).

DIRITHROMYCIN

BRAND NAME
Dynabac
Generic Not Available

ABOUT THIS DRUG
Dirithromycin is an antibiotic often prescribed to treat bronchitis, certain types of pneumonia, skin infections, and tonsillitis or other throat infections. This drug prevents bacteria from producing the special proteins they need to survive.

SIDE EFFECTS
Contact your doctor if your child experiences any side effects that are persistent or troubling, including any that are not listed here.

- *Most common:* none
- *Less common/rare:* diarrhea (mild), dizziness, fatigue, headache, nausea (mild), stomach upset, unusual fatigue, vomiting

HOW TO USE THIS DRUG

Dirithromycin is available in tablets. The dosages given here
are ones that are usually recommended for children. However, your doctor will determine the most appropriate dose
and schedule for your child.

- Children younger than 12 years: not recommended
- Children 12 years and older: 500 mg once daily for 5
  to 14 days; your doctor will determine the length of
  treatment based on the infection

Dirithromycin should be taken with food or within 1 hour
of eating. It is best to take dirithromycin at the same time
each day. If your child misses a dose, give it as soon as you
remember. If it is nearly time for the next dose, skip the
missed dose and continue with the regular dosing schedule.
Never give a double dose.

TIME UNTIL IT TAKES EFFECT

Within 2 hours, with the full effect typically occurring in 2
to 5 days

POSSIBLE DRUG, FOOD, AND/OR SUPPLEMENT INTERACTIONS

Tell your doctor if your child is taking any prescription or
over-the-counter medications or any vitamins, herbs, or
other supplements. Possible interactions with dirithromycin
may include the following:

- Dirithromycin may react with the following medications: antacids, anti-ulcer medication, astemizole,
  bromocriptine, carbamazepine, cyclosporine, digoxin,
  disopyramide, ergotamine, felodipine, hexobarbital,
  phenytoin, theophylline, triazolam, valproate, and
  warfarin.
- Dirithromycin may interfere with the effectiveness of
  birth control pills.

SYMPTOMS OF OVERDOSE

No cases of overdose have been reported. However, symptoms would most likely include diarrhea, heartburn, nausea, and vomiting. If you believe an overdose has occurred, seek immediate medical attention and bring the drug container(s) with you.

THINGS TO TELL YOUR DOCTOR

- Tell your doctor if your child has had allergic reactions to any medications in the past or if he or she is taking any medications, herbal remedies, or supplements now.
- Let your doctor know if your child has any allergies or a blood or liver disorder.
- Consult your doctor if your child is pregnant or becomes pregnant during treatment.

IMPORTANT PRECAUTIONS

- Your child should drink lots of fluids while taking this medication.
- Your child should take this drug for the entire treatment course, even if he or she feels better before the scheduled course has ended.
- Because dirithromycin can interfere with the effectiveness of birth control pills, your child should use a backup form of birth control while taking this drug.
- Store dirithromycin in a tightly closed container and keep away from excess heat and moisture (e.g., the bathroom, near a stove or sink).

DOLASETRON—see *Antiemetics*

DOXEPIN—see *Tricyclic Antidepressants*

DOXYCYCLINE—see *Tetracycline Antibiotics*

EMEDASTINE

BRAND NAME
Emadine
Generic Not Available

ABOUT THIS DRUG
Emedastine is an ophthalmic antihistamine prescribed for the short-term treatment of itchy eyes associated with seasonal allergic conjunctivitis (inflammation of the whites of the eyes and the mucous membranes of the eyelids). This medication blocks the effects of histamine, a substance produced by the body that causes sneezing, itching, watery eyes, hives, and other symptoms associated with allergies.

SIDE EFFECTS
Contact your doctor if your child experiences any side effects that are persistent or troubling, including any that are not listed here.

- *Most common:* headache
- *Less common/rare:* abnormal dreams, bad taste in the mouth, blurry vision, burning or stinging eyes, dry eye, runny nose, rash, weakness

HOW TO USE THIS DRUG
Emedastine is available as eye drops. The dosages given here are ones that are usually recommended for children. However, your doctor will determine the most appropriate dose and schedule for your child.

- Children younger than 3 years: not recommended
- Children 3 years and older: 1 drop in the affected eye(s) up to 4 times daily, as prescribed by your doctor

If your child misses a dose, give it as soon as you remember. If it is nearly time for the next dose, skip the missed dose and continue with the regular dosing schedule. Never give a double dose.

TIME UNTIL IT TAKES EFFECT
Unknown

POSSIBLE DRUG, FOOD, AND/OR SUPPLEMENT INTERACTIONS
Tell your doctor if your child is taking any prescription or over-the-counter medications or any vitamins, herbs, or other supplements. No drug, food, or supplement interactions have been noted. However, tell your doctor if your child is using any other eye drops.

SYMPTOMS OF OVERDOSE
An overdose of emedastine is unlikely. However, if your child accidentally ingests the medication, or you believe an overdose has occurred, seek immediate medical attention and bring the drug container(s) with you.

THINGS TO TELL YOUR DOCTOR
- Tell your doctor if your child has had allergic reactions to any medications in the past or if he or she is taking any medications, herbal remedies, or supplements now.
- Consult your doctor if your child is pregnant or becomes pregnant during treatment.

IMPORTANT PRECAUTIONS
- If your child wears contact lenses, they need to be removed before the drops are used.
- Store emedastine in a tightly closed container and keep away from excess heat and moisture (e.g., the bathroom, near a stove or sink). Do not allow it to freeze.

ERYTHROMYCIN

BRAND NAMES
E-Base, E.E.S. Oral Suspension, E-Mycin, ERYC, EryPed, Ery-Tab, Erythro, Erythrocin, Erythrocot, Ilosone, Ilotycin, Ilotycin (ophthalmic), My-E, PCE, Wintrocin
Generics Available

ABOUT THIS DRUG

Erythromycin belongs to a class called macrolide antibiotics, which are used to treat bacterial infections that affect
the throat, ears, eyes, respiratory tract, urinary tract, intestinal tract, and heart. Erythromycins work by preventing the
bacteria from producing the specific proteins they need to
survive.

SIDE EFFECTS

Contact your doctor if your child experiences any side effects that are persistent or troubling, including any that are
not listed here.

- *Most common:* abdominal cramps, blurry vision (may
  last for up to 30 minutes after treatment; in ophthalmic
  product only), diarrhea, loss of appetite, nausea,
  vomiting
- *Less common/rare:* aching joints, blood in urine, fever,
  itching, jaundice, lower back pain, peeling and/or blis-
  tered skin, sore tongue or mouth, difficulty swallowing,
  swollen neck, vaginal discharge or itching, unusual
  bruising or bleeding; for ophthalmic solution only—
  eye irritation, itching, redness, swelling

HOW TO USE THIS DRUG

Erythromycin is available as capsules, tablets, and oral suspension and via an injection. (Information on the injectable
form is not provided here.) An ophthalmic ointment is also
available. The dosages given here are ones that are usually
recommended for children. However, your doctor will determine the most appropriate dose and schedule for your child.

For Streptococcal Infections of the Respiratory Tract

- Children weighing less than 44 lbs: 13.6 to 23 mg daily
  for each lb of body weight, divided into equal doses
  and given every 8 hours for at least 10 days
- Children weighing more than 44 lbs: 333 mg every 8
  hours or 500 mg every 12 hours for at least 10 days (the
  recommended adult dose)

For Rectal, Reproductive, or Urinary Infections
- Children weighing less than 44 lbs: 13.6 to 23 mg daily for each lb of body weight, divided into equal doses and given every 8 hours for at least 7 days
- Children weighing more than 44 lbs: 500 mg 4 times daily or 666 mg every 8 hours for at least 7 days (the recommended adult dose)

For Intestinal Infections
- Children weighing less than 44 lbs: 13.6 to 23 mg daily for each lb of body weight, divided into equal doses and given every 8 hours for 10 to 14 days
- Children weighing more than 44 lbs: 500 mg every 12 hours or 333 mg every 8 hours for 10 to 14 days (the recommended adult dose)

For Eye Infections
- Children of all ages: apply ointment to the affected eye up to 6 times daily, as instructed by your physician

The oral forms should be taken with a full glass of water at least 1 hour before or 2 hours after a meal. However, if the drug upsets your child's stomach, it can be taken with food.

If your child misses a dose, give it as soon as you remember. If it is nearly time for the next dose, do not give the missed dose. Continue with the regular dosing schedule. Never give a double dose.

TIME UNTIL IT TAKES EFFECT
Varies

POSSIBLE DRUG, FOOD, AND/OR SUPPLEMENT INTERACTIONS
Tell your doctor if your child is taking any prescription or over-the-counter medications or any vitamins, herbs, or other supplements. Possible interactions with erythromycin may include the following:

- Erythromycin should not be taken along with astemizole or pimozide.

- Various interactions may occur if erythromycin is taken along with any of the following: acetaminophen, amiodarone, antibiotics, azithromycin, carbamazepine, chloramphenicol, chloroquine, clarithyromycin, cyclosporine, dantrolene, disulfiram, divalproex, etretinate, hydroxychloroquine, lincomycin, methotrexate, mercaptopurine, methyldopa, phenothiazines, phenytoin, theophylline, valproic acid, warfarin, tacrolimus, disopyramide, lovastatin, or bromocriptine.
- Use of St. John's wort may cause an extreme reaction to sunlight.

SYMPTOMS OF OVERDOSE

Symptoms include diarrhea, nausea, stomach cramps, and vomiting. If overdose occurs, seek immediate medical attention and bring the drug container(s) with you.

THINGS TO TELL YOUR DOCTOR

- Tell your doctor if your child has had allergic reactions to any medications in the past or if he or she is taking any medications now. The ophthalmic form should not be used if your child has a history of allergy to azithromycin, clarithromycin, erythromycin, or lincomycin.
- Let your doctor know if your child has any of the following medical conditions: hearing problems, heart disease, liver disease, colitis or other stomach disorders, or any chronic illness.
- Consult your doctor if your child is pregnant or becomes pregnant during treatment. Oral erythromycin may cause liver damage in pregnant women, but there are no reports of birth defects.

IMPORTANT PRECAUTIONS

- Store erythromycin in a tightly closed container and keep away from excess heat and moisture (e.g., the bathroom, near a stove or sink). Do not allow the fluid forms or ointment to freeze.
- Long-term use of this drug may allow bacteria that are resistant to it to develop.

- Your child should take the entire treatment course as prescribed by your physician, even if he or she feels better before the scheduled end of treatment.

ERYTHROMYCIN PLUS SULFISOXAZOLE

BRAND NAMES
Eryzole, Pediazole
Generic Available

ABOUT THIS DRUG
Erythromycin + sulfisoxazole is a combination of an erythromycin antibiotic and a sulfonamide that is used to treat middle ear infections in children. The erythromycin prevents bacteria from manufacturing the specific proteins they need to survive, while the sulfisoxazole prevents bacteria from using folic acid, which it needs for growth and reproduction.

SIDE EFFECTS
Contact your doctor if your child experiences any side effects that are persistent or troubling, including any that are not listed here.

- *Most common:* abdominal discomfort and cramps, diarrhea, loss of appetite, nausea, vomiting
- *Less common/rare:* anxiety, blood in the urine, bluish discoloration of skin, chills, convulsions, cough, depression, difficulty urinating, dizziness, drowsiness, fatigue, fluid retention, gas, headache, hives, insomnia, inflammation of the mouth, itching, jaundice, low blood sugar, palpitations, ringing in the ears, sensitivity to light, shortness of breath, temporary hearing loss, vertigo, weakness

HOW TO USE THIS DRUG
This combination drug is available as an oral suspension. The dosages given here are ones that are usually recommended for children. However, your doctor will determine the most appropriate dose and schedule for your child.

(Note: All of the dosing instructions below should be followed for 10 days.)

- Children less than 18 lbs: to be determined by your physician
- Children 18 to 35 lbs: ½ teaspoon 4 times daily
- Children 36 to 53 lbs: 1 teaspoon 4 times daily
- Children 54 to 100 lbs: 1½ teaspoons 4 times daily
- Children more than 101 lbs: 2 teaspoons 4 times daily

An alternative dosing schedule is as follows:

- Children less than 13 lbs: to be determined by your physician
- Children 13 to 25 lbs: ½ teaspoon 3 times daily
- Children 26 to 39 lbs: 1 teaspoon 3 times daily
- Children 40 to 52 lbs: 1½ teaspoons 3 times daily
- Children 53 to 66 lbs: 2 teaspoons 3 times daily
- Children more than 66 lbs: 2½ teaspoons 3 times daily

This drug should be taken 1 hour before or 2 hours after meals with a full glass of water. If your child experiences stomach upset, the drug can be taken with food or milk. Make sure you use the special dosing spoon and not a kitchen spoon for dispensing this medication.

If your child misses a dose, give it as soon as you remember. If it is nearly time for the next dose, skip the missed dose and follow the regular dosing schedule. Never give a double dose.

TIME UNTIL IT TAKES EFFECT
Unknown

POSSIBLE DRUG, FOOD, AND/OR SUPPLEMENT INTERACTIONS
Tell your doctor if your child is taking any prescription or over-the-counter medications or any vitamins, herbs, or other supplements. Possible interactions with erythromycin + sulfisoxazole may include the following:

- Erythromycin + sulfisoxazole may interact with astemizole, blood thinners (e.g., warfarin), bromocriptine, carbamazepine, cyclosporine, digoxin, disopyramide, ergotamine, lovastatin, methotrexate, oral antidiabetic drugs, phenytoin, terfenadine, theophylline, and triazolam
- This drug combination should not be given with or immediately after your child has consumed carbonated beverages, fruit juices, or tea.

SYMPTOMS OF OVERDOSE
Symptoms include diarrhea, dizziness, drowsiness, fever, headache, loss of consciousness, severe nausea, and vomiting. If overdose occurs, seek immediate medical attention and bring the drug container(s) with you.

THINGS TO TELL YOUR DOCTOR
- Tell your doctor if your child has had allergic reactions to any medications in the past or if he or she is taking any medications now.
- Let your doctor know if your child has any of the following medical conditions: anemia, any blood condition, G6PD (glucose-6-phosphate dehydrogenase) deficiency, hearing loss, kidney disease, liver disease, porphyria
- Consult your doctor if your child is pregnant or becomes pregnant during treatment. Erythromycin may cause liver damage in pregnant women, but there are no reports of birth defects.

IMPORTANT PRECAUTIONS
- Because this drug combination can cause sensitivity to sunlight, make sure your child is protected against the sun by using sunscreen and wearing protective clothing.
- Long-term use of this drug may allow bacteria that are resistant to it to develop.
- Your child should take the entire treatment course as prescribed by your physician, even if he or she feels better before the scheduled end of treatment.
- Store erythromycin + sulfisoxazole in a tightly closed

container and keep in the refrigerator. Do not allow it
to freeze.

FEXOFENADINE

BRAND NAME
Allegra
No Generic Available

ABOUT THIS DRUG
Fexofenadine is an antihistamine that is used to relieve or prevent symptoms related to hay fever and other allergies, as well
as treat itchy skin and hives. It works by blocking the effects of
histamine, a naturally occurring substance that causes allergic
reactions such as sneezing, watery eyes, hives, and swelling,
among others. (See also fexofenadine-pseudoephedrine under
Antihistamine-Decongestant-(Antitussive) Combination.

SIDE EFFECTS
Contact your doctor if your child experiences any side effects that are persistent or troubling, including any that are
not listed here.

- *Most common:* none
- *Less common/rare:* drowsiness, fatigue, painful menstrual bleeding, stomach upset

HOW TO USE THIS DRUG
Fexofenadine is available as tablets, oral suspension, and
capsules. The dosages given here are ones that are usually
recommended for children. However, your doctor will determine the most appropriate dose and schedule for your
child.

Oral Suspension
- Children 6 monts to less than 2 years: 15 mg twice daily
- Children 2 to 11 years: 30 mg twice daily

Tablets and Capsules
- Children 6 to 11 years: 30 mg twice daily
- Children 12 years and older: 60 mg twice daily

Fexofenadine can be taken with or without food. If your child misses a dose, give it as soon as you remember. However, if it is nearly time for the next dose, skip the missed dose and resume the regular dosing schedule. Never give a double dose.

TIME UNTIL IT TAKES EFFECT
1 to 2 hours

POSSIBLE DRUG, FOOD, AND/OR SUPPLEMENT INTERACTIONS
Tell your doctor if your child is taking any prescription or over-the-counter medications or any vitamins, herbs, or other supplements. Possible interactions with fexofenadine may include the following:

- Use of antacids that contain aluminum or magnesium, such as Maalox, Milk of Magnesia, Mylanta, Pepcid Complete, and Rolaids, may decrease the effects of fexofenadine.
- Erythromycin or ketoconazole may increase the effects of fexofenadine.
- Fruit juices (e.g., apple, grapefruit, orange) may reduce the body's ability to use fexofenadine; therefore, take this drug with water.

SYMPTOMS OF OVERDOSE
Symptoms include extreme fatigue or drowsiness. If overdose occurs, seek immediate medical attention and bring the drug container(s) with you.

THINGS TO TELL YOUR DOCTOR
- Tell your doctor if your child has had allergic reactions to any medications in the past or if he or she is taking any medications now.

- Let your doctor know if your child has impaired kidney function.
- Consult your doctor if your child is pregnant or becomes pregnant during treatment.

IMPORTANT PRECAUTIONS
- Because fexofenadine may cause drowsiness, you should know how your child reacts to the drug before you allow him or her to participate in potentially dangerous activities, such as riding a bike, driving a car, or operating machinery.
- Store fexofenadine in a tightly closed container and keep away from excess heat and moisture (e.g., the bathroom, near a stove or sink).

FEXOFENADINE PLUS PSEUDOEPHEDRINE—see *Antihistamine-Decongestant-(Antitussive) Combination*

FLUNISOLIDE— see *Corticosteroids, Nasal Inhalants* and *Corticosteroids, Oral Inhalants*

FLUOCINOLONE— see *Corticosteroids, Topical*

FLUOCINONIDE— see *Corticosteroids, Topical*

FLUOXETINE

BRAND NAME
Prozac
Generic Available

ABOUT THIS DRUG
Fluoxetine is a selective serotonin reuptake inhibitor (SSRI) antidepressant that is prescribed for treatment of major depression, obsessive-compulsive disorder, and panic disorder.

This drug affects the level of serotonin, a chemical in the brain that has an effect on mood, emotions, and mental status.

SIDE EFFECTS
Contact your doctor if your child experiences any side effects that are persistent or troubling, including any that are not listed here.

- *Most common:* abnormal dreams, anxiety, dizziness, dry eyes, dry mouth, flulike symptoms, flushing, gas, headache, insomnia, itching, loss of appetite, nausea, nervousness, rash, sinusitis, sleepiness, sore throat, sweating, tremors, upset stomach, vision problems, vomiting, weakness, yawning
- *Less common:* especially in children and adolescents, they include agitation, excessive menstrual bleeding, frequent urination, hyperactivity, mania or hypomania, nosebleed, personality changes, thirst; others may include abnormal taste, bleeding problems, chills, confusion, ear pain, fever, high blood pressure, loss of memory, palpitations, ringing in the ears, weight gain

HOW TO USE THIS DRUG
Fluoxetine is available in capsules and as a syrup. The dosages given here are ones that are usually recommended for children. However, your doctor will determine the most appropriate dose and schedule for your child.

- Children younger than 12 years: not recommended
- Children 12 years and older: For depression, starting dose is 10 to 20 mg daily taken in the morning. Your physician may increase the dose as needed. It may take up to 4 weeks for this drug to be effective.
- Children 12 years and older: For obsessive-compulsive disorder, starting dose is 10 mg daily, which your physi-

cian may increase to 20 mg after 2 weeks. If no improvement is seen after several weeks, your physician may increase the dosage up to a maximum of 60 mg daily. It may take 5 weeks or longer for this drug to be effective.

If your child is underweight, has liver or kidney problems, or is taking other medications, your physician may need to adjust the fluoxetine dosages.

If your child misses a dose, give it as soon as you remember. If, however, it is nearly time for the next dose, skip the missed dose. Continue with the regular dosing schedule. Never give a double dose.

TIME UNTIL IT TAKES EFFECT
1 to 5 weeks

POSSIBLE DRUG, FOOD, AND/OR SUPPLEMENT INTERACTIONS
Tell your doctor if your child is taking any prescription or over-the-counter medications or any vitamins, herbs, or other supplements. Possible interactions with fluoxetine may include the following:

- Alcohol should be avoided while using fluoxetine.
- Monoamine oxidase (MAO) inhibitors should not be taken along with fluoxetine, and fluoxetine should not be taken within at least 14 days of stopping treatment with an MAO inhibitor. If use of an MAO inhibitor is indicated for any reason, your child must wait at least 5 weeks after stopping fluoxetine before starting the MAO inhibitor.
- Use of any of the following drugs along with or within 5 weeks of stopping fluoxetine may increase the chance of developing serotonin syndrome, a condition characterized by confusion, diarrhea, restlessness, shivering, sweating, twitching, and uncontrolled excitement: buspirone, bromocriptine, levodopa, dextromethorphan, lithium, meperidine, nefazodone, paroxetine, pentazocine, sertraline, sumatriptan, tramadol, trazodone, tryptophan, and venlafaxine.

- Fluoxetine may cause an increase in the levels of phenytoin and tricyclic antidepressants (e.g., amitriptyline, imipramine).
- Alprazolam may raise the blood levels of this drug and side effects may increase.
- Anticoagulants (e.g., warfarin) and digitalis may raise or lower levels of fluoxetine and these drugs.
- Do not take fluoxetine with grapefruit juice, as it may increase blood levels of the drug.
- Avoid use of herbs that produce a sedative effect, such as calendula, capsicum, catnip, goldenseal, gotu kola, hops, kava, lady's slipper, passionflower, sage, Siberian ginseng, skullcap, St. John's wort, and valerian, among others.

SYMPTOMS OF OVERDOSE
Symptoms include agitation, nausea, restlessness, seizures, and vomiting. If overdose occurs, seek immediate medical attention and bring the drug container(s) with you.

THINGS TO TELL YOUR DOCTOR
- Tell your doctor if your child has had allergic reactions to any medications in the past, especially similar drugs such as paroxetine or sertraline (Paxil, Zoloft), or if he or she is taking any medications now.
- Let your doctor know if your child has any of the following medical conditions: heart disease, diabetes, liver disease, history of seizures.
- If your child develops hives or a rash while taking fluoxetine, contact your physician immediately.
- Consult your doctor if your child is pregnant or becomes pregnant during treatment.

IMPORTANT PRECAUTIONS
- Fluoxetine is the only antidepressant approved by the U.S. Food and Drug Administration (FDA) for use in children and adolescents. However, a black box warning is required to appear on the packaging for this and other antidepressant medications. (See the introductory

material to this book for details.) In brief, use of fluoxetine may be associated with an increase in "suicidal
thinking or behavior . . . especially early in treatment."
Written information about fluoxetine and possible suicidality should be given to you with your prescription.

- Fluoxetine can cause dizziness and sleepiness, so make
  sure you know how your child reacts before allowing
  him or her to participate in potentially dangerous activities, such as riding a bike, driving a car, or operating
  machinery.
- Store fluoxetine in a tightly closed container and keep
  away from excess heat and moisture (e.g., the bathroom, near a stove or sink).

FLURANDRENOLIDE—
see *Corticosteroids, Topical*

FLUTICASONE—see *Corticosteroids, Nasal Inhalants; Corticosteroids, Oral Inhalants; and Corticosteroids, Topical*

FLUVOXAMINE

BRAND NAME
Luvox
Generic Available

ABOUT THIS DRUG
Fluvoxamine is a selective serotonin reuptake inhibitor
(SSRI) antidepressant that has been approved by the U.S.
Food and Drug Administration (FDA) for use in children
who have obsessive-compulsive disorder. Some physicians
also prescribe it for depression. This drug affects the levels
of serotonin, a chemical in the brain that is associated with
mood, emotions, and mental status.

SIDE EFFECTS
Contact your doctor if your child experiences any side effects that are persistent or troubling, including any that are not listed here.

- *Most common:* anxiety, decreased appetite, drowsiness, excessive sweating, headache, insomnia, nausea, nervousness
- *Less common/rare:* breathing problems, chills, decreased libido, diarrhea, dizziness, fainting, psychotic reactions, rapid heartbeat, difficulty swallowing, trembling, vomiting, weight gain

HOW TO USE THIS DRUG
Fluvoxamine is available in tablets. The dosages given here are ones that are usually recommended for children. However, your doctor will determine the most appropriate dose and schedule for your child.

- Children younger than 8 years: not recommended
- Children 8 to 17 years: starting dose is 25 mg as a single dose at bedtime. Your physician may increase it by 25 mg every 4 to 7 days as needed. The maximum daily dosage is 200 mg in divided doses.

Fluvoxamine can be taken with or without food. If your child misses a dose and he or she is taking one dose daily, take the missed dose if you remember the same day. However, skip the missed dose if you don't remember until the next day and return to the regular schedule. If your child is taking two doses daily and a dose is missed, skip the missed dose and return to your regular dosing schedule. Never give a double dose.

TIME UNTIL IT TAKES EFFECT
7 to 28 days

POSSIBLE DRUG, FOOD, AND/OR SUPPLEMENT INTERACTIONS
Tell your doctor if your child is taking any prescription or over-the-counter medications or any vitamins, herbs, or

other supplements. Possible interactions with fluvoxamine may include the following:

- Use of 5-HTP (5-hydroxytryptophan), St. John's wort, tryptophan, and grapefruit juice should be avoided while using this drug because they may increase the side effects of the drug.
- Herbs that produce a sedative effect may cause significant depressant symptoms if used along with fluvoxamine, including calendula, capsicum, catnip, goldenseal, gotu kola, hops, kava, lady's slipper, passionflower, sage, Siberian ginseng, skullcap, and valerian, among others.
- Monoamine oxidase (MAO) inhibitors (e.g., phenelzine) should not be taken at least 2 weeks before starting or 2 weeks after stopping fluvoxamine.
- Astemizole may cause potentially serious reactions.
- Benzodiazepines (e.g., diazepam, clonazepam) may accumulate in the blood and cause serious side effects.
- Theophylline and warfarin doses may need to be adjusted lower if your child is taking fluvoxamine.

SYMPTOMS OF OVERDOSE
Symptoms include dizziness, drowsiness, low blood pressure, rapid or slow heartbeat, seizures, severe diarrhea, and severe vomiting. If overdose occurs, seek immediate medical attention and bring the drug container(s) with you.

THINGS TO TELL YOUR DOCTOR
- Tell your doctor if your child has had allergic reactions to any medications in the past or if he or she is taking any medications, herbal remedies, or supplements now.
- Let your doctor know if your child has any of the following medical conditions: liver disease, seizures, history of mania.
- Consult your doctor if your child is pregnant or becomes pregnant during treatment.

IMPORTANT PRECAUTIONS

- A black box warning is required to appear on the packaging for this and other antidepressant medications (see the introductory material to this book for details). In brief, use of fluvoxamine may be associated with an increase in "suicidal thinking or behavior . . . especially early in treatment." Written information about fluvoxamine and possible suicidality should be given to you with your prescription.
- Withdrawal from fluvoxamine should be done under careful supervision of your physician to avoid withdrawal symptoms, which include dizziness, irritability, nausea, poor mood, tingling in the extremities, tiredness, and vivid dreams, and occur in up to 30 percent of cases.
- Because fluvoxamine can cause drowsiness, you should know how your child reacts to this drug before you allow him or her to participate in potentially dangerous activities, such as riding a bike, driving a car, or operating machinery.
- Store fluvoxamine in a tightly closed container and keep away from excess heat and moisture (e.g., the bathroom, near a stove or sink).

GABAPENTIN

BRAND NAME
Neurontin
Generic Available

ABOUT THIS DRUG

Gabapentin is an antiseizure medication used to control specific types of seizures associated with epilepsy. Although it is not certain how gabapentin works, many experts believe it inhibits firing of neurons in certain parts of the brain that cause convulsions. Gabapentin is also used to treat certain painful conditions.

SIDE EFFECTS
Contact your doctor if your child experiences any side effects that are persistent or troubling, including any that are not listed here.

* *Most common:* blurry vision, clumsiness or unsteadiness, dizziness, fatigue, nausea, sedation, tremor, vomiting
* *Less common/rare:* diarrhea, dry mouth, headache, irritability, muscle aches or weakness, sleep disturbances, slurred speech

HOW TO USE THIS DRUG
Gabapentin is available in tablets, capsules, and oral solution. The dosages given here are ones that are usually recommended for children. However, your doctor will determine the most appropriate dose and schedule for your child.

For Epilepsy
* Children 3 to 12 years: Starting dose is 4.5 to 6.8 mg per lb of body weight divided into 3 doses. Your doctor may then increase the dose as needed. For children 5 to 12 years, the usual dose is 11.3 to 15.9 mg per lb of body weight daily, divided into 3 doses. For children 3 to 4 years, the usual dose is 18.1 mg per lb of body weight daily, divided into 3 doses.
* Children 12 years and older: Starting dose is 300 mg 3 times daily. Your doctor may increase the dose, but dosage usually should not exceed 1,800 mg daily.

For Postherpetic Neuralgia
* Children 12 years and older: Starting dose is 300 mg on day 1, 300 mg 2 times daily on day 2, then 300 mg 3 times daily on day 3.

Gabapentin can be taken with food to help reduce stomach irritation. The capsules can be opened and the contents mixed with food if desired. Only mix one dose at a time.

If your child misses a dose, give it as soon as you remem-

ber. If it is nearly time for the next dose, skip the missed dose and continue with the regular dosing schedule. Never give a double dose.

TIME UNTIL IT TAKES EFFECT
Several hours

POSSIBLE DRUG, FOOD, AND/OR SUPPLEMENT INTERACTIONS
Tell your doctor if your child is taking any prescription or over-the-counter medications or any vitamins, herbs, or other supplements. Possible interactions with gabapentin may include the following:

- Antacids (e.g., Maalox, Mylanta) may reduce the effectiveness of gabapentin and should be taken at least 2 hours after taking gabapentin.
- Drugs that have depressive effects on the central nervous system may enhance the depressive effect and should be avoided. They include: anesthetics (including dental anesthetics), anticonvulsants, antihistamines, barbiturates, muscle relaxants, narcotics, sedatives, and tranquilizers.

SYMPTOMS OF OVERDOSE
Symptoms include diarrhea, double vision, drowsiness, lethargy, and slurred speech. If overdose occurs, seek medical attention immediately and bring the prescription container with you.

THINGS TO TELL YOUR DOCTOR
- Tell your doctor if your child has had allergic reactions to any medications in the past or if he or she is taking any medications now.
- Let your doctor know if your child has any of the following medical conditions: low blood pressure, history of kidney disease or impaired kidney function, pancreatitis.
- Consult your doctor if your child is pregnant or becomes pregnant during treatment. Although adequate

studies of the effects of gabapentin on pregnant women have not been done, other anticonvulsants have been proven to increase the risk of birth defects.

IMPORTANT PRECAUTIONS

- Do not suddenly withdraw this drug from your child, as seizures may occur. Only your physician can advise you on how to gradually reduce the dosage.
- Because gabapentin can cause dizziness and sleepiness, make sure you know how your child reacts to this drug before you allow him or her to participate in potentially dangerous activities, such as riding a bike, driving a car, or operating machinery.
- Store gabapentin in a tightly closed container and keep away from excess heat and moisture (e.g., the bathroom, near a stove or sink). Refrigerate the oral solution but do not allow it to freeze.

GENTAMICIN
(TOPICAL AND OPHTHALMIC)

BRAND NAMES

Garamycin, Genoptic, Genoptic SOP, Gentacidin, Gentak, G-Myticin
Generic Available

ABOUT THIS DRUG

Gentamicin is a topical antibacterial that is prescribed to treat bacterial infections of the skin and infections complicating rashes, eczema, dermatitis, and other inflammatory skin conditions. It is also available as an ophthalmic formula for eye infections. In both cases it works by preventing bacteria from manufacturing the proteins they need to grow and reproduce.

SIDE EFFECTS

Contact your doctor if your child experiences any side effects that are persistent or troubling, including any that are not listed here.

- *Most common:* none when used as directed
- *Less common/rare:* discomfort at the application site that was not present before treatment, increased redness, itching, swelling

HOW TO USE THIS DRUG
Gentamicin is available as cream, ointment, and eye drops. The dosages given here are ones that are usually recommended for children. However, your doctor will determine the most appropriate dose and schedule for your child.

- Children 1 year and older: for skin conditions, apply a thin layer to the affected site 3 or 4 times daily every 6 to 8 hours
- Children 1 year and older—Eye drops: 1 or 2 drops every 4 hours for mild to moderate infections; 1 to 2 drops every hour for severe infections or as directed

If your child misses a dose, apply the medication as soon as you remember. If it is nearly time for the next dose, skip the missed dose and continue with the regular dosing schedule. Do not double the dose or apply an excessive amount of the medication.

TIME UNTIL IT TAKES EFFECT
The drug begins to kill the causative bacteria shortly after it is applied, but other benefits may not be noticeable for several days.

POSSIBLE DRUG, FOOD, AND/OR SUPPLEMENT INTERACTIONS
Tell your doctor if your child is taking any prescription or over-the-counter medications or any vitamins, herbs, or other supplements. No drug interactions have been reported with gentamicin. If your child is using another topical medication, talk to your physician or pharmacist about any possible interactions and whether the other medication should be continued.

SYMPTOMS OF OVERDOSE
No specific symptoms of overdose have been reported. If your child accidentally ingests gentamicin, seek medical attention immediately and bring the prescription container with you.

THINGS TO TELL YOUR DOCTOR
- Tell your doctor if your child has had allergic reactions to any medications in the past or if he or she is taking any medications now.
- Let your doctor know if your child has any hearing problems, kidney disease, or a history of allergic reactions to antibiotics.
- Consult your doctor if your child is pregnant or becomes pregnant during treatment.

IMPORTANT PRECAUTIONS
- Gentamicin can make your child's skin more sensitive to sunlight. Make sure your child is adequately protected from the sun (e.g., sunscreen, long sleeves, long pants) while he or she is using this medication.
- Store gentamicin in a tightly closed container and keep at room temperature away from excess heat and moisture (e.g., the bathroom, near a stove or sink). Do not allow it to freeze.

GRANISETRON—see *Antiemetics*

GRISEOFULVIN

BRAND NAMES
Fulvicin U/F, Fulvicin P/G, Grifulvin V, Grisactin, Grisactin Ultra, Gris-PEG
Generic Available

ABOUT THIS DRUG
Griseofulvin is an antifungal used to treat various fungal infections, including ringworm, jock itch, athlete's foot, and

nail fungus. This drug prevents certain fungi from growing and reproducing.

SIDE EFFECTS
Contact your doctor if your child experiences any side effects that are persistent or troubling, including any that are not listed here.

- *Most common:* headache
- *Less common:* confusion, diarrhea, insomnia, itch, mouth or tongue irritation, nausea, rash, stomach pain, tiredness, vomiting
- *Rare:* cloudy urine, fever, jaundice, numbness or tingling in feet or hands, sore throat. These side effects are more likely to occur if your child uses high doses for a prolonged time.

HOW TO USE THIS DRUG
Griseofulvin is available as tablets, capsules, and oral suspension. The dosages given here are ones that are usually recommended for children. However, your doctor will determine the most appropriate dose and schedule for your child.

For Micro-size Capsules, Tablets, and Suspension
- Children younger than 12 years: for feet, nails, scalp, and groin—2.3 mg per lb of body weight every 12 hours, or 4.5 mg per lb of body weight once daily
- Children 12 years and older: for scalp, skin, and groin—250 mg every 12 hours or 500 mg once daily; for feet and nails—500 mg every 12 hours

Griseofulvin should be taken either with or after meals or milk. Fatty foods, such as whole milk or cheese, peanut butter, or avocados, increase the amount of the drug the body can absorb.

If your child misses a dose, give it as soon as you remember. However, if it is nearly time for the next dose, skip the missed dose and continue with the regular dosing schedule. Never give a double dose.

TIME UNTIL IT TAKES EFFECT

Symptoms may improve within a few days, but it takes longer for the infection to disappear. Typically it takes 2 to 4 weeks for skin infections, 4 to 6 weeks for scalp infections, 4 to 8 weeks for foot infections, 3 to 4 months for fingernail infections, and at least 6 months for toenail infections to heal.

POSSIBLE DRUG, FOOD, AND/OR SUPPLEMENT INTERACTIONS

Tell your doctor if your child is taking any prescription or over-the-counter medications or any vitamins, herbs, or other supplements. Possible interactions with griseofulvin may include the following:

- Anticoagulants, cyclosporine, phenobarbital, and oral contraceptives may cause negative reactions if taken with griseofulvin.
- Griseofulvin may decrease the effectiveness of oral contraceptives. Your child should use a backup form of birth control while taking griseofulvin.
- Alcohol should be avoided while taking griseofulvin.

SYMPTOMS OF OVERDOSE

Symptoms include diarrhea, nausea, and vomiting. If overdose occurs, seek immediate medical attention and bring the drug container(s) with you.

THINGS TO TELL YOUR DOCTOR

- Tell your doctor if your child has had allergic reactions to any medications in the past or if he or she is taking any medications, herbal remedies, or supplements now.
- Let your doctor know if your child has lupus, kidney disease, or porphyria.
- Griseofulvin causes birth defects and should not be used during pregnancy. Consult your doctor if your child is pregnant or becomes pregnant during treatment.

IMPORTANT PRECAUTIONS

- Griseofulvin may make your child's skin more likely to burn in sunlight. Make sure your child's skin is protected against the sun (e.g., sunscreen, long sleeves and long pants) while he or she is using this drug.
- Store griseofulvin in a tightly closed container and keep away from excess heat and moisture (e.g., the bathroom, near a stove or sink). Keep the liquid form refrigerated, but do not allow it to freeze.

GUAIFENESIN

BRAND NAMES

Amonidrin, Anti-Tuss, Breonesin, Fenesin, Gee-Gee, Genatuss, GG-Cen, Glyate, Glycotuss, Glytuss, Guaifenesin, Guiatuss, Halotussin, Humibid LA, Humibid Sprinkle, Hytuss, Hytuss 2X, Malotuss, Mytussin, Robitussin, Scottussin Expectorant, Sinumist-SR Capsulets, Uni-tussin. Guaifenesin appears in many combination products for cold/flu/cough.
Generic Available/Over-the-Counter Available

ABOUT THIS DRUG

Guaifenesin is an expectorant, a product that is designed to reduce phlegm and thick mucus and ultimately make it easier for an individual to cough up these substances from the lungs. To accomplish this, guaifenesin reportedly increases the production of fluid in the respiratory tract, which in turn thins out mucus and makes it easier to expel.

SIDE EFFECTS

Contact your doctor if your child experiences any side effects that are persistent or troubling, including any that are not listed here.

- Most common: none
- *Less common/rare:* abdominal pain, diarrhea, dizziness, headache, hives, itching, nausea, rash

HOW TO USE THIS DRUG

Guaifenesin is available in tablets, capsules, oral solution, syrup, and extended-release forms. The dosages given here are ones that are usually recommended for children. However, your doctor will determine the most appropriate dose and schedule for your child.

- Children 2 to 6 years: 50 to 100 mg every 4 hours
- Children 7 to 12 years: 100 to 200 mg every 4 hours
- Children 13 years and older: 200 to 400 mg every 4 hours of short-acting capsules, tablets, oral solution, or syrup. The maximum intake is 2,400 mg daily. For extended-release capsules and tablets, 600 to 1,200 mg every 12 hours to a maximum of 2,400 mg daily

Your child should drink extra fluids while using this drug, as it helps clear mucus from the lungs. Capsules and tablets should not be chewed and should be taken with a full glass of water.

If your child misses a dose, give it as soon as you remember. However, if it is nearly time for the next dose, skip the missed dose and continue with the regular dosing schedule. Never give a double dose.

TIME UNTIL IT TAKES EFFECT
Within several hours

POSSIBLE DRUG, FOOD, AND/OR SUPPLEMENT INTERACTIONS
Tell your doctor if your child is taking any prescription or over-the-counter medications or any vitamins, herbs, or other supplements. No drug, food, or supplement interactions with guaifenesin have been reported.

SYMPTOMS OF OVERDOSE
No specific overdose symptoms have been noted. However, if you think an overdose has occurred, seek immediate medical attention and bring the drug container(s) with you.

THINGS TO TELL YOUR DOCTOR
- Tell your doctor if your child has had allergic reactions to any medications in the past or if he or she is taking any medications, herbal remedies, or supplements now.
- If your child is younger than 12 years of age and has had a persistent cough, talk to your doctor before giving your child guaifenesin.
- Consult your doctor if your child is pregnant or becomes pregnant during treatment.

IMPORTANT PRECAUTIONS
- Guaifenesin is found in many nonprescription cough and cold medications, so be sure to ask your pharmacist or physician about any other medications your child is taking before you give your child guaifenesin.
- Store guaifenesin in a tightly closed container and keep away from excess heat and moisture (e.g., the bathroom, near a stove or sink). The liquid forms can be refrigerated but do not allow them to freeze.

HALCINONIDE—see *Corticosteroids, Topical*

HALOBETASOL— see *Corticosteroids, Topical*

HALOPERIDOL

BRAND NAME
Haldol
Generic Available

ABOUT THIS DRUG
Haloperidol is an antipsychotic drug prescribed primarily to reduce severe anxiety, agitation, psychotic behavior, and behavior problems in children, to treat infantile autism, and to reduce the symptoms of Tourette's syndrome. It works by blocking the

effects of dopamine, a chemical in the brain that facilitates the transmission of nerve signals. When these signals are blocked, the result is a calming effect on the individual.

SIDE EFFECTS
Contact your doctor if your child experiences any side effects that are persistent or troubling, including any that are not listed here.

- *Most common:* blurry vision, drowsiness, intermittent spasms of the facial muscles or muscles of the body, involuntary or jerky movements (especially in the tongue, lips, or face), slow tremor of the limbs or head, lack of facial expression, restlessness
- *Less common/rare:* breast pain or swelling, constipation, difficult urination, dry mouth, dizziness, heart palpitations, increased sensitivity to sunlight, itching, low blood pressure, sedation

Use of this drug may also cause a rare but life-threatening syndrome called neuroleptic malignant syndrome (NMS). Symptoms include fever, difficulty breathing, rapid heartbeat, rigid muscles, mental changes, increased sweating, irregular blood pressure, and convulsions. If your child displays these symptoms, seek immediate medical attention.

Very rarely in young people, a disorder known as tardive dyskinesia may occur. Characteristics include wormlike movements of the tongue, lip smacking, and slow, rhythmical, involuntary movements, which may become permanent. If your child experiences these side effects, contact your doctor immediately, and he or she will likely advise you to stop giving your child the medication.

HOW TO USE THIS DRUG
Haloperidol is available in tablets and liquid and via injection. (Injection information is not provided here.) The dosages given here are ones that are usually recommended for children. However, your doctor will determine the most appropriate dose and schedule for your child.

For Psychotic Disorders

- Children 3 to 12 years weighing 33 to 88 lbs: 0.011 to 0.07 mg per lb of body weight in 2 to 3 divided doses
- Children 13 years and older: 0.5 to 5 mg 2 or 3 times daily, based on the severity of symptoms. The usual maximum dose is 100 mg daily.

For Tourette's Syndrome and Behavior Problems

- Children 3 to 12 years: 0.034 mg per lb of body weight
- Children 13 years and older: 0.5 to 5 mg 2 to 3 times daily, based on the severity of symptoms

Haloperidol should be taken with food or a full glass of water or milk, never with coffee, tea, or carbonated beverages. To help prevent stomach irritation when taking the oral solution, you can mix the medication into apple or orange juice or milk.

If your child misses a dose, give it as soon as you remember, then take the remaining doses for the day at equally spaced intervals. Continue with the regular dosing schedule. Never give a double dose.

TIME UNTIL IT TAKES EFFECT

Sedation typically occurs within minutes, but antipsychotic effects may take hours, days, or even weeks.

POSSIBLE DRUG, FOOD, AND/OR SUPPLEMENT INTERACTIONS

Tell your doctor if your child is taking any prescription or over-the-counter medications or any vitamins, herbs, or other supplements. Possible interactions with haloperidol may include the following:

- Increased sedation may occur if your child takes antidepressants (e.g., amitriptyline, fluoxetine), antihistamines (e.g., clemastine, cetirizine), barbiturates (e.g., amobarbital), narcotics (e.g., codeine), or procarbazine.
- Antihypertensive drugs (e.g., clonidine, guanfacine) may cause a severe decrease in blood pressure.

- Bupropion may increase the risk of seizures.
- Lithium and clozapine may cause toxic effects.
- Methyldopa may cause psychosis.
- Haloperidol may decrease the effects of levodopa, pergolide, and guanethidine.

SYMPTOMS OF OVERDOSE
Symptoms include confusion, coma, deep sleep, dizziness, muscle weakness or tremor, shallow breathing, weak or rapid pulse. If overdose occurs, seek immediate medical attention and bring the drug container(s) with you.

THINGS TO TELL YOUR DOCTOR
- Tell your doctor if your child has had allergic reactions to any medications in the past or if he or she is taking any medications, herbal remedies, or supplements now.
- Let your doctor know if your child has any of the following medical conditions: any type of movement disorder, glaucoma, epilepsy, liver or kidney disease.
- Consult your doctor if your child is pregnant or becomes pregnant during treatment.

IMPORTANT PRECAUTIONS
- Haloperidol can alter your child's temperature-regulating system, which means he or she may become overheated more easily during exercise or hot weather. Avoid extreme temperatures.
- Haloperidol can increase your child's sensitivity to sunlight. Make sure he or she wears sunscreen and/or long sleeves and long pants when exposed to the sun.
- Store haloperidol in a tightly closed container and keep at room temperature away from excess heat and moisture (e.g., the bathroom, near a stove or sink).

HYDROCODONE PLUS CHLORPHENIRAMINE

BRAND NAME
Tussionex
Generic Not Available

ABOUT THIS DRUG
Hydrocodone + chlorpheniramine brings together a narcotic and an antihistamine for treatment of coughs and upper respiratory symptoms of allergies and colds. The narcotic, hydrocodone, works by suppressing the cough center in the brain, while the antihistamine, chlorpheniramine, reduces swelling and itching and helps dry up secretions from the throat, eyes, and nose.

SIDE EFFECTS
Contact your doctor if your child experiences any side effects that are persistent or troubling, including any that are not listed here.

- *Most common:* chills, dizziness, drowsiness, dry mouth, increased sweating, itching, lightheadedness, nausea, sensitivity to bright lights, vomiting
- *Less common/rare:* agitation, anemia, blurry vision, disorientation, euphoria, hallucinations, low blood sugar, palpitations, ringing in the ears, urinary problems, wheezing

HOW TO USE THIS DRUG
Hydrocodone + chlorpheniramine is available as a syrup. The dosages given here are ones that are usually recommended for children. However, your doctor will determine the most appropriate dose and schedule for your child.

- Children younger than 6 years: not recommended
- Children 6 years and older: one-half teaspoon every 12 hours, not exceeding 1 teaspoon in 24 hours

Your child can take this medication with food to help prevent stomach upset.

If your child misses a dose, give it as soon as you remember. If it is nearly time for the next dose, do not give the missed dose. Continue with the regular dosing schedule. Never give a double dose.

TIME UNTIL IT TAKES EFFECT
30 to 60 minutes

POSSIBLE DRUG, FOOD, AND/OR SUPPLEMENT INTERACTIONS
Tell your doctor if your child is taking any prescription or over-the-counter medications or any vitamins, herbs, or other supplements. Possible interactions with hydrocodone + chlorpheniramine may include the following:

- Use of antidepressants (e.g., amitriptyline, fluoxetine), antihistamines (e.g., clemastine, loratadine), phenothiazines (e.g., chlorpromazine, promazine), sedatives, tranquilizers, sleeping pills, or tramadol may increase the sedative effects.
- Alcohol should be avoided, as the combination increases the intoxicating effects.
- Other narcotics (e.g., codeine, oxycodone), sotalol, nonsteroidal anti-inflammatory drugs (NSAIDs; e.g., aspirin, naproxen), and molindone may increase narcotic effects.
- Naltrexone may cause respiratory arrest, coma, and death.
- Phenytoin and rifampin may decrease the narcotic effects.
- Sertraline may increase the depressive effects.
- Selegiline may cause severe toxicity, characterized by seizures, coma, and difficulty breathing.

SYMPTOMS OF OVERDOSE
Symptoms include bluish skin, cardiac arrest, cold and clammy skin, extreme sleepiness leading to stupor or coma,

low blood pressure, slow heartbeat, and temporary cessation of breathing. If overdose occurs, seek immediate medical attention and bring the drug container(s) with you.

THINGS TO TELL YOUR DOCTOR

- Tell your doctor if your child has had allergic reactions to any medications in the past or if he or she is taking any medications, herbal remedies, or supplements now.
- Let your doctor know if your child has any of the following medical conditions: asthma, convulsions, diabetes, glaucoma, heart disease, hypertension, intestinal disorder, liver or kidney disease, lung disease, thyroid or adrenal gland disorders, urinary difficulties.
- Consult your doctor if your child is pregnant or becomes pregnant during treatment. This drug combination should not be used during pregnancy, as overuse can cause drug dependence in the fetus.

IMPORTANT PRECAUTIONS

- Because this drug combination can cause dizziness, drowsiness, and lightheadedness, make sure you know how your child reacts to these drugs before you allow him or her to participate in potentially dangerous activities, such as riding a bike, driving a car, or operating machinery.
- This drug combination contains a narcotic that can cause tolerance and dependence if it is taken for several weeks. Such a response is unlikely, however, if your child uses it for a short time for cough.
- Store hydrocodone + chlorpheniramine in a tightly closed container and keep at room temperature away from excess heat and moisture (e.g., the bathroom, near a stove or sink). Do not refrigerate.

HYDROCORTISONE—
see *Corticosteroids, Oral* and *Corticosteroids, Topical*

HYDROXYZINE

BRAND NAMES
Anxanil, Atarax, E-Vista, Hydroxacen, Hyzine-50, Vistaject-25, Vistaject-50, Vistaril, Vistazine 50
Generic Available

ABOUT THIS DRUG
Hydroxyzine is an antihistamine and mild sedative that is used to treat several conditions, including insomnia and agitation; itching, hives, and other allergic symptoms; and nausea and vomiting. It is also used as a mild sedative before dental procedures. Consequently, hydroxyzine acts in several ways. As an antihistamine it blocks the effects of histamine, a naturally occurring substance in the body that causes sneezing, watery eyes, hives, and other allergy symptoms. It also suppresses activity in some parts of the brain and spinal cord that are associated with nausea and emotional distress.

SIDE EFFECTS
Contact your doctor if your child experiences any side effects that are persistent or troubling, including any that are not listed here.

- *Most common:* drowsiness; dry mouth, nasal passages, and other mucous membranes
- *Less common/rare:* difficult urination, dizziness, increased sensitivity to sunlight, loss of appetite, nightmares, rash, restlessness, sore throat, stomach upset

HOW TO USE THIS DRUG
Hydroxyzine is available in tablets and syrup and via injection. (Injection information is not provided here.) The dosages given here are ones that are usually recommended for children. However, your doctor will determine the most appropriate dose and schedule for your child.

For Allergy
- Children younger than 6 years: 12.5 mg every 6 hours as needed
- Children 6 years and older: 12.5 to 25 mg every 6 hours as needed

For Nausea and Vomiting
- Children: 0.27 mg per lb of body weight daily

The tablets can be crushed and mixed with food or liquid if your child has difficulty swallowing a tablet. If your child misses a dose, give it as soon as you remember. However, if it is nearly time for the next dose, skip the missed dose and continue with the regular dosing schedule. Do not give a double dose.

TIME UNTIL IT TAKES EFFECT
15 to 30 minutes

POSSIBLE DRUG, FOOD, AND/OR SUPPLEMENT INTERACTIONS
Tell your doctor if your child is taking any prescription or over-the-counter medications or any vitamins, herbs, or other supplements. Possible interactions with hydroxyzine may include the following:

- Tricyclic antidepressants (e.g., imipramine) and narcotics (e.g., codeine) may increase the effects of both drugs.
- Antihistamines (e.g., cetirizine, loratadine) may increase the effect of hydroxyzine.
- Sedatives, antidepressants, and barbiturates may cause greater depression of the central nervous system.
- Clozapine may be toxic to the central nervous system.
- Fluoxetine and sertraline may cause increased depressant effects of both drugs.
- Alcohol may increase sedation and intoxication.
- Excessive sedation may occur if hydroxyzine is taken along with GABA (gamma-aminobutynic acid), 5-

HTP (5-hydroxytryptophan), valerian, melatonin, melissa, or kava.

- Both hydroxyzine and St. John's wort can cause increased sensitivity to sunlight. Consult your physician before combining these two elements.

SYMPTOMS OF OVERDOSE

Symptoms include difficulty breathing; extreme drowsiness; fainting; hallucinations; loss of coordination; severe dry mouth, nose, and throat; and tremors. If overdose occurs, seek medical attention immediately and bring the prescription container with you to the hospital.

THINGS TO TELL YOUR DOCTOR

- Tell your doctor if your child has had allergic reactions to any medications in the past or if he or she is taking any medications now.
- Let your doctor know if your child has asthma or kidney disease or plans to undergo surgery (including dental surgery) within the next 2 months that will require spinal or general anesthesia.
- Consult your doctor if your child is pregnant or becomes pregnant during treatment.

IMPORTANT PRECAUTIONS

- Store hydroxyzine in a tightly closed container and keep it away from heat and moisture (e.g., in the bathroom, near a stove or sink). Do not allow the syrup to freeze.
- Long-term use of hydroxyzine results in tolerance and reduced effectiveness.
- Because hydroxyzine can cause drowsiness and dizziness, make sure you know how your child reacts to it before you allow him or her to participate in potentially dangerous activities, such as riding a bike, driving a car, or operating machinery.

IBUPROFEN

BRAND NAMES
Advil, Children's Advil Suspension, Children's Motrin Chewable Tablets, Children's Motrin Drops, Children's Motrin Oral Suspension, Ibuprin, Medipren, Midol 200, Motrin, Motrin IB, Nuprin, PediaCare Fever Drops, Pediatric Advil Drops, Pamprin-IB, Q-Profen
Generic Available/Over-the-Counter Available

ABOUT THIS DRUG
Ibuprofen is a nonsteroidal anti-inflammatory drug (NSAID) that is used to treat mild to moderate pain and inflammation caused by a variety of conditions, including but not limited to arthritis, bursitis, gout, menstrual cramps, migraine and other vascular headache, and tendonitis. It is also used to reduce fever. This drug works on pain and inflammation in several ways, one of which is to interfere with the formation of prostaglandins, substances that cause inflammation and make nerves more sensitive to pain signals.

SIDE EFFECTS
Contact your doctor if your child experiences any side effects that are persistent or troubling, including any that are not listed here.

- *Most common:* constipation, diarrhea, dizziness, headache, heartburn, nausea, sleepiness, vomiting
- *Less common/rare:* blistering of skin, blurry vision, depression, rash, ringing in the ears, sores or ulcers in mouth, unusual tingling or numbness

HOW TO USE THIS DRUG
Ibuprofen is available as tablets, chewable tablets, and oral solution. The dosages given here are ones that are usually recommended for children. However, you should consult your doctor about the specific brand or prescription of ibuprofen you have and allow him or her to determine the most appropriate dose and schedule for your child.

For Fever
- Children 6 months to 12 years: 2.3 mg per lb of body weight if temperature is less than 102.5° F or 4.5 mg per lb of body weight if temperature is 102.5° F or greater.
- Children 13 years and older: 200 to 400 mg every 4 to 6 hours but not more than 1,200 mg daily

For Mild to Moderate Pain
- Children 6 months to 12 years: 4.5 mg per lb of body weight every 6 to 8 hours but not more than 4 such doses per day
- Children 13 years and older: 200 to 400 mg every 4 to 6 hours but not more than 1,200 mg daily

For Juvenile Arthritis
- Typical dose is 13.6 to 18 mg per lb of body weight divided into 3 or 4 doses daily; some children need only 9 mg per lb

Ibuprofen can be taken with food, milk, or an antacid to help prevent stomach irritation.

If your child misses a dose, give it as soon as you remember. However, if it is nearly time for the next dose, skip the missed dose and continue with the regular dosing schedule. Do not give a double dose.

TIME UNTIL IT TAKES EFFECT
When treating pain and fever, 30 minutes; for juvenile arthritis, up to 3 weeks for full effect

POSSIBLE DRUG, FOOD, AND/OR SUPPLEMENT INTERACTIONS
Tell your doctor if your child is taking any prescription or over-the-counter medications or any vitamins, herbs, or other supplements. Possible interactions with ibuprofen may include the following:

- Other NSAIDs (e.g., naproxen, fenoprofen) and dipyridamole, sulfinpyrazone, valproic acid, and blood thin-

ners should not be taken along with ibuprofen, as they increase the risk of bleeding.
- Ibuprofen taken along with cyclosporine may increase the negative effects on the kidney from both drugs.
- Lithium or methotrexate may reach toxic levels in the body.
- Use of alcohol along with ibuprofen can increase the risk of stomach bleeding and ulcers.
- Do not combine ibuprofen with clove oil, feverfew, garlic, ginkgo, or ginseng, as they can affect clotting.

SYMPTOMS OF OVERDOSE

Symptoms include abdominal pain, agitation, disorientation, diarrhea, drowsiness, nausea, rapid breathing, rapid heartbeat, ringing in the ears, stupor, and seizures. If overdose occurs, seek immediate medical attention and bring the drug container(s) with you.

THINGS TO TELL YOUR DOCTOR

- Tell your doctor if your child has had allergic reactions to any medications in the past or if he or she is taking any medications, herbal remedies, or supplements now.
- Let your doctor know if your child has any of the following medical conditions: asthma, colitis, high blood pressure, heart problems, history of ulcers, gastrointestinal bleeding, liver or kidney problems.
- If your child needs to undergo any dental procedures or surgery, tell your physician or dentist that your child is taking ibuprofen.
- Consult your doctor if your child is pregnant or becomes pregnant during treatment. Ibuprofen may be safe to use during early pregnancy if ordered by your doctor, but it should be avoided during the last trimester.

IMPORTANT PRECAUTIONS

- Ibuprofen may increase your child's sensitivity to sunlight. Make sure he or she wears sunscreen and/or protective clothing when outside.

- Store ibuprofen in a tightly closed container and keep away from excess heat and moisture (e.g., the bathroom, near a stove or sink).

IBUPROFEN PLUS PSEUDOEPHEDRINE

BRAND NAMES
Advil Cold and Sinus, Children's Motrin Cold, DayQuil Pressure and Pain Caplet, Dimetapp Sinus, Dristan Sinus, Motrin Cold and Flu, Motrin IB Sinus, Sine-Aid IB
Generic Available

ABOUT THIS DRUG
Ibuprofen + pseudoephedrine is a combination drug used to relieve symptoms of cold and flu. Ibuprofen is a non-steroidal anti-inflammatory drug (NSAID), which reduces pain and inflammation by reducing the hormones that cause these symptoms. Pseudoephedrine is a decongestant, which helps relieve congestion associated with allergies, sinus irritation, the common cold, and hay fever.

SIDE EFFECTS
Contact your doctor if your child experiences any side effects that are persistent or troubling, including any that are not listed here.

- *Most common:* constipation, diarrhea, dizziness, headache, heartburn, nausea, sleepiness, vomiting
- *Less common/rare:* blistering of skin, blurry vision, depression, rash, ringing in the ears, sores or ulcers in mouth, unusual tingling or numbness

HOW TO USE THIS DRUG
Ibuprofen + pseudoephedrine is available as tablets, caplets, and oral suspension. The dosages given here are ones that are usually recommended for children. However, your doctor will determine the most appropriate dose and schedule for your child.

- Children younger than 12 years: generally not recommended, although some brand names may be specially formulated for younger children. Check individual package instructions and talk to your doctor.
- Children 12 years and older: 1 tablet or caplet every 4 to 6 hours, not to exceed 6 tablets or caplets in a 24-hour period

Your child can take ibuprofen + pseudoephedrine with food to prevent stomach irritation. If your child misses a dose, give it as soon as you remember. If it is nearly time for the next dose, skip the missed dose and continue with the regular dosing schedule. Never give a double dose.

TIME UNTIL IT TAKES EFFECT
About 30 minutes

POSSIBLE DRUG, FOOD, AND/OR SUPPLEMENT INTERACTIONS
Tell your doctor if your child is taking any prescription or over-the-counter medications or any vitamins, herbs, or other supplements. Possible interactions with ibuprofen + pseudoephedrine may include the following:

- Monoamine oxidase (MAO) inhibitors should not be taken within at least 14 days of using ibuprofen + pseudoephedrine, as serious side effects may occur.
- Other NSAIDs (e.g., naproxen, fenoprofen) and dipyridamole, sulfinpyrazone, valproic acid, and blood thinners should not be taken, as they increase the risk of bleeding.
- Cyclosporine may increase the negative effects on the kidney from both drugs.
- Lithium or methotrexate may reach toxic levels in the body.
- Use of alcohol can increase the risk of stomach bleeding and ulcers.
- Do not allow your child to use clove oil, feverfew, garlic, ginkgo, or ginseng, as these substances can affect clotting.

SYMPTOMS OF OVERDOSE

Symptoms include blurry vision, dizziness, headache, nausea, ringing in the ears, seizures, slowed breathing, slowed heartbeat, and vomiting. If overdose occurs, seek immediate medical attention and bring the drug container(s) with you.

THINGS TO TELL YOUR DOCTOR

- Tell your doctor if your child has had allergic reactions to any medications in the past, especially aspirin and other NSAIDs, or if he or she is taking any medications, herbal remedies, or supplements now.
- Let your doctor know if your child has any of the following medical conditions: diabetes, heart disease, high blood pressure, thyroid problems, difficulty urinating.
- This medication should not be taken for more than 7 days. Consult your doctor if symptoms do not improve, are accompanied by fever that lasts for more than 3 days, or if new symptoms appear.
- Consult your doctor if your child is pregnant or becomes pregnant while taking ibuprofen + pseudoephedrine. This combination may be safe during early pregnancy, but it should be avoided during the last trimester.

IMPORTANT PRECAUTIONS

- Your child should not lie down for about 30 minutes after taking a dose of this drug combination, as irritation may cause trouble with swallowing.
- Store ibuprofen + pseudoephedrine in a tightly closed container and keep away from excess heat and moisture (e.g., the bathroom, near a stove or sink).

IMIPRAMINE—
see *Tricyclic Antidepressants*

INSULIN

TYPES
(1) Intermediate-acting, NPH, Lente; (2) Glargine (rDNA origin); (3) Lispro (rDNA origin); (4) Long-acting, Ultralente; (5) Regular, rapid-acting, or Semilente

BRAND NAMES
(1) Humulin L, Humulin N, Humulin R, Insulatar NPH, Mixtard, Novolin, Velosulin; (2) Lantus; (3) Humalog; (4) Humulin U Ultralente; (5) Humulin BR, Humulin R, Novolin R, Novolin R PenFill Cartridges, Regular Iletin I, Semilente Insulin, Velosulin Human, Velosulin
Generic Available on (1), (4), and (5)

ABOUT THIS DRUG
Insulin is an antidiabetic agent prescribed for diabetes mellitus when the condition cannot be controlled using oral antidiabetic medications, diet, and/or exercise. In young people, insulin is prescribed for type 1 diabetes, which is characterized by the failure of the pancreas to produce insulin naturally. Prescribed insulin acts like natural insulin, which helps sugar (glucose) enter cells, where it is used by the body to produce energy.

SIDE EFFECTS
Contact your doctor if your child experiences any side effects that are persistent or troubling, including any that are not listed here.

- *Most common:* itching, redness, or swelling at the injection site
- *Less common/rare:* fast pulse, low blood pressure, perspiration, rash, shallow breathing, shortness of breath, wheezing

HOW TO USE THIS DRUG
Insulin is available in injectable form. Dosage of insulin is very individualized; therefore, your physician will determine the most appropriate dose and schedule for your child.

TIME UNTIL IT TAKES EFFECT
Glargine, 1 to 2 hours; intermediate-acting insulin, within 1 hour, but the peak effect occurs within 8 to 12 hours; Lispro, within 30 to 45 minutes and peaks within 1 hour; long-acting Ultralente, within 6 to 8 hours and peaks within 10 to 20; regular, rapid-acting, or Semilente, within 45 minutes and peaks within 2 to 4 hours

POSSIBLE DRUG, FOOD, AND/OR SUPPLEMENT INTERACTIONS
Tell your doctor if your child is taking any prescription or over-the-counter medications or any vitamins, herbs, or other supplements. Possible interactions with insulin may include the following:

- The effects of insulin may increase if taken with acarbose, aspirin and other salicylates, some beta-blockers, clofibrate, disopyramide, fenfluramine, MAO inhibitors, or oral antidiabetic drugs.
- Use of alcohol can lead to severe hypoglycemia and cause brain damage.
- The effects of insulin may decrease if taken with oral contraceptives, chlorthalidone, cortisone-like drugs (e.g., betamethasone, cortisone), furosemide, phenytoin, thiazide diuretics, or thyroid preparations.

SYMPTOMS OF OVERDOSE
An overdose of insulin can cause hypoglycemia (low blood sugar), characterized by abnormal behavior and personality changes, blurry vision, cold sweat, confusion, depression, dizziness, drowsiness, headache, hunger, lightheadedness, nausea, nervousness, rapid heartbeat, sleep problems, slurred speech, tingling (in the tongue, lips, hands, or feet), and tremor. Severely low blood sugar can result in disorientation and coma. If overdose occurs and your child can safely eat or drink, give him or her something that is high in sugar (e.g., candy, orange juice), seek immediate medical attention, and bring the drug container with you.

THINGS TO TELL YOUR DOCTOR

- Tell your doctor if your child has had allergic reactions to any medications in the past or if he or she is taking any medications, herbal remedies, or supplements now.
- Certain medical conditions or events can increase or decrease your child's need for insulin. Let your doctor know whenever your child has any of the following: an infection, excessive stress, uncontrolled hyperthyroidism, underactive adrenal or pituitary glands, kidney disease.
- Consult your doctor if your child is pregnant or becomes pregnant during treatment. It is essential to maintain strict control of insulin levels during pregnancy to reduce the risk of birth defects and other complications.

IMPORTANT PRECAUTIONS

- Do not change the brand or type of insulin or the model of syringe or needle without first talking to your physician.
- Store insulin in a refrigerator, but do not allow it to freeze. It can be kept at room temperature for short amounts of time (e.g., if you are traveling), but do not expose it to high temperatures.

IPRATROPIUM BROMIDE

BRAND NAME
Atrovent
Generic Available

ABOUT THIS DRUG
Ipratropium is an anticholinergic/bronchodilator that is prescribed for treatment of bronchitis, chronic obstructive pulmonary disease, and emphysema. This drug inhibits the cough reflex by blocking the activity of acetylcholine, a chemical that causes the smooth muscles that surround the airways to constrict. Thus ipratropium causes the airways to dilate, which makes breathing easier.

SIDE EFFECTS

Contact your doctor if your child experiences any side effects that are persistent or troubling, including any that are not listed here.

- *Most common (associated with use of inhalation aerosol and inhalation solution):* blurry vision, cough, dizziness, dry mouth, fluttering heartbeat, gastrointestinal upset, headache, nausea, nervousness, rash
- *Most common (associated with use of nasal spray):* blurry vision, conjunctivitis, cough, dizziness, dry mouth, dry throat, eye irritation, headache, hoarseness, inflamed nasal ulcers, nasal congestion, nasal drip, nasal irritation, nausea, nosebleed, pounding heartbeat, rash, ringing in the ears, sore throat, swollen nose, thirst, upper respiratory infection
- *Less common (associated with use of inhalation aerosol and inhalation solution):* allergic reaction, constipation, drowsiness, eye pain, fatigue, flushing, hives, hoarseness, hair loss, itching, low blood pressure, mouth sores, swollen tongue, lips, and face, tight throat, tingling sensation, tremors, urinary difficulties

HOW TO USE THIS DRUG

Ipratropium is available as an inhalation aerosol, an inhalation solution, and a nasal spray. The dosages given here are ones that are usually recommended for children. However, your doctor will determine the most appropriate dose and schedule for your child.

Aerosol and Solution
- Children younger than 12 years: not recommended
- Children 12 years and older: starting dose is 2 inhalations 4 times daily, not exceeding 12

Nasal Spray—0.03%
- Children younger than 6 years: not recommended
- Children 6 years and older: 2 sprays in each nostril 2 or 3 times daily

Nasal Spray—0.06%
- Children younger than 6 years: not recommended
- Children 6 to 11 years: 2 sprays in each nostril 3 times daily
- Children 12 years and older: 2 sprays in each nostril 3 or 4 times daily

If your child misses a dose, give it as soon as you remember. If it is nearly time for the next dose, skip the missed dose and continue with the regular dosing schedule. Never give a double dose.

TIME UNTIL IT TAKES EFFECT
5 to 15 minutes

POSSIBLE DRUG, FOOD, AND/OR SUPPLEMENT INTERACTIONS
Tell your doctor if your child is taking any prescription or over-the-counter medications or any vitamins, herbs, or other supplements. Possible interactions with ipratropium may include the following:

- Use of anticholinergics (e.g., atropine, scopolamine) may cause an increased anticholinergic effect.
- Your child should not inhale a dose of ipratropium if there is food in his or her mouth.
- Use of fir or pine needle oil should be avoided when using ipratropium.

SYMPTOMS OF OVERDOSE
No specific symptoms of overdose have been reported. However, if you believe an overdose has occurred, seek immediate medical attention and bring the drug container(s) with you.

THINGS TO TELL YOUR DOCTOR
- Tell your doctor if your child has had allergic reactions to any medications in the past, including atropine, as well as aerosol propellants (fluorocarbons, in inhala-

tion form), benzalkonium chloride, edentate disodium
(in nasal form) or any belladonna derivatives, or if he
or she is taking any medications now.

- Let your doctor know if your child has a history of
glaucoma or has urinary retention.
- Consult your doctor if your child is pregnant or becomes pregnant during treatment.

IMPORTANT PRECAUTIONS

- If your child is allergic to peanuts, soy lecithin, or soy-
beans, do not allow him or her to use the inhalational
form of ipratropium.
- Because ipratropium can cause blurry vision, make
sure you know how your child reacts to this drug before he or she participates in potentially dangerous activities, such as riding a bike, driving a car, or operating
machinery.
- Store ipratropium in a tightly closed container and
keep away from excess heat and moisture (e.g., the
bathroom, near a stove or sink). Open bottles of the solution should be refrigerated, but do not allow them to
freeze.

ISOTRETINOIN

BRAND NAME
Accutane
Generic Not Available

ABOUT THIS DRUG
Isotretinoin is an antiacne drug that is related to retinol (vitamin A). It is used mainly to treat severe cystic and nodular
acne and other skin conditions caused by keratin disorders
such as keratinization and mycosis fungoides. Isotretinoin
works by reducing the size of the oil glands (sebaceous
glands), which in turn inhibits production of skin oils
(sebum) and reduces keratinization.

SIDE EFFECTS

Contact your doctor if your child experiences any side effects that are persistent or troubling, including any that are not listed here.

- *Most common:* dry mouth, dry nose, dry itchy skin, extreme increase in triglyceride levels (occurs in 25% of users), inflamed lips, liver inflammation (occurs in 15% of users), peeling of the palms and soles
- *Less common:* conjunctivitis, decreased night vision, fatigue, headache, indigestion, muscle and joint ache, rash, thinning hair
- *Rare:* abnormal acceleration of bone development in children, abnormal blood glucose control, depression, increased pressure in the head, kidney and liver toxicity, inflammatory bowel disorders, myopathy, nausea, opacities in the corner of the eye, pancreatitis, reduced red and white blood cell counts, seizures, tendonitis, vomiting

HOW TO USE THIS DRUG

Isotretinoin is available in capsules. The dosages given here are ones that are usually recommended for children. However, your doctor will determine the most appropriate dose and schedule for your child.

- Children younger than 12 years: not recommended
- Children 12 years and older: 0.23 to 0.45 mg per lb of body weight in 1 or 2 doses daily. Average length of treatment is 20 weeks. If your doctor decides treatment should be repeated, he or she will likely stop treatment for 2 months and then repeat it. Use of this drug needs to be closely monitored by your doctor.

Isotretinoin should always be taken with food. If your child misses a dose, give it as soon as you remember. If it is nearly time for the next dose, skip the missed dose and continue with the regular dosing schedule. Never give a double dose.

If your child has begun menstruation, dosing must be co-ordinated with her menstrual cycle. The first dose should be given on the second or third day of the next normal menstrual period.

TIME UNTIL IT TAKES EFFECT
Usually within several weeks

POSSIBLE DRUG, FOOD, AND/OR SUPPLEMENT INTERACTIONS
Tell your doctor if your child is taking any prescription or over-the-counter medications or any vitamins, herbs, or other supplements. Possible interactions with isotretinoin may include the following:

- Use of tetracycline along with isotretinoin has been associated with brain swelling.
- Consumption of foods or supplements that contain high amounts of vitamin A should be avoided or limited. Consult your physician about foods such as carrots and liver (high in vitamin A) and any supplements your child is taking.
- Use of St. John's wort can result in extreme photosensitivity to the sun.

SYMPTOMS OF OVERDOSE
Symptoms include elevated calcium levels in the blood, gastrointestinal bleeding, hallucinations, lethargy, nausea, psychosis, rise in blood pressure, and vomiting. If overdose occurs, seek immediate medical attention and bring the drug container(s) with you.

THINGS TO TELL YOUR DOCTOR
- Tell your doctor if your child has had allergic reactions to any medications in the past or if he or she is taking any medications now, or is allergic to parabens (preservatives used in this drug).
- Tell your doctor if your child has had an allergic reaction to vitamin A in the past or if he or she regularly

takes a vitamin A supplement or a multivitamin supplement that contains vitamin A.
- Let your doctor know if your child has any of the following medical conditions: diabetes, history of depression, liver or kidney disease, or a cholesterol or triglyceride disorder.

IMPORTANT PRECAUTIONS
- Isotretinoin causes severe birth defects, miscarriage, premature birth, and fetal death. Females capable of getting pregnant must be willing to take two forms of birth control at least 1 month before starting treatment, during treatment, and for at least 1 month after stopping treatment. Your physician will make sure your child is not pregnant before allowing her to start taking isotretinoin and will check each month while she is taking it. Female users of isotretinoin must read and sign a consent form that indicates they understand the dangers of the drug.
- If your child misses her period while using isotretinoin, stop the drug and call your doctor immediately.
- Because isotretinoin increases photosensitivity to sunlight, make sure your child wears sunscreen and/or protective clothing when he or she is outside.
- All patients who use isotretinoin should be observed for symptoms of depression or suicidal thoughts. You should report signs and symptoms such as irritability, anger, loss of pleasure or interest in social or sports activities, changes in weight or appetite, mood disturbances, or aggression to your doctor, as they may be indications of emotional problems. The U.S. Food and Drug Administration (FDA) assesses reports of suicide or suicide attempts associated with the use of isotretinoin.
- Store isotretinoin in a tightly closed container and keep away from excess heat and moisture (e.g., the bathroom, near a stove or sink).

KAOLIN PLUS PECTIN

BRAND NAMES
Kao-Spen, Kapectolin, K-P
Generic Available/Over-the-Counter Available

ABOUT THIS DRUG
Kaolin + pectin is an antidiarrheal medication used to treat diarrhea. This drug combination absorbs fluids in the intestinal tract and removes toxins and disease-causing bacteria from the digestive tract.

SIDE EFFECTS
Contact your doctor if your child experiences any side effects that are persistent or troubling, including any that are not listed here.

- *Most common:* none
- *Less common/rare:* constipation

HOW TO USE THIS DRUG
Kaolin + pectin is available as an oral suspension. The dosages given here are ones that are usually recommended for children. However, your doctor will determine the most appropriate dose and schedule for your child.

- Children 3 to 6 years: 1 to 2 tablespoons (15 to 30 mL) after each loose bowel movement
- Children 7 to 12 years: 2 to 4 tablespoons (30 to 60 mL) after each loose bowel movement
- Children 13 years and older: 4 to 8 tablespoons (60 to 120 mL) after each loose bowel movement

If your child misses a dose, give it as soon as you remember. If it is nearly time for the next dose, skip the missed dose and continue with the regular dosing schedule. Never give a double dose.

TIME UNTIL IT TAKES EFFECT
Unknown

POSSIBLE DRUG, FOOD, AND/OR SUPPLEMENT INTERACTIONS

Tell your doctor if your child is taking any prescription or over-the-counter medications or any vitamins, herbs, or other supplements. Possible interactions with kaolin + pectin may include the following:

- Do not give your child any medications or supplements within 2 to 3 hours of taking kaolin + pectin.
- Talk to your doctor if your child is taking anticholinergics, digitalis drugs, phenothiazines, or any other oral medications.
- Your child should avoid fried or spicy foods, bran, caffeine, fruits, and candy while being treated for diarrhea, as they can make the diarrhea worse.

SYMPTOMS OF OVERDOSE

The main symptom of an overdose is constipation. If overdose occurs, seek immediate medical attention and bring the drug container(s) with you.

THINGS TO TELL YOUR DOCTOR

- Tell your doctor if your child has had allergic reactions to any medications in the past or if he or she is taking any medications, herbal remedies, or supplements now.
- Let your doctor know if your child's diarrhea may be caused by dysentery or parasites, or if your child has allergies, heart disease, or bowel problems.
- If your child has a fever or has mucus or blood in the stool, contact your doctor before you administer this drug. This drug should not be given in these circumstances.

IMPORTANT PRECAUTIONS

- It is important to replace lost fluids while your child has diarrhea and is taking kaolin + pectin. Choose caffeine-free liquids such as water, broth, ginger ale, and herbal tea. Younger children may benefit from an oral electrolyte maintenance solution; check with your doctor.

- Store kaolin + pectin in a tightly closed container and keep away from excess heat and moisture (e.g., the bathroom, near a stove or sink).

KETOCONAZOLE

BRAND NAME
Nizoral
Generic Available

ABOUT THIS DRUG
Ketoconazole is an antifungal medication used to treat serious fungal infections that affect the lungs, skin (e.g., athlete's foot, jock itch), and other parts of the body. The drug works by preventing the fungi from producing the crucial substances they need to grow and reproduce.

SIDE EFFECTS
Contact your doctor if your child experiences any side effects that are persistent or troubling, including any that are not listed here.

- *Most common:* none
- *Less common:* constipation, diarrhea, dizziness, flushed or red skin, headache, nausea, vomiting

HOW TO USE THIS DRUG
Ketoconazole is available in tablets. (There is a topical form that is not recommended for children.) The dosages given here are ones that are usually recommended for children. However, your doctor will determine the most appropriate dose and schedule for your child.

- Children 2 to 12 years: 1.5 to 3.0 mg per lb of body weight once daily
- Children 13 years and older: 200 to 400 mg once daily

Taking ketoconazole with food aids absorption and helps prevent stomach irritation. If your child misses a dose, give it as soon as you remember. However, if it is nearly time for the next dose, skip the missed dose and continue with the regular dosing schedule. Never give a double dose.

TIME UNTIL IT TAKES EFFECT
Unknown

POSSIBLE DRUG, FOOD, AND/OR SUPPLEMENT INTERACTIONS
Tell your doctor if your child is taking any prescription or over-the-counter medications or any vitamins, herbs, or other supplements. Possible interactions with ketoconazole may include the following:

- Antacids (e.g., Maalox, Mylanta), anticholinergics (e.g., atropine, scopolamine), histamine H2 blockers (e.g., cimetidine), omeprazole, and sucralfate should be taken at least 2 hours after taking ketoconazole.
- Astemizole, terfenadine, and cisapride may cause serious side effects that affect the heart and should not be taken with ketoconazole.
- Alcohol and any medications or products that contain it should be avoided.
- Ketoconazole may decrease the effects of amphotericin B, didanosine, and theophylline.
- Ketoconazole may increase the effects of benzodiazepines (e.g., alprazolam, diazepam), carbamazepine, cortisone-like drugs (e.g., cortisone, prednisone), cyclosporine, delavirdine, some calcium channel blockers (e.g., nifedipine), oral antidiabetes drugs (e.g., glyburide), guanidine, ritonavir, tretinoin, warfarin, and trimexate.
- Taking phenytoin along with ketoconazole may change the levels of both drugs.

SYMPTOMS OF OVERDOSE
Symptoms include diarrhea, nausea, and vomiting. If overdose occurs, seek immediate medical attention and bring the drug container(s) with you.

THINGS TO TELL YOUR DOCTOR
- Tell your doctor if your child has had allergic reactions to any medications in the past or if he or she is taking any medications now.
- Let your doctor know if your child has a low amount of stomach acid or has liver or kidney disease.
- Consult your doctor if your child is pregnant or becomes pregnant during treatment.

IMPORTANT PRECAUTIONS
- Ketoconazole may make your child's eyes more sensitive to sunlight. Make sure your child wears sunglasses and avoids exposure to bright light.
- Your child should take ketoconazole for the entire treatment period prescribed by your physician, even if he or she feels better before treatment has been completed. Stopping the drug too soon may allow the infection to return.
- Long-term use of ketoconazole can interfere with your child's steroid hormone functioning and cause menstruation to stop.
- Store ketoconazole in a tightly closed container and keep away from excess heat and moisture (e.g., the bathroom, near a stove or sink).

CLASS: LEUKOTRIENE ANTAGONIST/INHIBITORS

GENERICS
(1) montelukast; (2) zafirlukast

BRAND NAMES
(1) Singulair; (2) Accolate
Generics Not Available

ABOUT THESE DRUGS
Leukotriene antagonist/inhibitors are prescribed to help prevent asthma attacks. They are not effective in the treatment

of sudden asthma episodes. Montelukast is also prescribed to prevent exercise-induced asthma. Both of the leukotrienes are also used to treat symptoms of seasonal allergies.

The leukotriene antagonist/inhibitors help prevent the body's allergic response by blocking leukotrienes from binding to receptors.

SIDE EFFECTS
Contact your doctor if your child experiences any side effects that are persistent or troubling, including any that are not listed here.

Montelukast
- *Most common:* headache
- *Less common:* abdominal pain, cough, dental pain, dizziness, fatigue, fever, heartburn, rash, stuffy nose, weakness

Zafirlukast
- *Most common:* dizziness, headache
- *Less common/rare:* abdominal pain, back pain, diarrhea, infections, liver inflammation, muscle aches, overall pain, stomach upset, weakness, vomiting

HOW TO USE THESE DRUGS
Leukotriene antagonist/inhibitors are available in tablets and granules. The dosages given here are ones that are usually recommended for children. However, your doctor will determine the most appropriate dose and schedule for your child.

Montelukast
- Children 6 to 23 months: for perennial allergy—one 4-mg packet oral granules
- Children 12 to 23 months: for asthma—one 4-mg packet oral granules
- Children 2 to 5 years: for asthma or allergic rhinitis—one 4-mg tablet or one 4-mg packet oral granules
- Children 6 to 14 years: for asthma or allergic rhinitis—one 5-mg tablet daily

- Children 15 years and older: for asthma or allergic rhinitis—one 10-mg tablet daily

Zafirlukast
- Children 7 to 11 years: 10 mg twice daily
- Children 12 years and older: 20 mg twice daily

Montelukast should be taken in the morning. The oral granules can be dissolved in baby formula or breast milk only, no other liquid. They can, however, be mixed into applesauce, carrots, rice, or ice cream. Zafirlukast should be taken on an empty stomach, 1 hour before or 2 hours after meals.

These drugs are used to prevent asthma attacks, so they need to be taken regularly. If your child misses a dose, give it as soon as you remember. However, if it is nearly time for the next dose, skip the missed dose. Continue with the regular dosing schedule. Never give a double dose.

TIME UNTIL THEY TAKE EFFECT
Response by montelukast is variable; zafirlukast takes effect within 3 to 14 days

POSSIBLE DRUG, FOOD, AND/OR SUPPLEMENT INTERACTIONS
Tell your doctor if your child is taking any prescription or over-the-counter medications or any vitamins, herbs, or other supplements. Possible interactions with leukotriene antagonist/inhibitors may include the following:

- Phenobarbital or rifampin may reduce montelukast blood levels.
- Aspirin significantly increases zafirlukast blood levels.
- Erythromycin, terfenadine, and theophylline reduce zafirlukast blood levels.
- Zafirlukast may increase the thinning of the blood if taken with warfarin.
- Zafirlukast should be taken with caution with the following drugs: alprazolam, amitriptyline, amlodipine,

astemizole, carbamazepine, cisapride, cyclosporine, diclofenac, diltiazem, erythromycin, felodipine, ibuprofen, imipramine, isradipine, lovastatin, nicardipine, phenytoin, quinidine, simvastatin, tolbutamide, trizolam, and verapamil.

- Herbal remedies for asthma, such as ephedra, should be avoided.

SYMPTOMS OF OVERDOSE

No symptoms of overdose have been reported. If you believe an overdose has occurred, seek immediate medical attention and bring the drug container(s) with you.

THINGS TO TELL YOUR DOCTOR

- Tell your doctor if your child has had allergic reactions to any medications in the past or if he or she is taking any medications now.
- Let your doctor know if your child has liver or kidney disease or elevated liver enzymes.
- Contact your physician if your child's need for other asthma drugs increases while he or she is taking a leukotriene antagonist/inhibitor.
- Consult your doctor if your child is pregnant or becomes pregnant during treatment.

IMPORTANT PRECAUTIONS

- Because these drugs can cause dizziness, make sure you know how your child reacts to them before you allow him or her to participate in potentially dangerous activities, such as riding a bike, driving a car, or operating machinery.
- Store leukotriene antagonist/inhibitors in a tightly closed container and keep at room temperature away from excess heat and moisture (e.g., the bathroom, near a stove or sink).
- Chewable montelukast contains aspartame and 0.842 mg phenylalanine per tablet, which should be avoided by children who have phenylketonuria.

LEVOTHYROXINE—
see *Thyroid Hormone Replacements*

LINDANE

BRAND NAMES
G-well, Kwell, Scabene
Generic Available

ABOUT THIS DRUG
Lindane is a topical medication used to treat scabies and lice infestations that have not responded to other treatments. The medication is absorbed into the bodies of these insects and affects the nervous system, resulting in their deaths.

SIDE EFFECTS
Contact your doctor if your child experiences any side effects that are persistent or troubling, including any that are not listed here.

- *Most common:* none
- *Less common/rare:* rash, redness, or skin irritation

HOW TO USE THIS DRUG
Lindane is available as a lotion, cream, and shampoo. The lotion and cream are used to treat scabies; the shampoo is for lice. The instructions given here are for children of all ages. However, it should be used very cautiously on children who weigh less than 110 pounds. Talk to your doctor about the best way to treat your child, especially if you are treating a child who weighs less than 110 pounds.

- Cream and lotion: Your child's skin should be washed, rinsed, and dried before you apply the medication. Apply the cream or lotion to the entire body from the neck to the soles of the feet and rub it in well. Leave it on for no more than 8 hours, then wash it off thoroughly. Do not allow lindane to get near the mouth or eyes.

- Shampoo: After the lindane has been washed off your child's body, apply the shampoo to the hair and scalp. Allow the medication to remain on the hair for 4 minutes, then lather. Rinse thoroughly and dry with a clean towel. Use a fine-tooth comb to remove nits.

This treatment may be repeated after 7 days if necessary, but only after consultation with your doctor.

TIME UNTIL IT TAKES EFFECT
Unknown

POSSIBLE DRUG, FOOD, AND/OR SUPPLEMENT INTERACTIONS
Tell your doctor if your child is taking any prescription or over-the-counter medications or any vitamins, herbs, or other supplements. Possible drug interactions include the following:

- Some medications may increase the chance of experiencing a seizure, including antidepressants, chlorpromazine or other antipsychotics, chloroquine, ciprofloxacin, corticosteroids, methocarbamol, penicillins, promethazine, theophylline.

SYMPTOMS OF OVERDOSE
Symptoms include dizziness, seizures, and vomiting. If swallowed, lindane can be fatal. If overdose occurs, seek immediate medical attention and bring the drug container(s) with you.

THINGS TO TELL YOUR DOCTOR
- Tell your doctor if your child has had allergic reactions to any medications in the past or if he or she is taking any medications now.
- Let your doctor know if your child has a rash or skin disorder, diabetes, liver disease, or a seizure disorder.
- Consult your doctor if your child is pregnant or becomes pregnant during treatment.

IMPORTANT PRECAUTIONS

- Lindane is a toxic medication that should be used only if other medications designed to eliminate scabies and lice have not successfully eliminated them.
- It is very important to use lindane as directed. Seizures and death have occurred in patients who have used too much of the medication or who have used it a second time.
- Store lindane in a tightly closed container and keep at room temperature away from excess heat and moisture (e.g., the bathroom, near a stove or sink).

LIOTHYRONINE—
see *Thyroid Hormone Replacements*

LIOTRIX—
see *Thyroid Hormone Replacements*

LITHIUM

BRAND NAMES
Cibalith-S, Eskalith, Lithane, Lithonate, Lithotabs
Generic Available

ABOUT THIS DRUG
Lithium is an antimanic medication used to treat the manic phase of bipolar disorder and to enhance the benefits of other antidepressant medications. The drug interferes with the synthesis and reuptake of chemicals (neurotransmitters) in the brain that allow nerves to communicate with each other. It especially affects the neurotransmitters serotonin and tryptophan, which are associated with mood.

SIDE EFFECTS
Contact your doctor if your child experiences any side effects that are persistent or troubling, including any that are not listed here.

- *Most common:* diarrhea, fatigue, hand tremors, increased thirst, increased urination, loss of appetite, metallic taste in mouth, unexpected weight gain
- *Less common/rare:* acne, hair loss, rash

HOW TO USE THIS DRUG

Lithium is available as capsules, tablets, extended-release tablets, and syrup. Your doctor will determine the most appropriate dose and schedule for your child. The dose is determined by measuring the blood level of the drug 12 hours after it is administered.

Short-Acting Lithium
- Children younger than 12 years: 6.8 to 9 mg per lb of body weight per day given in 2 or 3 smaller doses
- Children 12 years and older: 300 to 600 mg 3 times per day to start

Longer-Acting Lithium
- Children younger than 12 years: to be determined by your doctor
- Children 12 years and older: 300 to 600 mg 3 times per day or 450 to 900 mg twice a day

Your child should take lithium with food to reduce stomach irritation. He or she should also drink 8 to 10 glasses of water or other caffeine-free beverages daily. If your child misses a dose, give it as soon as you remember. If it is nearly time for the next dose, skip the missed dose and continue with the regular dosing schedule. Never give a double dose.

TIME UNTIL IT TAKES EFFECT

When treating mania, 1 to 2 weeks; when enhancing the effects of antidepressants, within a few days

POSSIBLE DRUG, FOOD, AND/OR SUPPLEMENT INTERACTIONS

Tell your doctor if your child is taking any prescription or over-the-counter medications or any vitamins, herbs, or

other supplements. Possible interactions with lithium may include the following:

- Taking lithium along with other antipsychotic drugs may increase the risk of side effects of all drugs used.
- In rare cases, lithium taken along with haloperidol has caused nervous system damage, including irreversible tardive dyskinesia and severe rigidity.
- Diuretics can cause serious side effects.
- Over-the-counter medications that contain iodides should be avoided because they can increase lithium's antithyroid effect.
- Lithium may increase absorption of warfarin, which can increase the risk of bleeding.
- Lithium may increase blood levels of insulin. If your child is a diabetic, his or her insulin therapy may need to be adjusted.
- Lithium may increase the effects of tricyclic antidepressants.
- Carbamazepine, methyldopa, nonsteroidal anti-inflammatory drugs (NSAIDs; e.g., aspirin, ibuprofen), loop and thiazide diuretics, and selective serotonin re-uptake inhibitors (e.g., fluoxetine) may increase the absorption of lithium.
- Acetazolamide, mannitol, sodium bicarbonate, theophylline drugs, and verapamil may reduce the absorption of lithium.
- Avoid herbs that have a sedative effect, such as catnip, goldenseal, gotu kola, hops, kava, lemon balm, skullcap, St. John's wort, and valerian.

SYMPTOMS OF OVERDOSE
Symptoms include confusion, disorientation, drowsiness, loss of consciousness, muscle weakness, slurred speech, tremor, twitching, and vomiting. If overdose occurs, seek immediate medical attention and bring the drug container(s) with you.

THINGS TO TELL YOUR DOCTOR

- Tell your doctor if your child has had allergic reactions to any medications in the past or if he or she is taking any medications now.
- Let your doctor know if your child has any of the following medical conditions: heart or blood vessel disease, leukemia, kidney disease, epilepsy, urination difficulties, psoriasis, history of brain disease, thyroid disease, diabetes, or any infection.
- Before your child undergoes any type of surgery, including dental surgery, tell the physician or dentist that your child is taking lithium.
- Contact your physician if your child develops diarrhea, vomiting, or sweating, as he or she may need to stop taking lithium until the condition clears.
- Consult your doctor if your child is pregnant or becomes pregnant during treatment. Lithium can have negative effects on the fetus, especially if taken during the first trimester.

IMPORTANT PRECAUTIONS

- Consult with your physician before you allow your child to stop taking this medication.
- Your child's blood levels of lithium should be monitored regularly by your physician to avoid toxicity.
- Monitor your child's diet and exercise while he or she is taking lithium. Caffeinated beverages and excessive salt should be avoided, and no drastic change in the amount of calories or types of foods should be made without consulting your physician. Be cautious of rigorous exercise or in hot weather that results in excessive sweating. Loss of salt and drinking excessive amounts of water can increase the risk of side effects.
- Store lithium in a tightly closed container and keep away from excess heat and moisture (e.g., the bathroom, near a stove or sink).

LODOXAMIDE

BRAND NAME
Alomide
Generic Not Available

ABOUT THIS DRUG
Lodoxamide is an antiallergy medication used to treat certain eye symptoms associated with allergy, such as watering, itching, swelling, and redness. It should not be used for bacterial, viral, or fungal infections of the eye. It works by inhibiting processes in the body that cause allergic symptoms.

SIDE EFFECTS
Contact your doctor if your child experiences any side effects that are persistent or troubling, including any that are not listed here.

- *Most common:* none
- *Less common/rare:* blurry vision, dry eyes, headache, increased eye tearing, sneezing, temporary stinging or burning in the eyes

HOW TO USE THIS DRUG
Lodoxamide is available in eye drops. The dosages given here are ones that are usually recommended for children. However, your doctor will determine the most appropriate dose and schedule for your child.

- Children younger than 2 years: not recommended
- Children 2 years and older: one drop in the affected eye 4 times a day for up to 3 months, as determined by your doctor

If your child misses a dose, give it as soon as you remember. If it is nearly time for the next dose, skip the missed dose and continue with the regular dosing schedule. Never give a double dose.

TIME UNTIL IT TAKES EFFECT
Unknown

POSSIBLE DRUG, FOOD, AND/OR SUPPLEMENT INTERACTIONS
Tell your doctor if your child is taking any prescription or over-the-counter medications or any vitamins, herbs, or other supplements. No drug, food, or supplement interactions with lodoxamide have been noted. However, if your child is using other eye drops, talk to your physician before giving lodoxamide to your child.

SYMPTOMS OF OVERDOSE
An overdose of this medication is highly unlikely to occur. If your child accidentally ingests the drops, symptoms may include diarrhea, dizziness, fatigue, lightheadedness, and nausea. Give your child plenty of water and contact a poison control center or other emergency medical facility for instructions.

THINGS TO TELL YOUR DOCTOR
- Tell your doctor if your child has had allergic reactions to any medications in the past or if he or she is taking any medications now.
- Consult your doctor if your child is pregnant or becomes pregnant during treatment.

IMPORTANT PRECAUTIONS
- Make sure you know how to properly administer this medication. The tip of the applicator is sterile; therefore, do not allow it to touch any surface, including your child's eye, or it will become contaminated. Keep the bottle tightly capped when not in use.
- If your child wears contact lenses, he or she should not wear them during the treatment period with lodoxamide, as this drug contains benzalkonium chloride, a preservative that can affect the lenses.
- Store lodoxamide in a tightly closed container and keep at room temperature away from excess heat and moisture (e.g., the bathroom, near a stove or sink).

LOPERAMIDE

BRAND NAMES
Imodium, Imodium A-D, Imodium Anti-Diarrheal Caplets,
Maalox Anti-Diarrheal Caplets, Pepto Diarrhea Control
Generic Available/Over-the-Counter Available

ABOUT THIS DRUG
Loperamide is an antidiarrheal medication used to treat diarrhea. It works by slowing the activity of the intestinal
tract.

SIDE EFFECTS
Contact your doctor if your child experiences any side effects that are persistent or troubling, including any that are
not listed here.

- *Most common:* none
- *Less common/rare:* dizziness, drowsiness, dry mouth,
  fatigue, stomach pain

HOW TO USE THIS DRUG
Loperamide is available as capsules, tablets, and oral solution. The dosages given here are ones that are usually recommended for children. However, your doctor will
determine the most appropriate dose and schedule for your
child.

- Children younger than 6 years: only if recommended
  by your doctor
- Children 6 to 8 years: capsules—2 mg twice daily; oral
  solution or tablets—2 mg after the first loose bowel
  movement, then 1 mg after each subsequent loose
  bowel movement, not exceeding 4 mg every 24 hours
- Children 9 to 12 years: capsules—2 mg 3 times daily;
  oral solution or tablets—2 mg after the first loose
  bowel movement, then 1 mg after each subsequent
  loose bowel movement, not exceeding 6 mg every 24
  hours

- Children 13 years and older: capsules—4 mg after the first loose bowel movement, then 2 mg after each subsequent loose bowel movement, not exceeding 16 mg every 24 hours; oral solution and tablets—4 mg after the first loose bowel movement, then 2 mg after each subsequent loose bowel movement, not exceeding 8 mg every 24 hours

TIME UNTIL IT TAKES EFFECT
Unknown

POSSIBLE DRUG, FOOD, AND/OR SUPPLEMENT INTERACTIONS
Tell your doctor if your child is taking any prescription or over-the-counter medications or any vitamins, herbs, or other supplements. Possible interactions with loperamide may include the following:

- Talk to your doctor if your child is taking antibiotics such as cephalosporin, erythromycin, or tetracycline.
- Cholestyramine reduces the effect of loperamide. At least 2 hours should separate the doses of these two drugs.
- Bethanechol, cisapride, metoclopramide, and erythromycin counteract the effects of loperamide.

SYMPTOMS OF OVERDOSE
Symptoms include constipation, depressed central nervous system, and gastrointestinal irritation. If overdose occurs, seek immediate medical attention and bring the drug container(s) with you.

THINGS TO TELL YOUR DOCTOR
- Tell your doctor if your child has had allergic reactions to any medications in the past or if he or she is taking any medications, especially antibiotics, or any herbal remedies or supplements now.
- Let your doctor know if your child has colitis or liver disease.

- If your child does not improve after taking loperamide for 2 days, and/or if he or she develops black or bloody stool, mucus in the stool, fever, or severe abdominal pain or swelling, call your doctor. Do not give loperamide to your child if he or she has a fever or there is blood or mucus in the stool.

IMPORTANT PRECAUTIONS
- Store loperamide in a tightly closed container and keep away from excess heat and moisture (e.g., the bathroom, near a stove or sink).

LORACARBEF

BRAND NAME
Lorabid
Generic Not Available

ABOUT THIS DRUG
Loracarbef is an antibiotic (similar to cephalosporin antibiotics) that is used to treat bacterial infections, including bronchitis, pneumonia, strep throat, and urinary tract infections. It kills the disease-causing bacteria by causing their cell walls to break down.

SIDE EFFECTS
Contact your doctor if your child experiences any side effects that are persistent or troubling, including any that are not listed here.

- *Most common:* mild diarrhea, loss of appetite, nausea, stomach pain, vomiting
- *Less common/rare:* dizziness, drowsiness, headache, insomnia, nervousness, vaginal discharge or itching

HOW TO USE THIS DRUG
Loracarbef is available in capsules and as an oral suspension. The dosages given here are ones that are usually rec-

ommended for children. However, your doctor will determine the most appropriate dose and schedule for your child.

All Uses
- Children 6 months to 12 years: as determined by your doctor

Urinary Tract Infections
- Children 13 years and older: 200 to 400 mg once or twice daily for 7 to 14 days

Bronchitis
- Children 13 years and older: 200 to 400 mg twice daily for 7 days

Pneumonia
- Children 13 years and older: 400 mg twice daily for 14 days

Skin and Soft Tissue Infections
- Children 13 years and older: 200 mg twice daily for 7 days

Strep Throat
- Children 13 years and older: 200 mg twice daily for 10 days

Loracarbef should be taken on an empty stomach at least 1 hour before or 2 hours after meals. If loracarbef causes stomach irritation, it can be taken with food. Make sure your child drinks plenty of fluids while taking this medication.

If your child misses a dose, give it as soon as you remember. However, if it is nearly time for the next dose, skip the missed dose and continue with the regular dosing schedule. Never give a double dose.

TIME UNTIL IT TAKES EFFECT
Unknown

POSSIBLE DRUG, FOOD, AND/OR SUPPLEMENT INTERACTIONS

Tell your doctor if your child is taking any prescription or over-the-counter medications or any vitamins, herbs, or other supplements. Possible interactions with loracarbef may include the following:

- Loracarbef may cause a depletion of vitamins B12 and K, biotin, riboflavin, and folic acid, as well as probiotic organisms
- Loracarbef may interact with alpha-lipoic acid, green tea, zinc, biotin, vitamin K, magnesium, and bromelain.
- Iron supplements may make loracarbef less effective. Give iron supplements at least 1 hour before or 2 hours after a loracarbef dose.

SYMPTOMS OF OVERDOSE

Symptoms include an unusual drop in blood pressure (causing dizziness, fainting, or lightheadedness) and an unusually rapid or slow heartbeat. If overdose occurs, seek immediate medical attention and bring the drug container(s) with you.

THINGS TO TELL YOUR DOCTOR

- Tell your doctor if your child has had allergic reactions to any medications in the past, including cephalosporin antibiotics, or if he or she is taking any medications now.
- Let your doctor know if your child has liver or kidney disease.
- Consult your doctor if your child is pregnant or becomes pregnant during treatment.

IMPORTANT PRECAUTIONS

- Your child should take the entire course of treatment as prescribed by your physician, even if he or she feels better before the medication is gone, as the infection may return if treatment is stopped too soon.
- Store loracarbef capsules in a tightly closed container

and keep away from excess heat and moisture (e.g., the bathroom, near a stove or sink). The oral suspension should be refrigerated, but do not allow it to freeze.

LORATADINE

BRAND NAMES
Alavert (OTC), Claritin, Claritin RediTabs
Generic Available/Over-the-Counter Available

ABOUT THIS DRUG
Loratadine is a long-acting antihistamine that is used to prevent or relieve symptoms of allergies and hay fever, such as sneezing, runny nose, itchy skin, and watery eyes. It blocks the effects of histamine, a naturally occurring substance that causes these and other allergy symptoms. A loratadine + pseudoephedrine combination is also available (see *Antihistamine-Decongestant-(Antitussive) Combination*).

SIDE EFFECTS
Contact your doctor if your child experiences any side effects that are persistent or troubling, including any that are not listed here.

- *Most common:* none
- *Less common/rare:* abdominal discomfort, dizziness, drowsiness, dry mouth, headache, itchy skin, nausea, nervousness

Because loratadine does not enter the brain through the bloodstream, it is much less likely to cause drowsiness like most other antihistamines.

HOW TO USE THIS DRUG
Loratadine is available in tablets, rapidly disintegrating tablets, and syrup. The dosages given here are ones that are usually recommended for children. However, your doctor will determine the most appropriate dose and schedule for your child.

- Children 2 to 9 years: 5 mg once daily
- Children 10 years and older: 10 mg once daily

It is best to take loratadine with food, as this may increase absorption of the drug by up to 40 percent. The disintegrating tablets can be taken with or without water. The regular tablets should be taken with 8 ounces of water.

If your child misses a dose, give it as soon as you remember. If it is nearly time for the next dose, skip the missed dose and continue with the regular dosing schedule. Never give a double dose.

TIME UNTIL IT TAKES EFFECT
Within 1 hour

POSSIBLE DRUG, FOOD, AND/OR SUPPLEMENT INTERACTIONS
Tell your doctor if your child is taking any prescription or over-the-counter medications or any vitamins, herbs, or other supplements. No drug, food, or supplement interactions have been reported. However, consult your doctor if your child is also taking clarithromycin, erythromycin, itraconazole, or ketoconazole.

SYMPTOMS OF OVERDOSE
Symptoms include drowsiness, headache, irregular heartbeat, nausea, and vomiting. If overdose occurs, seek immediate medical attention and bring the drug container(s) with you.

THINGS TO TELL YOUR DOCTOR
- Tell your doctor if your child has had allergic reactions to any medications in the past or if he or she is taking any medications now.
- Let your doctor know if your child has kidney or liver disease.
- The Alavert brand of loratadine disintegrating tablets contains phenylalanine. If your child has phenylketonuria, talk to your doctor before administering this product.

- Consult your doctor if your child is pregnant or becomes pregnant during treatment.

IMPORTANT PRECAUTIONS
- Store loratadine in a tightly closed container and keep away from excess heat and moisture (e.g., the bathroom, near a stove or sink). The syrup can be refrigerated, but do not allow it to freeze.

LORAZEPAM

BRAND NAMES
Ativan, Alzapam
Generic Available

ABOUT THIS DRUG
Lorazepam is a benzodiazepine tranquilizer and antianxiety drug used to treat anxiety and insomnia. It is also used before surgery to sedate patients before they are given anesthesia. This drug works by enhancing the effects of a chemical in the brain called gamma-aminobutyric acid (GABA), which inhibits the transmission of nerve signals and thus reduces nervous excitation.

SIDE EFFECTS
Contact your doctor if your child experiences any side effects that are persistent or troubling, including any that are not listed here.

- *Most common:* dizziness, drowsiness, lightheadedness, loss of coordination, sedation, slurred speech, unsteady gait
- *Less common/rare:* agitation, loss of appetite, depression, eye problems, nausea, sleep disturbances, stomach and intestinal disorders

HOW TO USE THIS DRUG
Lorazepam is available as tablets and oral solution and via injection (hospital only; injection dosage information is not

provided here). The dosages given here are ones that are usually recommended for children. However, your doctor will determine the most appropriate dose and schedule for your child.

- Children younger than 12 years: to be determined by your doctor
- Children 12 years and older (for anxiety): 1 to 2 mg every 8 to 12 hours, up to 6 mg daily
- Children 12 years and older (for insomnia): 1 to 2 mg taken at bedtime

Lorazepam can be taken with food to help prevent stomach irritation. If your child misses a dose, give it as soon as you remember. However, if it is nearly time for the next dose, skip the missed dose and continue with the regular dosing schedule. Never give a double dose.

TIME UNTIL IT TAKES EFFECT
Oral dose, 30 minutes to 2 hours

POSSIBLE DRUG, FOOD, AND/OR SUPPLEMENT INTERACTIONS
Tell your doctor if your child is taking any prescription or over-the-counter medications or any vitamins, herbs, or other supplements. Possible interactions with lorazepam may include the following:

- Use of central nervous system depressants can cause respiratory depression.
- The combination of lorazepam and clozapine may increase sedation and cause loss of muscle coordination.
- Birth control pills, theophylline, caffeine, and other stimulants can reduce the effects of lorazepam.
- Heparin, macrolide antibiotics, probenecid, quetiapine, and valproic acid may increase the effects of lorazepam.
- Lithium may cause your child's body temperature to drop.

- The combination of lorazepam and phenytoin may cause altered levels of both drugs in the body.
- Alcohol should be avoided, as the combination impairs mental function and coordination.
- Grapefruit juice should be avoided, as the juice slows the body's breakdown of the drug and can lead to dangerous concentrations in the blood.
- Herbs that have a sedative effect, including hops, kava, passionflower, and valerian, should be avoided, as they can increase the sedative effect.
- Caffeinated beverages should be avoided.

SYMPTOMS OF OVERDOSE
Symptoms include confusion, extreme drowsiness, loss of consciousness, poor coordination, slow reflexes, slowed breathing, slurred speech, and tremor. If overdose occurs, seek immediate medical attention and bring the drug container(s) with you.

THINGS TO TELL YOUR DOCTOR
- Tell your doctor if your child has had allergic reactions to any medications in the past or if he or she is taking any medications now.
- Let your doctor know if your child has any of the following medical conditions: asthma, depression or psychosis, epilepsy, emphysema, liver or kidney disease, low white blood cell count, narrow-angle glaucoma, or very low blood pressure.
- Consult your doctor if your child is pregnant or becomes pregnant during treatment. Lorazepam is associated with an increased risk of birth defects.

IMPORTANT PRECAUTIONS
- Long-term use (longer than 2 months) can lead to physical and/or psychological addiction.
- Do not stop treatment of lorazepam abruptly, as this can cause withdrawal symptoms in your child, including seizures, nervousness, irritability, diarrhea, abdominal cramps, and impaired memory. Talk to your doctor about gradually reducing your child's dose.

- Store lorazepam in a tightly closed container and keep at room temperature away from excess heat and moisture (e.g., the bathroom, near a stove or sink).

MEBENDAZOLE

BRAND NAME
Vermox
Generic Available

ABOUT THIS DRUG
Mebendazole is an anthelmintic medication used to treat intestinal infections of roundworm, hookworm, whipworm, and pinworm. It kills both immature and adult worms, but it does not kill the eggs. Therefore, two treatments are needed, about 2 weeks apart, with the second treatment needed to kill any worms that have hatched since the first treatment. It works by preventing the worms from absorbing glucose, which they need to survive.

SIDE EFFECTS
Contact your doctor if your child experiences any side effects that are persistent or troubling, including any that are not listed here.

- *Most common:* none
- *Less common/rare:* diarrhea, nausea, stomach pain, vomiting

HOW TO USE THIS DRUG
Mebendazole is available in chewable tablets. The dosages given here are ones that are usually recommended for children. However, your doctor will determine the most appropriate dose and schedule for your child.

For Roundworms, Whipworms, and Hookworms
- Children younger than 2 years: not recommended
- Children 2 years and older: 100 mg twice daily for 3 days; which may need to be repeated in 2 to 3 weeks

For Pinworms
- Children younger than 2 years: not recommended
- Children 2 years and older: 100 mg for 1 day, which may need to be repeated in 2 to 3 weeks

For Multiple Worm Infections
- Children younger than 2 years: not recommended
- Children 2 years and older: 100 mg 2 times daily for 3 days, which may need to be repeated in 2 to 3 weeks.

Mebendazole should be taken with a high-fat food (e.g., ice cream, peanut butter) to aid absorption. If your child misses a dose, give it as soon as you remember. If it is nearly time for the next dose, skip the missed dose and continue with the regular dosing schedule. Never give a double dose.

TIME UNTIL IT TAKES EFFECT
Unknown

POSSIBLE DRUG, FOOD, AND/OR SUPPLEMENT INTERACTIONS
Tell your doctor if your child is taking any prescription or over-the-counter medications or any vitamins, herbs, or other supplements. Possible interactions with mebendazole may include the following:

- Carbamazepine, ethotoin, mephenytoin, and phenytoin may decrease the effects of mebendazole.

SYMPTOMS OF OVERDOSE
Symptoms include gastrointestinal upset that lasts several hours, respiratory distress, or seizures. If overdose occurs, seek immediate medical attention and bring the drug container(s) with you.

THINGS TO TELL YOUR DOCTOR
- Tell your doctor if your child has had allergic reactions to any medications in the past or if he or she is taking any medications now.

- Let your doctor know if your child has liver disease, ulcerative colitis, or Crohn's disease.
- Consult your doctor if your child is pregnant or becomes pregnant during treatment. Mebendazole should not be used during pregnancy.

IMPORTANT PRECAUTIONS

- Mebendazole should be given for the entire treatment course prescribed by your doctor, even if your child feels better before the end of the scheduled therapy.
- If your child has whipworm or hookworm, anemia may also be present. Your doctor may want to prescribe iron supplements for your child, which should be taken as directed by your doctor.
- It may be necessary to treat family members and other individuals who are in close contact with an infected child, especially if the child has pinworm. Talk to your doctor.
- Store mebendazole in a tightly closed container and keep away from excess heat and moisture (e.g., the bathroom, near a stove or sink).

MECLIZINE

BRAND NAMES
Antivert, Antivert/25, Antivert/50, Bonine, Dramamine II, D-Vert 15, D-Vert 30, Meni-D
Generic Available/Over-the-Counter Available

ABOUT THIS DRUG
Meclizine is an antinausea, antivertigo medication that is used to treat and prevent nausea, vomiting, and dizziness that is caused by motion sickness and vertigo. The drug acts on the area of the brain that controls nausea, vomiting, and dizziness.

SIDE EFFECTS
Contact your doctor if your child experiences any side effects that are persistent or troubling, including any that are not listed here.

- *Most common:* drowsiness
- *Less common/rare:* blurry or double vision; constipation; diarrhea; dizziness; dry mouth, nose, and throat; fast heartbeat; headache; loss of appetite; nervousness; painful urination; restlessness; rash; upset stomach

HOW TO USE THIS DRUG

Meclizine is available in tablets, chewable tablets, and capsules. The dosages given here are ones that are usually recommended for children. However, your doctor will determine the most appropriate dose and schedule for your child.

- Children younger than 12 years: not recommended
- Children 12 years and older: to prevent and treat motion sickness—25 to 50 mg 1 hour before travel (dose may be repeated every 24 hours); to treat and prevent vertigo—25 to 100 mg daily as needed in divided doses.

This drug should be taken on an as-needed basis, based on the dosage guidelines given above or by your physician. It can be taken with food if it causes stomach upset.

TIME UNTIL IT TAKES EFFECT
Within 1 hour

POSSIBLE DRUG, FOOD, AND/OR SUPPLEMENT INTERACTIONS
Tell your doctor if your child is taking any prescription or over-the-counter medications or any vitamins, herbs, or other supplements. Possible interactions with meclizine may include the following:

- Avoid alcohol while taking meclizine.
- Barbiturates, digoxin, muscle relaxants, certain antibiotics given via injection, antianxiety medication, antidepressants, tranquilizers, sleep medications, and pain medications should be used with caution when taking meclizine. Talk to your doctor about multiple drug use.

SYMPTOMS OF OVERDOSE

Symptoms may include drowsiness, extreme excitability, hallucinations, and seizures. If you believe an overdose has occurred, seek immediate medical attention and bring the drug container(s) with you.

THINGS TO TELL YOUR DOCTOR

- Tell your doctor if your child has had allergic reactions to any medications in the past or if he or she is taking any medications now.
- Let your doctor know if your child has any of the following medical conditions: asthma, bronchitis, emphysema, glaucoma, heart failure, intestinal blockage, lung infection, or urinary tract blockage.
- Consult your doctor if your child is pregnant or becomes pregnant during treatment.

IMPORTANT PRECAUTIONS

- Because meclizine can cause drowsiness, make sure you know how your child reacts to it before you allow him or her to participate in potentially dangerous activities, such as riding a bike, driving a car, or operating machinery.
- If your child wears contact lenses, he or she may feel some discomfort while using meclizine. Lubricating eye drops may be needed.
- Store meclizine in a tightly closed container and keep away from excess heat and moisture (e.g., the bathroom, near a stove or sink).

MEPERIDINE

BRAND NAME
Demerol
Generic Available

ABOUT THIS DRUG

Meperidine is an opioid (narcotic) used to treat moderate to severe pain. It works by affecting specific areas of the brain and spinal cord that are involved in processing pain signals from the nerves throughout the body.

SIDE EFFECTS
Contact your doctor if your child experiences any side effects that are persistent or troubling, including any that are not listed here.

- *Most common:* constipation, dizziness or lightheadedness, itching, mild drowsiness, nausea, or vomiting
- *Less common/rare:* false sense of well-being, mood swings, redness or flushing of the face

HOW TO USE THIS DRUG
Meperidine is available in tablets and syrup and via injection. (Injection information is not provided here.) The dosages given here are ones that are usually recommended for children. However, your doctor will determine the most appropriate dose and schedule for your child.

- Children 1 year and older: 0.5 to 0.8 mg per lb of body weight every 3 to 4 hours

Meperidine tablets can be crushed and taken with food to help prevent stomach irritation. The syrup can be mixed with 4 ounces of water to reduce its numbing effect on the mouth and throat.

If your child misses a dose, give it as soon as you remember. However, if it is nearly time for the next dose, skip the missed dose and continue with the regular dosing schedule. Never give a double dose.

TIME UNTIL IT TAKES EFFECT
15 minutes

POSSIBLE DRUG, FOOD, AND/OR SUPPLEMENT INTERACTIONS
Tell your doctor if your child is taking any prescription or over-the-counter medications or any vitamins, herbs, or

other supplements. Possible interactions with meperidine may include the following:

- Monoamine oxidase (MAO) inhibitors should not be taken at the same time or within 14 days of taking meperidine.
- Tricyclic antidepressants increase the risk of respiratory depression.
- Cimetidine, famotidine, ranitidine, and omeprazole increase the blood levels of meperidine and thus its effects.
- Tramadol increases the risk of seizure.
- Use of other central nervous system depressants along with meperidine can cause excessive drowsiness.
- Atropine-like drugs raise the risk of urinary retention and impaired intestinal function.
- Naltrexone reduces the effects of meperidine.
- Alcohol should be avoided when using meperidine.
- Phenothiazines, phenytoin, sibutramine, and ritonavir should be used with caution with meperidine.
- Herbs such as hops, kava, passionflower, and valerian can increase sedative effects. Ginseng should be avoided completely.

SYMPTOMS OF OVERDOSE

Symptoms include breathing problems, coma, confusion, drowsiness, low blood pressure, sluggishness, stupor, and tremors. If overdose occurs, seek immediate medical attention and bring the drug container(s) with you.

THINGS TO TELL YOUR DOCTOR

- Tell your doctor if your child has had allergic reactions to any medications in the past or if he or she is taking any medications now.
- Let your doctor know if your child has any of the following medical conditions: abnormal heart rhythm, asthma, chronic bronchitis, chronic constipation, emphysema, epilepsy, glaucoma, head injury, kidney disease, lung disease, respiratory depression, or urinary problems.

- If your child is scheduled to undergo surgery or a dental procedure, tell your doctor or dentist that your child is taking meperidine.
- Consult your doctor if your child is pregnant or becomes pregnant during treatment. Excessive use during pregnancy can cause physical dependence in the fetus, and use right before delivery can cause difficulty breathing in the newborn.

IMPORTANT PRECAUTIONS
- Meperidine can lead to physical and/or psychological dependence; therefore, it should be used for a short term only.
- Because meperidine can cause drowsiness and dizziness, make sure you know how your child reacts to this drug before you allow him or her to participate in potentially dangerous activities, such as riding a bike, driving a car, or operating machinery.
- Store meperidine in a tightly closed container and keep away from excess heat and moisture (e.g., the bathroom, near a stove or sink).

METAPROTERENOL

BRAND NAMES
Alupent, Arm-a-Med Metaproterenol, Dey-Dose Metaproterenol, Metaprel, Prometa
Generic Available

ABOUT THIS DRUG
Metaproterenol is a bronchodilator medication used to prevent and treat shortness of breath, wheezing, and other breathing difficulties associated with asthma, bronchitis, emphysema, and other lung diseases. This drug works by dilating and relaxing constricted bronchial tubes, which opens the air passages in the lungs, making it easier to breathe.

SIDE EFFECTS

Contact your doctor if your child experiences any side effects that are persistent or troubling, including any that are not listed here.

- *Most common:* changes in taste, dry mouth, fast or irregular heartbeat, nervousness, throat irritation, trembling
- *Less common/rare:* bad taste in mouth, cough, diarrhea, dizziness, headache, heart rhythm disturbances, high blood pressure, insomnia, nausea, stomach upset, tiredness, tremors, worsening of asthma

HOW TO USE THIS DRUG

Metaproterenol is available as tablets, syrup, inhalation aerosol, and inhalation solution. The dosages given here are ones that are usually recommended for children. However, your doctor will determine the most appropriate dose and schedule for your child.

Syrup

- Children 6 to 9 years and weighing less than 60 lbs: 1 teaspoon (10 mg) 3 to 4 times daily
- Children 10 years and older and weighing more than 60 lbs: 2 teaspoons (20 mg) 3 to 4 times daily

Tablets

- Children 6 to 9 years and weighing less than 60 lbs: 10 mg 3 to 4 times daily
- Children 10 years and older and weighing more than 60 lbs: 20 mg 3 to 4 times daily

Inhalation Aerosol

- Children younger than 12 years: not recommended
- Children 12 years and older: 2 to 3 inhalations every 3 to 4 hours for a maximum of 12 inhalations

Inhalation Solution—5%

- Children younger than 6 years: not recommended
- Children 6 to 12 years: usual single dose is 0.1 mL

given by nebulizer; dosage can be increased by your physician to 0.2 mL 3 to 4 times daily.
- Children 13 years and older: the dosage range is 0.2 to 0.3 mL taken 3 to 4 times daily, as determined by your doctor

Metaproterenol should be taken exactly as prescribed by your doctor. Taking more than what is recommended can result in serious heart problems, including cardiac arrest. The oral form can be taken with or without food.

If your child misses a dose, give it as soon as you remember, then give the remaining doses for the day at evenly spaced intervals. Resume the regular dosing schedule the next day. Never give a double dose.

TIME UNTIL IT TAKES EFFECT
Inhalation forms, within 5 minutes; oral forms, 15 to 30 minutes

POSSIBLE DRUG, FOOD, AND/OR SUPPLEMENT INTERACTIONS
Tell your doctor if your child is taking any prescription or over-the-counter medications or any vitamins, herbs, or other supplements. Possible interactions with metaproterenol may include the following:

- Taking metaproterenol along with or within 14 days of monoamine oxidase (MAO) inhibitors can cause a dangerous increase in blood pressure.
- Use of other inhaled medications can result in increased cardiovascular side effects. Consult your doctor.
- Epinephrine should be taken at least 4 hours apart from metaproterenol.
- Many over-the-counter cold, flu, cough, allergy, sinus, and weight loss products can increase blood pressure. Talk to your doctor before you give your child any of these medications.
- Beta-blockers and phenothiazines may decrease the effects of metaproterenol.

- Tricyclic antidepressants should be used with caution.
- Avoid use of any herbs that increase blood pressure, such as ephedra, ginseng, goldenseal, licorice, and saw palmetto. Gotu kola can cause nervousness.
- Avoid use of caffeine, including colas, tea, coffee, and chocolate.

SYMPTOMS OF OVERDOSE
Symptoms include chest pain, dizziness, heart palpitations, severe headache, nervousness, rapid heart rate, severe weakness, sweating, tremor, and vomiting. If overdose occurs, seek immediate medical attention and bring the drug container(s) with you.

THINGS TO TELL YOUR DOCTOR
- Tell your doctor if your child has had allergic reactions to any medications in the past or if he or she is taking any medications, herbal remedies, or supplements now.
- Let your doctor know if your child has any of the following medical conditions: anxiety disorder, diabetes, glaucoma, heart disease, hyperthyroidism, irregular heartbeat, increased heart rate, high blood pressure, seizures.
- Consult your doctor if your child is pregnant or becomes pregnant during treatment.

IMPORTANT PRECAUTIONS
- If the dose prescribed by your doctor does not provide relief, do not increase the dosage, as too much of this medication can have serious and even fatal effects. Talk to your doctor about your child's lack of response.
- Store metaproterenol in a tightly closed container and keep away from excess heat and moisture (e.g., the bathroom, near a stove or sink). The inhalation forms should not be refrigerated.

METHENAMINE

BRAND NAMES
Hiprex, Mandelamine, Methenamine Hippurate, Methenamine Mandelate, Urex, Urised (combination form that also contains atropine and hyoscyamine)
Generic Available

ABOUT THIS DRUG
Methenamine is an anti-infective agent used to prevent and treat urinary tract infections. It kills bacteria in the urinary tract by forming ammonia and formaldehyde, which are toxic to these organisms.

SIDE EFFECTS
Contact your doctor if your child experiences any side effects that are persistent or troubling, including any that are not listed here.

- *Most common:* none (for methenamine alone)
- *Less common/rare:* nausea, vomiting (for methenamine alone)

For the combination product, unusual excitement, irritability, nervousness, and unusual warmth, dryness, and flushing skin are more likely to occur in children, who are usually sensitive to atropine and hyoscyamine. When the combination product is given to children during hot weather, a sudden increase in body temperature may occur.

HOW TO USE THIS DRUG
Methenamine is available in tablets, enteric-coated tablets, oral suspension, and granules for solution. The combination product is available in tablets. The dosages given here are ones that are usually recommended for children. However, your doctor will determine the most appropriate dose and schedule for your child.

Methenamine Hippurate Tablets
- Children younger than 6 years: to be determined by your physician
- Children 6 to 12 years: 500 to 1,000 mg twice daily, taken in the morning and evening
- Children 13 years and older: 1,000 mg twice daily, taken in the morning and evening

Methenamine Mandelate Oral Forms
- Children younger than 6 years: usual dose is 8.3 mg per lb of body weight 4 times daily, taken after meals and at bedtime
- Children 6 to 12 years: 500 mg 4 times daily, taken after meals and at bedtime
- Children 13 years and older: 1,000 mg 4 times daily, taken after meals and at bedtime

Urised Brand
- Children younger than 6 years: not recommended
- Children 6 to 12 years: to be determined by your physician
- Children 12 years and older: 1 to 2 tablets 4 times daily

Methenamine works best when urine is highly acidic, so give your child plenty of cranberry juice, cranberries, plums, or prunes. If this is not possible, give your child a vitamin C supplement. Talk to your doctor about the best amount of vitamin C to give. If using the granules form of methenamine, dissolve the contents of each packet in 2 to 4 ounces of cold water, stir well, and immediately give it to your child.

If your child misses a dose, give it as soon as you remember. If it is nearly time for the next dose, skip the missed dose and continue with the regular dosing schedule. Never give a double dose.

TIME UNTIL IT TAKES EFFECT
Within 1 hour

POSSIBLE DRUG, FOOD, AND/OR SUPPLEMENT INTERACTIONS

Tell your doctor if your child is taking any prescription or over-the-counter medications or any vitamins, herbs, or other supplements. Possible interactions with methenamine may include the following:

- Talk to your physician about using any of these drugs while taking methenamine, as they may decrease the effects of the drug: antacids, any antidiarrheal medicine that contains kaolin or attapulgite, thiazide diuretics, and urinary alkalizers, such as acetazolamide, potassium or sodium citrate, or sodium bicarbonate.
- Use of the combination form may reduce the effects of ketoconazole.
- Other anticholinergics may increase the effects of atropine and hyoscyamine (present in the combination product).
- Potassium chloride may worsen or cause lesions in the stomach or intestinal tract.
- Sulfa medications may increase the risk of crystals forming in the urine.
- Avoid milk products, citrus fruits and juices, and alkaline foods such as vegetables and peanuts while taking methenamine.

SYMPTOMS OF OVERDOSE

No specific symptoms have been reported with use of methenamine alone. With the combination product (Urised), symptoms may include abdominal pain, bloody diarrhea, bloody urine, burning in throat and mouth, circulatory collapse, coma, dilated pupils, dizziness, elevated blood pressure, extremely high body temperature, headache, painful and frequent urination, pounding heartbeat, rapid heartbeat, respiratory failure, sweating, vomiting, white sores in mouth. If overdose occurs, seek immediate medical attention and bring the drug container(s) with you.

THINGS TO TELL YOUR DOCTOR

- Tell your doctor if your child has had allergic reactions to any medications in the past or if he or she is taking any medications, herbal remedies, or supplements now. If your child will be taking the combination product, tell your doctor if your child has ever reacted to ingredients in this drug (atropine, hyoscyamine, benzoic acid, methylene blue, phenyl salicylate).
- Let your doctor know if your child has bleeding problems, brain damage, colitis, fever, hernia, glaucoma, heart disease, high blood pressure, hyperthyroidism, intestinal or stomach problems, lung disease, or liver or kidney disease or has ever experienced severe dehydration.
- Consult your doctor if your child is pregnant or becomes pregnant during treatment.

IMPORTANT PRECAUTIONS

- Your child should take this medication for the entire course prescribed by your doctor, even if he or she feels better before the scheduled end of treatment.
- Your child may need to undergo liver function tests if he or she takes this drug for an extended period of time.
- Store methenamine in a tightly closed container and keep away from excess heat and moisture (e.g., the bathroom, near a stove or sink).

METHOTREXATE

BRAND NAMES
Folex, Folex PFS, Mexate, Mexate-AQ, Rheumatrex, Trexall
Generic Available

ABOUT THIS DRUG
Methotrexate is an antimetabolic agent, which means it interferes with the metabolism of cells. For that reason it is used to treat conditions that involve abnormal cell growth,

such as cancer (e.g., breast, bone, blood, head, neck, lymph) and psoriasis. It is also used to treat rheumatoid arthritis. It is believed that methotrexate works by interfering with the activity of an enzyme required for the reproduction and maintenance of cells, including cancer cells and cells that make up bone marrow and line the bladder, mouth, and intestinal tract. It is uncertain how it helps relieve symptoms of rheumatoid arthritis except that it suppresses the immune system, which is believed to play a vital role in the progression of this disease.

SIDE EFFECTS
Contact your doctor if your child experiences any side effects that are persistent or troubling, including any that are not listed here.

- *Most common:* diarrhea, dizziness, increased risk of infection, liver and kidney problems, loss of appetite, mouth ulcers, nausea, vomiting
- *Less common/rare:* acne, birth defects, black or tarry stool, boils, fatigue, headache, infertility, inflammation of the gums and mouth, itching, miscarriage, pale skin, paralysis, rash

HOW TO USE THIS DRUG
Methotrexate is available in tablets and via injection. (Information on the injectable form is not provided here.) Use of methotrexate is highly individual and must be determined by your physician. Dosing can be as varied as once a day to once a week.

Tablets can be crushed and mixed with food to help prevent stomach irritation. If your child misses a dose, skip it and resume the regular dosing schedule. Never give a double dose.

TIME UNTIL IT TAKES EFFECT
Unknown

POSSIBLE DRUG, FOOD, AND/OR SUPPLEMENT INTERACTIONS

Tell your doctor if your child is taking any prescription or over-the-counter medications or any vitamins, herbs, or other supplements. Possible interactions with methotrexate may include the following:

- Do not take methotrexate with milk, as it reduces absorption of the drug.
- Alcohol should be avoided, as it can cause liver damage.
- Do not take medications for pain or inflammation, as they may increase the effects of methotrexate. They include aspirin and other salicylates, diclofenac, diflunisal, fenoprofen, ibuprofen, indomethacin, ketoprofen, meclofenamate, mefenamic acid, naproxen, phenylbutazone, piroxicam, sulindac, and tolmetin.
- Oral antibiotics, such as tetracycline, chloramphenicol, and broad-spectrum antibiotics, may reduce absorption of methotrexate.
- Penicillins may reduce the ability of the body to eliminate methotrexate and result in toxic levels of the drug.
- Methotrexate may reduce the ability of the body to eliminate theophylline and result in toxic levels of the drug.
- Use of drugs that can cause liver toxicity (e.g., azathioprine, retinoids, sulfasalazine) should be monitored closely if used along with methotrexate.

SYMPTOMS OF OVERDOSE

An overdose can cause severe damage to the liver, stomach, kidneys, intestines, lungs, and bone marrow, resulting in various symptoms. If overdose occurs, seek immediate medical attention and bring the drug container(s) with you.

THINGS TO TELL YOUR DOCTOR

- Tell your doctor if your child has had allergic reactions to any medications in the past or if he or she is taking any medications, herbal remedies, or supplements now.

- Let your doctor know if your child has any of the following medical conditions: chicken pox, colitis, any immune system disease, kidney stones, any infection, intestinal blockage, kidney disease, liver disease, mouth sores or inflammation, stomach ulcers.
- Consult your doctor if your child is pregnant or becomes pregnant during treatment. Methotrexate can cause birth defects and other serious problems if taken during pregnancy.

IMPORTANT PRECAUTIONS

- Methotrexate may cause serious lung problems. If your child experiences difficulty breathing, fever, or a dry cough, contact your doctor immediately.
- Your child should not receive any vaccinations while he or she is using methotrexate unless your physician approves.
- Methotrexate can cause birth defects if either the female or the male is using the drug at the time of conception.
- Use of methotrexate can reduce your child's resistance to infection. Your child should avoid contact with people who have infections.
- This drug may increase your child's sensitivity to the sun. Make sure your child is adequately protected from sunlight (e.g., sunscreen, long sleeves, long pants, hat) when he or she is exposed to the sun.
- Your physician may ask that your child drink extra fluids to increase urine production and stimulate elimination of the drug from the body to help prevent kidney damage.
- If your child vomits shortly after taking a dose, ask your doctor whether your child should immediately take another dose or wait until the next scheduled dose.
- Store methotrexate in a tightly closed container and keep away from excess heat and moisture (e.g., the bathroom, near a stove or sink).

METHYLPHENIDATE

BRAND NAMES
Concerta, Metadate CD, Methylphenidate Hydrochloride, Ritalin, Ritalin-SR
Generic Available

ABOUT THIS DRUG
Methylphenidate is a central nervous system stimulant that is used to treat attention deficit/hyperactivity disorder (ADHD). It is also used to treat narcolepsy. This drug is not considered to be appropriate treatment for children whose symptoms are related to a psychiatric condition or stress.

Methylphenidate appears to work by stimulating the release of various brain chemicals, including serotonin, dopamine, and norepinephrine, which are involved in behavior, mood, and thought, and also promotes the transmission of nerve signals in the brain. This drug increases attention and decreases restlessness in both children and adults who have ADHD.

SIDE EFFECTS
Contact your doctor if your child experiences any side effects that are persistent or troubling, including any that are not listed here.

- *Common:* abnormal heart rhythms, insomnia, loss of appetite, stomach pain, weight loss
- *Less common/rare:* dizziness, drowsiness, headache, nausea

HOW TO USE THIS DRUG
Methylphenidate is available in tablets and extended-release tablets. The dosages given here are ones that are usually recommended for children. However, your doctor will determine the most appropriate dose and schedule for your child.

ADHD
- Children 6 to 12 years: for tablets—5 mg twice daily (your doctor may increase the dose by 5 to 10 mg a

week); for extended-release tablets, 20 mg 2 to 3 times daily
- Children 13 years and older: for tablets—5 to 20 mg 2 to 3 times daily, taken with or after meals; for extended-release tablets, 20 mg 1 to 3 times daily, every 8 hours

Narcolepsy
- Children 13 years and older: for tablets—5 to 20 mg 3 or 4 times daily; for extended-release tablets—20 mg 2 to 3 times daily

Methylphenidate should be taken with meals or after meals when used to treat ADHD; it should be taken 30 to 45 minutes before meals when treating narcolepsy.

If your child misses a dose, give it as soon as you remember. If it is nearly time for the next dose, skip the missed dose and continue with the regular dosing schedule. Never give a double dose.

TIME UNTIL IT TAKES EFFECT
Tablets, within 30 minutes; extended-release tablets, between 30 and 60 minutes

POSSIBLE DRUG, FOOD, AND/OR SUPPLEMENT INTERACTIONS
Tell your doctor if your child is taking any prescription or over-the-counter medications or any vitamins, herbs, or other supplements. Possible interactions with methylphenidate may include the following:

- Methylphenidate may increase the effects of tricyclic antidepressants.
- Methylphenidate reduces the effectiveness of guanethidine.
- Methylphenidate may alter the effects of blood thinners such as warfarin and of seizure medications including phenobarbital, phenytoin, and primidone.
- Avoid alcohol and caffeinated beverages, such as coffee, tea, and colas.

- Food rich in the amino acid tyramine should be avoided while methylphenidate is being used. Such foods include but are not limited to aged cheeses, bologna, chicken liver, chocolate, pepperoni, raisins, salami, soy sauce, and yeast extracts.
- Herbs that affect the central nervous system should be avoided, including ephedra, St. John's wort, guarana, and gotu kola.

SYMPTOMS OF OVERDOSE

Symptoms include agitation, confusion, convulsions, delirium, dry mucous membranes, elevated blood pressure and body temperature, enlarged pupils, euphoria, flushing, hallucinations, headache, muscle twitching, rapid or irregular heartbeat, tremors, and vomiting. If overdose occurs, seek immediate medical attention and bring the drug container(s) with you.

THINGS TO TELL YOUR DOCTOR

- Tell your doctor if your child has had allergic reactions to any medications in the past or if he or she is taking any medications, herbal remedies, or supplements now.
- Let your doctor know if your child has any of the following medical conditions: severe anxiety or tension, glaucoma or other visual problems, high blood pressure, motor tics or spasms, a seizure disorder, or Tourette's syndrome.
- Before any type of surgical or dental procedure is performed, tell the doctor or dentist that your child is taking methylphenidate.
- Consult your doctor if your child is pregnant or becomes pregnant during treatment.

IMPORTANT PRECAUTIONS

- Long-term use of this drug can lead to dependence. Your physician should carefully monitor your child during treatment.
- Store methylphenidate in a tightly closed container and keep at room temperature away from excess heat and moisture (e.g., the bathroom, near a stove or sink).

METHYLPREDNISOLONE—
see *Corticosteroids, Oral*

METRONIDAZOLE

BRAND NAMES
Flagyl, MetroGel, Protostat
Generic Available

ABOUT THIS DRUG
Metronidazole is an antibiotic that is effective against anaerobic bacteria and some parasites that cause conditions including but not limited to bacterial peritonitis, amebic dysentery, giardiasis, and *Trichomonas* vaginal infections, as well as abscesses in the pelvis, abdomen, brain, colon, and liver. It is believed to work by interfering with the organisms' production of DNA, thus resulting in their death.

SIDE EFFECTS
Contact your doctor if your child experiences any side effects that are persistent or troubling, including any that are not listed here.

- *Most common (oral and injection forms):* diarrhea, dizziness, headache, loss of appetite, stomach pain, vomiting
- *Most common (vaginal gel):* burning urination, itching of genital area, painful intercourse, thick vaginal discharge
- *Less common/rare (oral and injection forms):* change in taste, dry mouth, sharp metallic taste in mouth
- *Less common/rare (vaginal gel):* diarrhea, dizziness, furry tongue, lightheadedness, loss of appetite, metallic taste in mouth, nausea, vomiting
- *Less common/rare (vaginal cream):* dry skin, irritated skin, watery eyes that burn or sting

HOW TO USE THIS DRUG

Metronidazole is available in capsules, tablets, cream, and gel and via injection. (Information on the injectable form is not provided here.) The dosages given here are ones that are usually recommended for children. However, your doctor will determine the most appropriate dose and schedule for your child.

Bacterial Infections

- Children younger than 12 years (dose is based on body weight): for capsules and tablets—the usual dose is 3.4 mg per lb of body weight every 6 hours; or 4.5 mg per lb every 8 hours
- Children 12 years and older (dose is based on body weight): for capsules and tablets—the usual dose is 3.4 mg per lb of body weight every 6 hours for at least 7 days.

Amebiasis Infections

- Children younger than 12 years (dose is based on body weight): for capsules and tablets—the usual dose is 5.3 to 7.6 mg per lb of body weight 3 times daily for 10 days
- Children 12 years and older: for capsules and tablets— 500 to 750 mg 3 times daily for 5 to 10 days

Trichomoniasis Infections

- Children younger than 12 years (dose is based on body weight): for capsules and tablets—the usual dose is 2.3 mg per lb of body weight 3 times daily for 7 days
- Children 12 years and older: for capsules and tablets— 1 dose of 2 g or 1 g twice daily for 1 day; or 250 mg 3 times daily for 7 days

Bacterial Vaginosis

- Children younger than 12 years: to be determined by your doctor
- Children 12 years and older: for extended-release tablets—750 mg once daily for 7 days

Metronidazole can be taken with food or milk to help prevent stomach irritation. If your child misses a dose, give it as soon as you remember. If it is nearly time for the next dose, skip the missed dose and continue with the regular dosing schedule. Never give a double dose.

TIME UNTIL IT TAKES EFFECT
Unknown

POSSIBLE DRUG, FOOD, AND/OR SUPPLEMENT INTERACTIONS
Tell your doctor if your child is taking any prescription or over-the-counter medications or any vitamins, herbs, or other supplements. Possible interactions with metronidazole may include the following:

- Metronidazole may increase the blood levels and effects of lithium and phenytoin.
- Use of alcohol may result in cramps, flushing, headache, nausea, and vomiting.
- Disulfiram may cause increased nervous system effects such as confusion and psychotic reactions.
- Cimetidine may increase the effects of metronidazole.
- Barbiturates (e.g., phenobarbital) may reduce the effects of metronidazole.
- Use of blood thinners (e.g., warfarin) may increase the risk of bleeding.
- Use of vitamin B6 (pyridoxine) along with metronidazole may increase nervous system side effects.

SYMPTOMS OF OVERDOSE
Symptoms include loss of muscle coordination, nausea, and vomiting. If overdose occurs, seek immediate medical attention and bring the drug container(s) with you.

THINGS TO TELL YOUR DOCTOR
- Tell your doctor if your child has had allergic reactions to any medications in the past or if he or she is taking any medications, herbal remedies, or supplements now.

- Let your doctor know if your child has any of the following medical conditions: epilepsy, heart disease, high blood pressure, liver or kidney problems, oral thrush, or a vaginal yeast infection.
- Consult your doctor if your child is pregnant or becomes pregnant during treatment. Use of the oral forms of metronidazole should be avoided during the first trimester.

IMPORTANT PRECAUTIONS
- Your child should complete the prescribed treatment course even if he or she feels better before the course is completed, because stopping the medication too soon may allow the infection to recur.
- Because metronidazole can cause dizziness, make sure you know how your child reacts to it before you allow him or her to participate in potentially hazardous activities, such as riding a bike, driving a car, or operating machinery.
- Store metronidazole in a tightly closed container and keep away from excess heat and moisture (e.g., the bathroom, near a stove or sink).

MINOCYCLINE–
see *Tetracycline Antibiotics*

MOMETASONE–
see *Corticosteroids, Nasal Inhalants* and *Corticosteroids, Topical*

MONTELUKAST–
see *Leukotriene Antagonist/Inhibitors*

MORPHINE

BRAND NAMES
AVINZA, MS Contin, MSIR, Oramorph SR, Roxanol, Roxanol SR
Generic Available

ABOUT THIS DRUG
Morphine is an opioid (narcotic) painkiller that is used to relieve severe pain. It works by acting on specific areas of the brain and spinal cord that process pain messages from nerves throughout the body.

SIDE EFFECTS
Contact your doctor if your child experiences any side effects that are persistent or troubling, including any that are not listed here.

- *Most common:* constipation, dizziness, drowsiness, itching, nausea, vomiting
- *Less common/rare:* euphoria, hallucinations, jerking body movements, mood swings, sweating

HOW TO USE THIS DRUG
Morphine is available as tablets, capsules, suppositories, and oral solution and via injection. (Information on the injectable form is not provided here.) Dosing is highly individual for morphine; therefore, your physician will determine the most appropriate dose and schedule for your child's needs.

Oral morphine can be taken with food to help prevent stomach irritation. If your child misses a dose, give it as soon as you remember. However, if it is nearly time for the next dose, skip the missed dose and continue with the regular dosing schedule. Never give a double dose.

TIME UNTIL IT TAKES EFFECT
Oral forms, within 60 minutes; suppositories, 20 to 60 minutes; injection, 10 to 30 minutes

POSSIBLE DRUG, FOOD, AND/OR SUPPLEMENT INTERACTIONS

Tell your doctor if your child is taking any prescription or over-the-counter medications or any vitamins, herbs, or other supplements. Possible interactions with morphine may include the following:

- Alcohol, tranquilizers, sleep medications, and other drugs that affect the central nervous system should not be used along with morphine because serious depressant effects may occur.
- Antihypertensives, beta-blockers, and other drugs that reduce blood pressure should not be used along with morphine because abnormally low blood pressure may result.
- Cimetidine use may result in breathing problems, confusion, disorientation, and seizures.
- Morphine may increase the blood levels of zidovudine.
- Herbs that cause sedation may cause potentially dangerous depressant effects when used with morphine. Some of those herbs include calendula, capsicum, catnip, goldenseal, gotu kola, hops, kava, lady's slipper, passionflower, sage, Siberian ginseng, skullcap, St. John's wort, and valerian.

SYMPTOMS OF OVERDOSE

Symptoms include cold clammy skin, confusion, loss of consciousness, pinpoint pupils, seizures, severe drowsiness or dizziness, slowed breathing, and weakness. If overdose occurs, seek immediate medical attention and bring the drug container(s) with you.

THINGS TO TELL YOUR DOCTOR

- Tell your doctor if your child has had allergic reactions to any medications in the past, especially other opioids, or if he or she is taking any medications, herbal remedies, or supplements now.
- Let your doctor know if your child has any of the following medical conditions: brain disorder, colitis, gall-

stones, head injury, heart disease, kidney or liver disease, lung disease, seizures, or thyroid disease.
- Consult your doctor if your child is pregnant or becomes pregnant during treatment. Use of morphine during pregnancy should be avoided.

IMPORTANT PRECAUTIONS
- Regular and long-term use of morphine can lead to physical dependence, which may result in withdrawal symptoms if the morphine is discontinued abruptly.
- Store morphine in a tightly closed container and keep away from excess heat and moisture (e.g., the bathroom, near a stove or sink). Do not allow the liquid form to freeze.

NAFCILLIN—see *Penicillin Antibiotics*

NEDOCROMIL SODIUM (INHALANT)

BRAND NAME
Tilade
Generic Not Available

ABOUT THIS DRUG
Nedocromil is a respiratory inhalant that is prescribed to prevent the symptoms of asthma and to prevent bronchospasm. It is designed to be taken on a regular basis and cannot stop an asthma attack once it has started. This drug prevents inflammatory cells in the lungs from releasing substances that cause bronchospasm or symptoms of asthma.

SIDE EFFECTS
Contact your doctor if your child experiences any side effects that are persistent or troubling, including any that are not listed here.

- *Most common:* chest pain, cough, fever, headache, inflamed nose and sinuses, nausea, sore throat, unpleasant taste, upper respiratory tract infection, wheezing
- *Less common/rare:* abdominal pain, bronchitis, conjunctivitis, diarrhea, difficulty breathing, dizziness, dry mouth, fatigue, indigestion, rash, viral infection, vomiting

HOW TO USE THIS DRUG

Nedocromil is available as an inhalation aerosol. The dosages given here are ones that are usually recommended for children. However, your doctor will determine the most appropriate dose and schedule for your child.

- Children younger than 6 years: not recommended
- Children 6 years and older: 2 inhalations (3.5 to 4 mg total of both inhalations) 2 to 4 times daily (for a total not to exceed 14 to 16 mg daily)

If your child misses a dose, give it as soon as you remember. However, if it is nearly time for the next dose, skip the missed dose and continue with the regular dosing schedule. Never give a double dose. If your child's asthma is well controlled on the recommended dosage, your doctor may reduce the dose.

TIME UNTIL IT TAKES EFFECT

Several days or up to 4 weeks

POSSIBLE DRUG, FOOD, AND/OR SUPPLEMENT INTERACTIONS

Tell your doctor if your child is taking any prescription or over-the-counter medications or any vitamins, herbs, or other supplements. No interactions have been reported.

SYMPTOMS OF OVERDOSE

No specific overdose symptoms have been noted. However, if you suspect an overdose has occurred, seek immediate medical attention and bring the drug container(s) with you.

THINGS TO TELL YOUR DOCTOR
- Tell your doctor if your child has had allergic reactions to any medications in the past or if he or she is taking any medications, herbal remedies, or supplements now.
- Consult your doctor if your child is pregnant or becomes pregnant during treatment.

IMPORTANT PRECAUTIONS
- The inhaler should be cleaned at least twice a week to keep it functioning properly.
- Store nedocromil away from excess heat and direct light (e.g., near a stove or sink), as the aerosol canister is under pressure and can burst.

NEDOCROMIL SODIUM (OPHTHALMIC)

BRAND NAME
Alocril
Generic Not Available

ABOUT THIS DRUG
Nedocromil ophthalmic is an antihistamine solution used for temporary relief of itchy eyes caused by allergic conjunctivitis. The drug interferes with the release of histamine and blocks its effects, which include sneezing, watery eyes, swelling, and other allergic reactions.

SIDE EFFECTS
Contact your doctor if your child experiences any side effects that are persistent or troubling, including any that are not listed here.

- *Most common:* blurry vision, burning and stinging of the eye (temporary), headache, nasal congestion, unpleasant taste
- *Less common/rare:* asthma, conjunctivitis, eye redness, increased eye sensitivity to light, runny nose

HOW TO USE THIS DRUG

Nedocromil ophthalmic is available in eye drops. The dosage for children older than 3 years is usually 1 or 2 drops in each affected eye twice daily. However, your doctor may determine a different dose and schedule for your child.

If your child misses a scheduled dose, give it as soon as you remember. If it is nearly time for the next dose, skip the missed dose and continue with the regular dosing schedule. Never give a double dose.

TIME UNTIL IT TAKES EFFECT

Unknown

POSSIBLE DRUG, FOOD, AND/OR SUPPLEMENT INTERACTIONS

Tell your doctor if your child is taking any prescription or over-the-counter medications or any vitamins, herbs, or other supplements. No drug, food, or supplement interactions have been noted. However, do not give your child any other eye drops without first talking with your doctor.

SYMPTOMS OF OVERDOSE

An overdose is unlikely to occur. However, if your child applies an excessive amount of nedocromil or accidentally ingests the medication, seek immediate medical attention and bring the drug container(s) with you.

THINGS TO TELL YOUR DOCTOR

- Tell your doctor if your child has had allergic reactions to any medications in the past or if he or she is taking any medications, herbal remedies, or supplements now.
- Let your doctor know if your child has a bacterial, viral, or fungal eye infection.
- Consult your doctor if your child is pregnant or becomes pregnant during treatment.

IMPORTANT PRECAUTIONS

- Do not give your child nedocromil if he or she has a bacterial, fungal, or viral eye infection unless you have the permission of your doctor.

- Because nedocromil can cause blurry vision, make sure you know how your child reacts to the drug before he or she participates in potentially dangerous activities, such as riding a bike, driving a car, or operating machinery.
- Your child should not wear his or her contacts while being treated with nedocromil.
- Store nedocromil in a tightly closed container and keep away from heat, moisture, and direct light. Do not allow it to freeze.

NEOMYCIN PLUS POLYMYXIN B PLUS GRAMICIDIN (OPHTHALMIC)

BRAND NAMES
Ak-Spore Ophthalmic Solution, Neocidin Ophthalmic Solution, Neosporin Ophthalmic Solution, Ocu-Spor-G, Ocutricin Ophthalmic Solution, PN Ophthalmic, Tribiotic, Tri-Ophthalmic, Triple Antibiotic
Generic Available

ABOUT THIS DRUG
This combination of neomycin + polymyxin B + gramicidin is an antibiotic used to treat eye infections. It works by destroying common bacteria that are responsible for eye infections.

SIDE EFFECTS
Contact your doctor if your child experiences any side effects that are persistent or troubling, including any that are not listed here.

- *Most common:* eye irritation, itching, redness, swelling
- *Less common/rare:* allergic reaction, burning, development of secondary eye infection, stinging

HOW TO USE THIS DRUG
Neomycin + polymyxin B + gramicidin is available as eye drops. The dosage given here is the one usually recom-

mended for children. However, your doctor will determine the most appropriate dose and schedule for your child.

- Children: apply 1 to 2 drops to the affected eye(s) 2 to 4 times daily

If your child wears contact lenses, he or she needs to remove them when using this drug. The lenses can be reinserted 15 minutes after the drops have been applied.

If your child misses a dose, give it as soon as you remember. If it is nearly time for the next dose, skip the missed dose and continue with the regular dosing schedule. Never give a double dose.

To avoid contamination and infection, do not touch the dropper to the eye or to any other surface.

TIME UNTIL IT TAKES EFFECT
Unknown

POSSIBLE DRUG, FOOD, AND/OR SUPPLEMENT INTERACTIONS
Tell your doctor if your child is taking any prescription or over-the-counter medications or any vitamins, herbs, or other supplements. No specific drug, food, or supplement interactions have been reported with this combination product. However, tell your physician if your child is using any other eye drops.

SYMPTOMS OF OVERDOSE
An overdose is unlikely to occur. However, if you believe an overdose has occurred, or if your child accidentally ingests the eye drops, seek immediate medical attention and bring the drug container(s) with you.

THINGS TO TELL YOUR DOCTOR
- Tell your doctor if your child has had allergic reactions to any medications in the past, including other antibiotics or eye drops, or if he or she is taking any medications, herbal remedies, or supplements now.

- If the infection does not begin to improve within a few days of starting treatment or if symptoms get worse, call your doctor.
- Tell your doctor if your child wears contact lenses, as he or she may be asked to stop wearing them for the duration of treatment.
- Consult your doctor if your child is pregnant or becomes pregnant during treatment.

IMPORTANT PRECAUTIONS
- Store neomycin + polymyxin B + gramicidin in a tightly closed container and keep away from heat, moisture, and direct light. Do not allow it to freeze.

NEOMYCIN PLUS POLYMYXIN B PLUS HYDROCORTISONE (OTIC)

BRAND NAMES
AK-Spore HC Otic, Antibiotic Ear, Cortatrigen Ear, Cort-Biotic, Ear-Eze, Masporin, Octicair, Octigen, Otic, Otic-Care, Otocidin, Otocort, Pediotic, and others
Generic Available

ABOUT THIS DRUG
Neomycin + polymyxin B + hydrocortisone is a combination antibiotic and cortisone-like medication used to treat infections of the ear canal and to relieve symptoms of various ear problems, including mastoid cavity infection.

SIDE EFFECTS
Contact your doctor if your child experiences any side effects that are persistent or troubling, including any that are not listed here.

- *Most common:* itching, rash, redness, swelling (or other signs of irritation) near the ear that was not present before treatment

HOW TO USE THIS DRUG

Neomycin + polymyxin B + hydrocortisone is available as ear drops. The dosages given here are ones that are usually recommended for children. However, your doctor will determine the most appropriate dose and schedule for your child.

For Ear Canal Infection
- Children: 3 drops in the affected ear 3 or 4 times daily

For Mastoid Cavity Infection
- Children: 4 or 5 drops in the affected ear every 6 to 8 hours

If your child misses a dose, give it as soon as you remember. However, if it is nearly time for the next dose, skip the missed dose and continue with the regular dosing schedule. Never give a double dose.

TIME UNTIL IT TAKES EFFECT
Unknown

POSSIBLE DRUG, FOOD, AND/OR SUPPLEMENT INTERACTIONS

Tell your doctor if your child is taking any prescription or over-the-counter medications or any vitamins, herbs, or other supplements. No drug, food, or supplement interactions have been reported. However, tell your doctor if your child is using any other ear medications.

SYMPTOMS OF OVERDOSE
An overdose is unlikely. However, if you suspect an overdose or if your child has accidentally ingested the ear drops, seek immediate medical attention and bring the drug container(s) with you.

THINGS TO TELL YOUR DOCTOR
- Tell your doctor if your child has had allergic reactions to any medications in the past or if he or she is taking any medications, herbal remedies, or supplements now.

- Let your doctor know if your child has any other ear infection or condition, such as a punctured ear drum.

IMPORTANT PRECAUTIONS
- Your child needs to take the entire course of treatment as prescribed by your doctor. If treatment is stopped before the scheduled time, the infection may return.
- This drug should not be used for longer than 10 days without the permission of your doctor.
- Store neomycin + polymyxin B + hydrocortisone in a tightly closed container and keep away from heat, direct light, and extremes in temperature.

NITROFURANTOIN

BRAND NAMES
Furadantin, Macrobid, Macrodantin
Generic Available

ABOUT THIS DRUG
Nitrofurantoin is an antiinfective agent used to treat urinary tract infections. It works by interfering with the metabolism and cell wall formation of the offending bacteria, eventually leading to their death.

SIDE EFFECTS
Contact your doctor if your child experiences any side effects that are persistent or troubling, including any that are not listed here.

- *Most common:* abdominal pain or discomfort, diarrhea, loss of appetite, nausea, vomiting
- *Less common/rare:* brown or dark yellow urine

HOW TO USE THIS DRUG
Nitrofurantoin is available in capsules, extended-release capsules, oral suspension, and tablets. The dosages given here are ones that are usually recommended for children.

However, your doctor will determine the most appropriate dose and schedule for your child.

To Prevent Urinary Tract Infections

- Children 1 month to 12 years: dose is based on body weight and usually is 0.44 mg per lb of body weight, given as 1 or 2 divided doses per day
- Children 13 years and older: for capsules, tablets, and oral suspension—50 to 100 mg once daily at bedtime

To Treat Urinary Tract Infections

- Children 1 month to 12 years: dose is based on body weight and usually is 2.3 to 3.1 mg per lb of body weight, divided into 4 doses over 24 hours
- Children 13 years and older: for capsules, tablets, and oral suspension—50 to 100 mg every 6 hours; for extended-release capsules—100 mg every 12 hours for 7 days

Nitrofurantoin can be taken with food to improve absorption and to prevent stomach irritation.

If your child misses a dose, give it as soon as you remember. If it is nearly time for the next dose, skip the missed dose and continue with the normal dosing schedule. Never give a double dose.

TIME UNTIL IT TAKES EFFECT
Within 60 minutes

POSSIBLE DRUG, FOOD, AND/OR SUPPLEMENT INTERACTIONS
Tell your doctor if your child is taking any prescription or over-the-counter medications or any vitamins, herbs, or other supplements. Possible interactions with nitrofurantoin may include the following:

- Many drugs may increase the side effects of nitrofurantoin, including those that affect the blood. Examples include acetohydroxamic acid, dapsone, furazolidone, methyldopa, primaquine, procainamide, quinidine, sulfa drugs, and oral antidiabetic medications.

- Many drugs increase the risk of nervous system side effects, including carbamazepine, chloroquine, cisplatin, DTaP vaccine, disulfiram, hydroxychloroquine, lindane, lithium, mexiletine, phenytoin, and vincristine.
- Probenecid and sulfinpyrazone may reduce the effectiveness of nitrofurantoin and increase the risk of side effects.
- Nitrofurantoin may interact with nutritional supplements, especially vitamins B6 and K, and the mineral magnesium. Talk to your doctor before giving these supplements and nitrofurantoin to your child.

SYMPTOMS OF OVERDOSE
Symptoms include diarrhea, loss of appetite, severe nausea, and vomiting. If overdose occurs, seek medical attention immediately and bring the prescription container with you to the hospital.

THINGS TO TELL YOUR DOCTOR
- Tell your doctor if your child has had allergic reactions to any medications in the past or if he or she is taking any medications now.
- Let your doctor know if your child has any of the following medical conditions, as they can increase the risk of side effects: asthma, diabetes, kidney or lung disease, vitamin B6 deficiency, or G6PD (glucose-6-phosphate dehydrogenase) deficiency.
- Tell your doctor if your child has diarrhea, as it may be an indication of serious intestinal inflammation.
- If your child's symptoms do not improve within a few days of starting treatment or if they become worse, call your doctor.
- Consult your doctor if your child is pregnant or becomes pregnant during treatment. Nitrofurantoin should not be taken within a few weeks of delivery or during labor.

IMPORTANT PRECAUTIONS

- Your child should take nitrofurantoin for the entire time prescribed by your doctor even if he or she feels better before treatment is scheduled to end. Stopping too soon may cause the infection to recur.
- Nitrofurantoin may cause your child's skin to be more sensitive to sunlight. Make sure your child is protected against the sun with sunscreen and protective clothing.
- Store nitrofurantoin in a tightly sealed container away from heat and moisture (e.g., in the bathroom, near a stove or sink). Do not allow the liquid form to freeze.

NYSTATIN

BRAND NAMES

Mycostatin, Nilstat, Nystex, Nystop, Pedi-Dri
Generic Available

ABOUT THIS DRUG

Nystatin is an antifungal medication used to treat fungal infections of the skin, mouth, vagina, and intestinal tract. It works by preventing the fungi from producing the components it needs to survive.

SIDE EFFECTS

Contact your doctor if your child experiences any side effects that are persistent or troubling, including any that are not listed here.

- *Most common:* burning sensation, cramps, headache, hives, irritation, rash, vaginal itching
- *Less common/rare:* diarrhea, nausea, stomach pain, vomiting

HOW TO USE THIS DRUG

Nystatin is available as ointment, cream, lozenges, oral tablets, oral suspension, powder for oral suspension, and vaginal tablets. The dosages given here are ones that are usually recommended for children. However, your doctor will determine the most appropriate dose and schedule for your child.

Oral Tablets and Lozenges
- Children 5 years and older: 1 to 2 lozenges or tablets 3 to 5 times daily for up to 14 days. The lozenges should be allowed to dissolve in the mouth, not swallowed. It may take 15 to 30 minutes for them to dissolve.

Cream and Ointment
- All ages: Apply a small amount to the affected skin several times daily, as directed by your physician

Oral Suspension
- Children 1 to 4 years: 2 mL 4 times daily
- Children 5 years and older: 4 to 6 mL (1 teaspoon) 4 times daily

Vaginal Tablets
- Females 13 years and older: insert one 100,000-unit tablet into the vagina 1 or 2 times daily for 14 days

If your child misses a dose, give it as soon as you remember. If it is nearly time for the next dose, skip the missed dose and continue with the regular dosing schedule. Never give a double dose.

TIME UNTIL IT TAKES EFFECT
Unknown

POSSIBLE DRUG, FOOD, AND/OR SUPPLEMENT INTERACTIONS
Tell your doctor if your child is taking any prescription or over-the-counter medications or any vitamins, herbs, or other supplements. Possible interactions with nystatin may include the following:

- Use of iron supplements may make nystatin less effective. Iron supplements should be taken 2 hours before or after a dose of nystatin.

- Use of other antifungal creams, ointments, or vaginal tablets may interact with nystatin. Talk to your physician before giving your child nystatin.

SYMPTOMS OF OVERDOSE

Symptoms include diarrhea, nausea, and vomiting. If overdose occurs, seek immediate medical attention and bring the drug container(s) with you.

THINGS TO TELL YOUR DOCTOR

- Tell your doctor if your child has had allergic reactions to any medications in the past or if he or she is taking any medications, herbal remedies, or supplements now.
- Consult your doctor if your child is pregnant or becomes pregnant during treatment.

IMPORTANT PRECAUTIONS

- Make sure your child takes nystatin for the entire time prescribed by your doctor. Stopping treatment too soon may cause the infection to recur.
- Nystatin lozenges can be given to children 5 years and older only if they are able to allow the lozenge to dissolve over 15 to 30 minutes without swallowing it.
- Store nystatin in a tightly closed container and keep away from excess heat and moisture (e.g., the bathroom, near a stove or sink). The lozenges should be refrigerated. Do not allow the liquid form to freeze.

OLANZAPINE

BRAND NAMES

Zydis, Zyprexa
Generic Not Available

ABOUT THIS DRUG

Olanzapine is an atypical antipsychotic drug that is approved for short-term treatment of schizophrenia or of acute mania associated with bipolar disorder and as maintenance treatment in bipolar disorder. It is increasingly prescribed by physicians for treatment of these disorders in children and adolescents.

This drug works by blocking the action of dopamine and serotonin, two nerve transmitters in the brain that correct an imbalance that is believed to cause or contribute to various mental disorders.

SIDE EFFECTS
Contact your doctor if your child experiences any side effects that are persistent or troubling, including any that are not listed here.

- *Common:* agitation, dizziness, fatigue, headache, hostility, runny nose, sleeplessness, weight gain
- *Less common/rare:* abdominal pain, anxiety, back pain, constipation, cough, dizziness or fainting upon rising, dry mouth, fever, increased appetite, low blood pressure, memory loss, muscle stiffness, personality changes, rapid heart rate, restlessness, rigid neck, stuttering, swelling in the arms or legs, trouble swallowing, vaginal infection, vision problems, vomiting

In rare cases, Parkinson's disease–like reactions (e.g., uncontrollable jerking movements), symptoms of tardive dyskinesia (e.g., lip smacking, wormlike movements of the tongue, or slow, rhythmical, involuntary movements), and symptoms of neuroleptic malignant syndrome (e.g., difficulty breathing, rapid heartbeat, rigid muscles, mental changes, increased sweating, irregular blood pressure, convulsions) have occurred. Contact your doctor immediately if your child exhibits any of these symptoms.

HOW TO USE THIS DRUG
Olanzapine is available as regular tablets and as oral disintegrating tablets that dissolve in the mouth without water. The dosages given here are ones that are usually recommended for children. However, your doctor will determine the most appropriate dose and schedule for your child.

- Children younger than 6 years: not recommended
- Children 6 years and older: starting dose is usually 5 to 10 mg once daily; your doctor may increase the dose as needed

Olanzapine can be taken with or without food. If your child misses a dose, give it as soon as you remember. If it is nearly time for the next dose, do not give the missed dose and continue with the regular dosing schedule. Never give a double dose.

TIME UNTIL IT TAKES EFFECT
At least 1 week to be effective

POSSIBLE DRUG, FOOD, AND/OR SUPPLEMENT INTERACTIONS
Tell your doctor if your child is taking any prescription or over-the-counter medications or any vitamins, herbs, or other supplements. Possible interactions with olanzapine may include the following:

- Medications that lower blood pressure (e.g., antihypertensives, beta-blockers) may cause very low blood pressure if taken along with olanzapine.
- Use of antianxiety benzodiazepines (e.g., diazepam) may increase the risk of very low blood pressure.
- Fluoroquinolone antibiotics or fluvoxamine may result in olanzapine toxicity.
- Carbamazepine reduces the amount of olanzapine that the body absorbs.
- Omeprazole and rifampin may reduce the effects of olanzapine.
- Use of lithium along with olanzapine increases the risk of serious nerve side effects. Do not use these two medications together.
- Use of any sedatives may cause increased drowsiness.
- Olanzapine should not be taken with grapefruit juice, as it can lead to toxic amounts of the drug in the blood.
- Herbs that cause sedation should not be used along

with olanzapine, such as catnip, goldenseal, gotu kola, hops, kava, lemon balm, skullcap, St. John's wort, and valerian.

SYMPTOMS OF OVERDOSE

Symptoms of overdose include drowsiness and slurred speech. If overdose occurs, seek immediate medical attention and bring the prescription container(s) with you.

THINGS TO TELL YOUR DOCTOR

- Tell your doctor if your child has had allergic reactions to any medications in the past or if he or she is taking any medications, herbal remedies, or supplements now.
- Tell your doctor if your child has heart disease, seizures, liver disease, a bowel obstruction, low blood pressure, dehydration, constipation, trouble swallowing, glaucoma, or a family history of diabetes.
- Let your doctor know if your child is pregnant or becomes pregnant while taking this drug.
- Tell your doctor if your child smokes cigarettes, as smoking may decrease the effectiveness of the drug.
- Olanzapine can increase blood sugar (hyperglycemia), even if your child does not have diabetes. Contact your doctor immediately if your child develops any of the following symptoms while taking olanzapine: extreme thirst, frequent urination, blurry vision, weakness, or extreme hunger.

IMPORTANT PRECAUTIONS

- Do not allow your child to get overheated (e.g., from exercise, taking a hot bath, or using a sauna), as olanzapine increases sweating and may lead to dehydration, dizziness, fainting, and vomiting.
- Because olanzapine can cause dizziness and drowsiness, know how your child reacts to this drug before you allow him or her to participate in potentially hazardous activities, such as riding a bike, driving a car, or operating machinery.
- When your child begins treatment with olanzapine or

has a dose increase, he or she may experience dizziness or faintness when rising quickly from a seated or reclined position. Advise your child to get up slowly.

• Store olanzapine in a tightly closed container and keep away from excess heat and moisture (e.g., the bathroom, near a stove or sink).

ONDANSETRON—see *Antiemetics*

OXACILLIN—see *Penicillin Antibiotics*

OXCARBAZEPINE

BRAND NAME
Trileptal
Generic Not Available

ABOUT THIS DRUG
Oxcarbazepine is an anticonvulsant medication used to control partial seizures, either alone or along with other anticonvulsant medications. It is believed oxcarbazepine works by inhibiting the activity of certain areas of the brain and suppressing the abnormal firing of neurons that are associated with seizures.

SIDE EFFECTS
Contact your doctor if your child experiences any side effects that are persistent or troubling, including any that are not listed here.

• *Most common:* abdominal pain, abnormal gait, coordination problems, dizziness, double vision, drowsiness, fatigue, indigestion, nausea, tremor, vomiting
• *Less common/rare:* acne, impaired hand-eye coordination, insomnia, muscle weakness, nervousness, speech and language difficulties

HOW TO USE THIS DRUG

Oxcarbazepine is available in tablets and oral suspension. The dosages given here are ones that are usually recommended for children. However, your doctor will determine the most appropriate dose and schedule for your child.

- Children younger than 4 years: not recommended
- Children 4 to 16 years: start with 3.7 to 4.5 mg per lb of body weight, but do not exceed 600 mg daily. Oxcarbazepine should be taken in 2 equal doses daily. Your doctor may adjust your child's dose.

Oxcarbazepine can be taken with or without food. If your child misses a dose, give it as soon as you remember. If it is nearly time for the next dose, skip the missed dose and continue with the regular dosing schedule. Never give a double dose.

TIME UNTIL IT TAKES EFFECT

A minimum of 2 to 3 days

POSSIBLE DRUG, FOOD, AND/OR SUPPLEMENT INTERACTIONS

Tell your doctor if your child is taking any prescription or over-the-counter medications or any vitamins, herbs, or other supplements. Possible interactions with oxcarbazepine may include the following:

- Oxcarbazepine interacts with many of the other drugs used to treat seizures.
- Oxcarbazepine interferes with the effectiveness of birth control pills. A second form of birth control should be used during treatment with oxcarbazepine.
- Oxcarbazepine may increase the effects of antidepressants, alcohol, antihistamines, antianxiety medications, muscle relaxants, pain relievers, and sedatives.

SYMPTOMS OF OVERDOSE

Overdoses with oxcarbazepine have not been reported. However, if you believe an overdose has occurred, seek immediate medical attention and bring the drug container(s) with you.

THINGS TO TELL YOUR DOCTOR
- Tell your doctor if your child has had allergic reactions to any medications in the past or if he or she is taking any medications, herbal remedies, or supplements now.
- Let your doctor know if your child has reduced kidney function or severe liver disease.
- In rare cases, a life-threatening rash or other skin reaction can appear. Contact your physician immediately if your child develops a rash or other skin condition.
- Consult your doctor if your child is pregnant or becomes pregnant during treatment. Although no studies have been done on the impact of oxcarbazepine on pregnant women, this drug is closely related to carbamazepine, which can cause birth defects.

IMPORTANT PRECAUTIONS
- Your child should wear medical identification stating that he or she is taking oxcarbazepine, in case of an emergency.
- Your doctor may periodically monitor your child's serum sodium levels, as oxcarbazepine can lower sodium levels.
- Your child should not stop taking oxcarbazepine suddenly, as it could result in increased seizures. If your child stops taking oxcarbazepine for any reason, contact your doctor before you restart the medication, as the dose may need to be adjusted.
- Because oxcarbazepine can cause dizziness and drowsiness, make sure you know how your child reacts to it before he or she participates in potentially dangerous activities, such as riding a bike, driving a car, or operating machinery.
- Store oxcarbazepine in a tightly closed container and keep at room temperature away from excess heat and moisture (e.g., the bathroom, near a stove or sink).

OXTRIPHYLLINE—
see *Xanthine Bronchodilators*

OXYBUTYNIN

BRAND NAME
Ditropan
Generic Available

ABOUT THIS DRUG
Oxybutynin is an antispasmodic drug used to reduce muscle spasms in the bladder and to manage certain urinary problems, including urgency, painful urination, and urinary leakage. The drug works in two ways. It blocks the release of acetylcholine, a substance that causes the smooth muscle of the bladder to contract, and it relaxes the bladder's outer muscles. Together these actions control muscle spasms.

SIDE EFFECTS
Contact your doctor if your child experiences any side effects that are persistent or troubling, including any that are not listed here.

- *Most common:* constipation; decreased sweating; drowsiness; dry mouth, throat, and nose
- *Less common/rare:* difficulty urinating, dizziness, impotence, nausea, palpitations, photosensitivity, rapid heart rate, rash, restlessness, sleep disturbances, visual disturbances, weakness

HOW TO USE THIS DRUG
Oxybutynin is available in syrup, tablets, and extended-release tablets and as a patch. The dosages given here are ones that are usually recommended for children. However, your doctor will determine the most appropriate dose and schedule for your child.

- Children 5 to 12 years: 5 mg 2 times daily (daily total intake usually should not exceed 15 mg)
- Children 13 years and older: 5 mg 2 to 3 times daily; for the patch—apply a new patch every 3 to 4 days

Oxybutynin can be taken with or without food. The safety and effectiveness of the extended-release tablets have not been determined for children under the age of 18.

If your child misses a dose, give it as soon as you remember. If it is nearly time for the next dose, skip the missed dose and continue with the regular dosing schedule. If the patch falls off, reapply it. If it will not stay on, throw it away and apply a new one. When using the patch always change it on the same two days each week.

TIME UNTIL IT TAKES EFFECT
30 to 60 minutes

POSSIBLE DRUG, FOOD, AND/OR SUPPLEMENT INTERACTIONS
Tell your doctor if your child is taking any prescription or over-the-counter medications or any vitamins, herbs, or other supplements. Possible interactions with oxybutynin may include the following:

- Use of oxybutynin may enhance the effects of central nervous system depressants, including antihistamines, barbiturates, muscle relaxants, narcotics, sedatives, tranquilizers, and sleeping pills.
- Amantadine and atenolol may increase the effects of oxybutynin.
- Oxybutynin may disrupt the activity of digoxin, haloperidol, levodopa, phenothiazine drugs, and nitrofurantoin.
- Alcohol should not be consumed while taking this drug.
- Herbs that have a sedative effect should be avoided, including catnip, goldenseal, gotu kola, hops, kava, lemon balm, skullcap, St. John's wort, and valerian.

SYMPTOMS OF OVERDOSE

Symptoms include difficulty breathing, clumsiness, confusion, drowsiness, fever, flushing, hallucinations, irritability, rapid heartbeat, restlessness, and unusual nervousness. If overdose occurs, seek immediate medical attention and bring the drug container(s) with you.

THINGS TO TELL YOUR DOCTOR

- Tell your doctor if your child has had allergic reactions to any medications in the past or if he or she is taking any medications, herbal remedies, or supplements now.
- Let your doctor know if your child has any of the following medical conditions: severe bleeding, colitis, severe and persistent dry mouth, glaucoma, heart disease, hiatal hernia, high blood pressure, hyperthyroidism, intestinal or stomach problems, liver or kidney disease, urinary difficulties.
- Consult your doctor if your child is pregnant or becomes pregnant during treatment.

IMPORTANT PRECAUTIONS

- Do not allow your child to get overheated, as oxybutynin decreases sweating and may lead to heat stroke.
- Because oxybutynin can cause drowsiness, know how your child reacts to this drug before you allow him or her to participate in potentially hazardous activities, such as riding a bike, driving a car, or operating machinery.
- Store oxybutynin in a tightly closed container and keep away from excess heat and moisture (e.g., the bathroom, near a stove or sink). The syrup can be refrigerated, but do not allow it to freeze.

OXYMETAZOLINE

BRAND NAMES

Afrin, Afrin Children's Strength Nose Drops, Allerest 12 Hour, Dristan Long-Acting, Duramist Plus 12 Hour, Duration 12 Hour 4-Way Long Acting, Genasal, Neo-Synephrine

12 Hour, Oxymeta-12, Sinarest 12 Hour, Vicks Sinex Long
Acting
Generic Available/Over-the-Counter Available

ABOUT THIS DRUG
Oxymetazoline is a decongestant that is used to relieve nasal
congestion caused by allergies, sinus conditions, or colds.
This drug constricts the blood vessels to reduce the flow of
blood to swollen nasal passages, which in turn reduces the
amount of nasal secretions and improves airflow.

SIDE EFFECTS
Contact your doctor if your child experiences any side effects that are persistent or troubling, including any that are
not listed here.

- *Most common:* burning, dryness, or stinging inside the
  nose
- *Less common/rare:* excitability, headache, rapid or irregular heartbeat, restlessness

HOW TO USE THIS DRUG
Oxymetazoline is available as nasal spray and nasal drops.
The dosages given here are ones that are usually recommended for children. However, your doctor will determine
the most appropriate dose and schedule for your child.

- Children younger than 2 years: not recommended
- Children 2 to 6 years: 2 or 3 drops of the 0.025% solution in each nostril twice daily, in the morning and
  evening
- Children 7 years and older: 2 or 3 drops or sprays of
  0.05% solution in each nostril twice daily, in the morning and evening

If your child misses a dose, give it as soon as you remember. If it is nearly time for the next dose, skip the missed
dose and continue with the regular dosing schedule. Never
give a double dose.

TIME UNTIL IT TAKES EFFECT
5 to 30 minutes

POSSIBLE DRUG, FOOD, AND/OR SUPPLEMENT INTERACTIONS
Tell your doctor if your child is taking any prescription or over-the-counter medications or any vitamins, herbs, or other supplements. Possible interactions with oxymetazoline may include the following:

- Oxymetazoline may interact with tricyclic antidepressants or maprotiline and cause an increase in blood pressure.
- Alcohol should be avoided.

SYMPTOMS OF OVERDOSE
Symptoms include dizziness, headache, increased sweating, nervousness, paleness, rapid irregular heartbeat, and trembling. If overdose occurs, seek immediate medical attention and bring the drug container(s) with you.

THINGS TO TELL YOUR DOCTOR
- Tell your doctor if your child has had allergic reactions to any medications in the past or if he or she is taking any medications, herbal remedies, or supplements now.
- Let your doctor know if your child has blood vessel disease, diabetes, heart disease, hypothyroidism.
- Do not give this drug to your child for more than 3 days without first consulting your doctor. Prolonged use may result in rebound congestion (severe congestion caused by the body's adaptation to the drug).
- Consult your doctor if your child is pregnant or becomes pregnant during treatment.

IMPORTANT PRECAUTIONS
- Store oxymetazoline in a tightly closed container and keep away from excess heat and moisture (e.g., the bathroom, near a stove or sink). Do not allow it to freeze.

OXYTETRACYCLINE—
see *Tetracycline Antibiotics*

PALONOSETRON—see *Antiemetics*

PANCRELIPASE

BRAND NAMES
Cotazym, Cotazym-S, Ilozyme, Ku-Zyme HP, Pancrease, Pancrease MT, Protilase, Ultrase MT, Viokase, Zymase
Generic Available

ABOUT THIS DRUG
Pancrelipase is a pancreatic enzyme that is prescribed to replace the enzymes not being produced by a patient's pancreas. This drug contains the enzymes a healthy pancreas produces to digest fats, starches, and proteins.

SIDE EFFECTS
Contact your doctor if your child experiences any side effects that are persistent or troubling, including any that are not listed here.

* *Most common:* none
* *Less common/rare:* hives or rash

HOW TO USE THIS DRUG
Pancrelipase is available in capsules, delayed-release capsules, powder, and tablets. The dosages given here are ones that are usually recommended for children. However, your doctor will determine the most appropriate dose and schedule for your child.

Delayed-Release Capsules
* Infants 6 months to 1 year: contents of half a capsule per meal

- Children 1 to 6 years: contents of 1 to 2 capsules with meals
- Children older than 6 years: contents of 1 to 4 capsules with meals

Capsules
- Children 6 months to 12 years: contents of 1 to 3 capsules sprinkled on food with each meal
- Children 13 years and older: contents of 1 to 3 capsules before or with meals and snacks

Powder
- Children 6 months to 12 years: ¼ teaspoon with meals
- Children 13 years and older: ¼ teaspoon with meals and snacks

Tablets
- Children 6 months to 12 years: 1 to 2 tablets with meals
- Children 13 years and older: 1 to 3 tablets before or with meals and snacks

The contents of the capsules should be taken with liquid or in a small amount of soft food, such as applesauce, and swallowed without chewing. If your child misses a dose, give it as soon as you remember. If it is nearly time for the next dose, skip the missed dose and continue with the regular dosing schedule. Never give a double dose.

TIME UNTIL IT TAKES EFFECT
Variable

POSSIBLE DRUG, FOOD, AND/OR SUPPLEMENT INTERACTIONS
Tell your doctor if your child is taking any prescription or over-the-counter medications or any vitamins, herbs, or other supplements. Possible interactions with pancrelipase may include the following:

- Antacids that contain calcium carbonate and/or magnesium hydroxide may reduce the effectiveness of pancrelipase and should be avoided.
- Do not mix the contents of the capsules with alkaline foods (e.g., milk, ice cream) because the protective coating may dissolve prematurely and reduce its effect.

SYMPTOMS OF OVERDOSE

Symptoms include abdominal cramps, diarrhea, nausea, and vomiting. If overdose occurs, seek immediate medical attention and bring the drug container(s) with you.

THINGS TO TELL YOUR DOCTOR

- Tell your doctor if your child has had allergic reactions to any medications in the past or if he or she is taking any medications, herbal remedies, or supplements now.
- Let your doctor know if your child has pancreatitis.
- Consult your doctor if your child is pregnant or becomes pregnant during treatment.

IMPORTANT PRECAUTIONS

- Your doctor should monitor your child regularly while he or she is taking pancrelipase.
- Make sure your child or others who are around the powder or capsules do not inhale the powder or powder in the capsules, as it may cause shortness of breath, wheezing, tightness in the chest, and a stuffy nose.
- Store pancrelipase in a tightly closed container and keep away from excess heat and moisture (e.g., the bathroom, near a stove or sink).

PENICILLIN V POTASSIUM—
see *Penicillin Antibiotic*

CLASS: **PENICILLIN ANTIBIOTICS**

GENERICS
(1) amoxicillin; (2) ampicillin; (3) cloxacillin; (4) dicloxacillin; (5) nafcillin; (6) oxacillin; (7) penicillin V potassium

BRAND NAMES
(1) Amoxil, Biomox, Polymox, Trimox, Utimox, Wymox,
and available in combination with clavulanic acid (Aug-
mentin); (2) Ampicillin, D-Amp, Omnipen, Polycillin,
Principen, Totacillin; (3) Cloxapen; (4) Dycill, Dy-
cloxacillin sodium, Dynapen, Pathocil; (5) Unipen; (6) Bactocill, Prostaphlin, Oxacillin; (7) Beepen-VK, Betapen-VK,
Ledercillin VK, Penicillin VK, Pen-Vee K, Robicillin VK,
Uticillin VK, V-Cillin K, Veetids
Generic Available except for nafcillin

ABOUT THESE DRUGS
Penicillin antibiotics are a class of drugs used to treat various infections that affect the ears, sinuses, throat, respiratory
tract, heart, and genitourinary tract, which can include conditions such as pneumonia, ulcers, middle ear infections, sinusitis, strep throat, scarlet fever, and dental abscesses.
These drugs work by destroying the cell walls of the
disease-causing bacteria. They are not effective against
viruses, parasites, or fungi. Some bacteria are resistant to
penicillin antibiotics.

SIDE EFFECTS
Contact your doctor if your child experiences any side effects that are persistent or troubling, including any that are
not listed here.

- *Most common:* abdominal pain, coated tongue, colitis,
  diarrhea, nausea, oral or rectal fungal infection, sore
  mouth, upset stomach, vaginal irritation, vomiting
- *Less common/rare:* abnormally low white blood cell
  count, anemia, black tongue, bleeding abnormalities,

itchy eyes, jaundice, loss of appetite, severe skin reactions, superinfection

HOW TO USE THESE DRUGS

Penicillin antibiotics are available in many forms, including tablets, capsules, and oral suspension, and via intravenous injection. (Information on the injectable form is not provided here.) The dosages given here are ones that are usually recommended for children. However, your doctor will determine the most appropriate dose and schedule for your child.

Amoxicillin
- Children older than 3 months and weighing up to 88 lbs: the usual dose is 6.7 to 13.3 mg per lb of body weight every 8 hours or 5.7 to 10.2 mg per lb of body weight every 12 hours
- Children weighing more than 88 lbs: 250 mg every 8 hours for ear, nose, throat, skin, genital, and urinary tract infections; 500 mg every 8 hours for lower respiratory tract infections

Ampicillin
- Children weighing up to 44 lbs: the usual dose is 5.7 to 11.4 mg per lb of body weight every 6 hours or 7.6 to 15 mg per lb of body weight every 8 hours
- Children weighing more than 44 lbs: 250 to 500 mg given every 6 hours

Cloxacillin
- Children weighing up to 44 lbs: usual dose is 2.8 to 5.7 mg per lb of body weight every 6 hours
- Children weighing more than 44 lbs: 250 to 500 mg every 6 hours

Dicloxacillin
- Children weighing less than 88 lbs: dose to be determined by your doctor; the usual dose is 1.4 to 2.8 mg per lb of body weight given every 6 hours
- Children weighing 88 lbs or more: 125 to 250 mg

every 6 hours, for a total dosage of 500 to 1,000 mg daily

Nafcillin
- Given by injection, as determined by your doctor

Oxacillin
- Children weighing up to 88 lbs: 5.7 to 11.4 mg per lb of body weight every 6 hours
- Children weighing more than 88 lbs: 500 to 1,000 mg every 4 to 6 hours

Penicillin V Potassium
- Children 12 years and younger: dose is based on body weight and must be determined by your physician; the usual dose is 1.1 to 7.6 mg per lb of body weight every 4 to 8 hours
- Children 13 years and older: 125 to 500 mg every 6 or 8 hours
- To prevent infection after dental surgery, the usual dose is 1 g 30 to 60 minutes before the procedure and then 500 mg 6 hours after the procedure

Most penicillin antibiotics are best absorbed on an empty stomach. If your child experiences stomach upset, however, he or she can take them with food. If your child misses a dose, give it as soon as you remember. If it is nearly time for the next dose, skip the missed dose and continue with the regular dosing schedule. Never give a double dose.

TIME UNTIL THEY TAKE EFFECT
When oral forms are taken, it usually takes several days for them to affect the infection. Injectable forms usually provide an immediate response.

POSSIBLE DRUG, FOOD, AND/OR SUPPLEMENT INTERACTIONS
Tell your doctor if your child is taking any prescription or over-the-counter medications or any vitamins, herbs, or

other supplements. Possible interactions with penicillin antibiotics may include the following:

- Probenecid, rifampin, and warfarin may cause adverse effects.
- Other antibiotics, as well as cholestyramine, colestipol, and antacids, may decrease the effects of penicillin antibiotics.
- Amoxicillin increases the effects of methotrexate and allopurinol.
- Penicillin antibiotics may decrease the effectiveness of oral contraceptives.
- Iron supplements may make penicillin antibiotics less effective. Your child should take iron supplements at least 2 hours before or after the antibiotic dose.
- Penicillin antibiotics should not be taken with carbonated beverages or fruit juices.

SYMPTOMS OF OVERDOSE
Symptoms include severe diarrhea, nausea, stomach upset, and vomiting. If overdose occurs, seek immediate medical attention and bring the drug container(s) with you.

THINGS TO TELL YOUR DOCTOR
- Tell your doctor if your child has had allergic reactions to any medications in the past, especially to other penicillins or cephalosporin antibiotics, or if he or she is taking any medications, herbal remedies, or supplements now.
- Let your doctor know if your child has any of the following medical conditions: asthma, eczema, infectious mononucleosis, kidney disease, liver disease, stomach problems, other chronic conditions.
- Consult your doctor if your child is pregnant or becomes pregnant during treatment.

IMPORTANT PRECAUTIONS
- It is important that your child take the medication for the entire course of treatment, even if he or she feels better before scheduled treatment is complete. Stop-

ping treatment too soon may result in a serious, drug-resistant infection.

- Store any nonliquid form of penicillin antibiotics in a tightly closed container and keep away from excess heat and moisture (e.g., the bathroom, near a stove or sink). Generally, the liquid forms of these drugs are effective for only 7 days at room temperature, but 14 days if refrigerated. Do not freeze.

PERMETHRIN

BRAND NAMES
Acticin, Elimite, Nix, Rid
Generic Available

ABOUT THIS DRUG
Permethrin is an antiparasitic medication used to treat head lice and scabies. The lotion kills both the lice and their eggs, whereas the cream destroys the mites that cause scabies. In both cases, the parasites are eliminated because the drug interferes with their nervous systems.

SIDE EFFECTS
Contact your doctor if your child experiences any side effects that are persistent or troubling, including any that are not listed here.

- *Most common:* burning, itching, stinging
- *Less common/rare:* numbness, rash, redness, swelling, tingling

HOW TO USE THIS DRUG
Permethrin is available in 1% lotion to treat head lice in children 2 years and older and 5% cream to treat scabies in children 2 months and older. The instructions given here are ones that are usually recommended for children. However, your doctor will determine whether alternative action should be taken.

Head Lice

- Shampoo your child's hair and scalp with regular shampoo, rinse, and towel dry the hair and scalp.
- Allow the hair to air dry for several minutes.
- Shake the bottle of permethrin well. With your child's head over a sink (not in the shower or bathtub), apply the permethrin, thoroughly wetting the hair and scalp and covering the skin behind the ears and on the back of the neck.
- Leave the permethrin on the hair for 10 minutes.
- Rinse the hair thoroughly and towel dry.
- Use a fine-toothed comb to remove any lice eggs from the hair.
- Wash your hands to remove any residue of permethrin.

Scabies

- Give your infant (age 2 months or older) or child (or have your child take) a bath or shower.
- Apply the cream over the entire body, including the head, and massage it in well.
- Leave the cream on for 8 to 14 hours. It is recommended that you apply the cream before bedtime so it can work while your child sleeps. Any clothing your child will wear while the cream is on should be thoroughly cleaned in hot water and dried in a hot dryer to rid them of scabies prior to cream application.
- Wash off the cream using warm, soapy water in a shower or bath.

See "Important Precautions" for instructions on preventing reinfestation.

TIME UNTIL IT TAKES EFFECT
Shampoo, within 10 minutes; cream, 8 to 14 hours.

POSSIBLE DRUG, FOOD, AND/OR SUPPLEMENT INTERACTIONS
Tell your doctor if your child is taking any prescription or over-the-counter medications, especially other topical med-

ications, or any vitamins, herbs, or other supplements. No drug, food, or supplement interactions have been noted.

SYMPTOMS OF OVERDOSE
No overdose information is available. If your child accidentally ingests permethrin, seek immediate medical attention and bring the drug container(s) with you.

THINGS TO TELL YOUR DOCTOR
- Tell your doctor if your child has had allergic reactions to any medications in the past or if he or she is taking any medications, herbal remedies, or supplements now.
- Consult your doctor if your child is pregnant or becomes pregnant during treatment.

IMPORTANT PRECAUTIONS
- Permethrin should not be applied around the mouth, nose, or eyes. If you accidentally get the medication into the eyes, flush them immediately with lots of water. If eye irritation persists, call your physician.
- Because parasites are easily transferred from one person to another either through direct contact or by touching or using clothing or other items such as bed linens, hair brushes, and combs, it is critical that you take steps to prevent infection or reinfection. Therefore, wash clothing, bedding, and towels in very hot water, soak hair brushes and combs in hot water, and do not allow anyone to share these items. If there are items that cannot be washed, place them in an airtight plastic bag for one week. This deprives the parasites of oxygen and they die.
- Store permethrin in a tightly closed container and keep at room temperature away from excess heat and moisture (e.g., the bathroom, near a stove or sink).

PHENYLEPHRINE (NASAL)

BRAND NAMES
Alconefrin, Doktors, Duration, Neo-Synephrine, Nostril Spray Pump, Rhinall, Vicks Sinex
Generic Available/Over-the-Counter Available

ABOUT THIS DRUG
Phenylephrine (nasal) is a decongestant used to relieve nasal congestion caused by allergies, sinus conditions, and colds and to relieve congestion that can accompany ear infections. It works by constricting the blood vessels, which in turn reduces blood flow to swollen nasal tissues and improves nasal air flow.

SIDE EFFECTS
Contact your doctor if your child experiences any side effects that are persistent or troubling, including any that are not listed here.

- *Most common:* burning, dryness, or stinging inside the nose
- *Less common/rare:* excitability, headache, rapid or irregular heartbeat, restlessness

HOW TO USE THIS DRUG
Phenylephrine (nasal) is available as a nasal jelly, nasal drops, and nasal spray. The dosages given here are ones that are usually recommended for children. However, your doctor will determine the most appropriate dose and schedule for your child.

- Children younger than 6 years: 2 to 3 drops of 0.125% solution every 4 hours
- Children 6 to 12 years: 2 to 3 drops or 1 to 2 sprays of the 0.25% solution in each nostril every 4 hours
- Children 13 years and older: 2 to 3 drops of 0.25% to 0.5% solution or 1 to 2 sprays, or a small amount of jelly in each nostril every 4 hours

TIME UNTIL IT TAKES EFFECT
Within minutes

POSSIBLE DRUG, FOOD, AND/OR SUPPLEMENT INTERACTIONS
Tell your doctor if your child is taking any prescription or over-the-counter medications or any vitamins, herbs, or other supplements. Possible interactions with phenylephrine may include the following:

- Monoamine oxidase (MAO) inhibitors (e.g., phenelzine, isocarboxazid) should not be taken within 14 days of using phenylephrine, as serious side effects could occur.
- Tricyclic antidepressants (e.g., amitriptyline, imipramine), medications used to treat diabetes, high blood pressure, or heart disease, or any other decongestant could have a negative effect if taken along with phenylephrine.

SYMPTOMS OF OVERDOSE
Symptoms include dizziness; headache; increased sweating; insomnia; nervousness; paleness; rapid, irregular, or pounding heartbeat; and trembling. If overdose occurs, seek immediate medical attention and bring the drug container(s) with you.

THINGS TO TELL YOUR DOCTOR
- Tell your doctor if your child has had allergic reactions to any medications in the past or if he or she is taking any medications, herbal remedies, or supplements now.
- Let your doctor know if your child has a history of blood vessel disease, diabetes, heart disease, high blood pressure, or hypothyroidism.

IMPORTANT PRECAUTIONS
- There are special instructions on how to administer each form of this drug. Ask your doctor, pharmacist, or nurse practitioner how to correctly give the form you have chosen.

- Store phenylephrine in a tightly closed container and keep away from excess heat and moisture (e.g., the bathroom, near a stove or sink).

PHENYLEPHRINE (OPHTHALMIC)

BRAND NAMES
Ak-Dilate, Ak-Nefrin, Dilatair, I-Phrine, Isopto Frin, Mydfrin, Neo-Synephrine Ophthalmic, Ocugestrin, Ocu-Phrin, Phenoptic, Prefrin Liquifilm, Relief Eye Drops for Red Eyes
Generic Available/Over-the-Counter Available

ABOUT THIS DRUG
Phenylephrine (ophthalmic) is an adrenergic agent that is used to treat certain eye conditions. Your child may also receive this drug when he or she undergoes an eye examination, as it is used to dilate the pupils to facilitate examination. Ophthalmic phenylephrine affects the muscles that control the pupils and causes them to dilate, and it also constricts the superficial blood vessels in the whites of the eye to reduce redness.

SIDE EFFECTS
Contact your doctor if your child experiences any side effects that are persistent or troubling, including any that are not listed here.

- *Most common:* burning, stinging, or watering of the eyes, eyes that are overly sensitive to light; headache; unusually large pupils
- *Less common/rare:* eye irritation that was not present before treatment

HOW TO USE THIS DRUG
Phenylephrine (ophthalmic) is available in 2.5% and 10% solution. The dosages given here are ones that are usually recommended for children. However, your doctor will determine the most appropriate dose and schedule for your child.

- Children younger than 12 years: one drop of 2.5% solution in the affected eye 1 to 3 times daily, depending on the eye condition and the age of the child; your doctor will determine the dose
- Children 12 years and older: one drop of 2.5% or 10% solution in the affected eye 1 to 3 times daily, depending on the eye condition

If your child misses a dose, give it as soon as you remember. If it is nearly time for the next dose, skip the missed dose and continue with the regular dosing schedule. Never give a double dose.

TIME UNTIL IT TAKES EFFECT
Within minutes

POSSIBLE DRUG, FOOD, AND/OR SUPPLEMENT INTERACTIONS
Tell your doctor if your child is taking any prescription or over-the-counter medications, especially other eye drops, or any vitamins, herbs, or other supplements. No specific drug, food, or supplement interactions have been noted.

SYMPTOMS OF OVERDOSE
Symptoms include coma; dizziness; paleness; rapid, irregular, or pounding heartbeat; profuse sweating; trembling; and vomiting. If overdose occurs, seek immediate medical attention and bring the drug container(s) with you.

THINGS TO TELL YOUR DOCTOR
- Tell your doctor if your child has had allergic reactions to any medications in the past or if he or she is taking any medications, herbal remedies, or supplements now.
- Let your doctor know if your child has a history of blood vessel disease, closed-angle glaucoma, diabetes, heart disease, high blood pressure, or idiopathic orthostatic hypotension.
- Consult your doctor if your child is pregnant or becomes pregnant during treatment.

IMPORTANT PRECAUTIONS

- Because phenylephrine causes the pupils to become unusually large, your child's eyes will be especially sensitive to light while using this drug. He or she should wear sunglasses that block ultraviolet rays both outdoors (even when cloudy) and indoors if there are bright lights.
- Store phenylephrine in a tightly closed container and keep at room temperature away from excess heat and moisture (e.g., the bathroom, near a stove or sink). Do not allow the medicine to freeze.

PHENYTOIN

BRAND NAMES
Dilantin, Dilantin Infatabs, Diphenylan
Generic Available

ABOUT THIS DRUG
Phenytoin is a hydantoin anticonvulsant used to relieve epileptic seizures. It works by inhibiting activity in the area of the brain that is associated with grand mal seizures. Phenytoin usually is taken along with other anticonvulsants.

SIDE EFFECTS
Contact your doctor if your child experiences any side effects that are persistent or troubling, including any that are not listed here. Side effects usually are more common at the start of treatment but tend to disappear over time. If symptoms are prolonged or severe, contact your doctor.

- *Most common:* dizziness, drowsiness, irritability, impaired coordination, mental confusion, nervousness, unusual eye movements
- *Less common/rare:* excessive hair growth on the body or face, breast development in males, clumsiness, confusion, diarrhea, fever, headache, inflamed or bleeding

gums, itching, learning difficulties, nausea, rash, sensitivity to light, shallow breathing, slurred speech, stuttering, swollen glands, vomiting, weight gain

HOW TO USE THIS DRUG

Phenytoin is available as chewable tablets, immediate-release and extended-release capsules, and oral suspension. Dosages of phenytoin are highly individualized to a person's unique needs. The dosage given here is a generally accepted starting point; however, your doctor will determine the most appropriate dose and schedule for your child.

- Infants and Children: 2.5 mg per lb of body weight to start, which your doctor may increase gradually as needed to a usual maximum daily dosage of 300 mg; dosing may be 1 to 3 times daily

Phenytoin can be taken with food to prevent stomach irritation. If your child misses a dose, give it as soon as you remember. If it is within 4 hours of the next dose, skip the missed dose and continue with the regular dosing schedule. Never give a double dose.

TIME UNTIL IT TAKES EFFECT
Several hours

POSSIBLE DRUG, FOOD, AND/OR SUPPLEMENT INTERACTIONS
Tell your doctor if your child is taking any prescription or over-the-counter medications or any vitamins, herbs, or other supplements. Possible interactions with phenytoin may include the following:

- Phenytoin may increase the effectiveness of other anticonvulsants.
- Use of sedatives, antidepressants, tranquilizers, or narcotics may cause increased sedation and drowsiness.
- Phenytoin reduces the effectiveness of many drugs, including but not limited to amiodarone, carbamazepine,

    corticosteroids, digitalis drugs, disopyramide, doxycycline, estrogens, haloperidol, methadone, oral contraceptives, quinine, theophylline, and valproic acid.

- Because phenytoin may reduce the effectiveness of oral contraceptives, a backup method of birth control should be used if your child is taking phenytoin.
- Antacids, antidiarrheal drugs, and calcium supplements should be taken at least 2 to 3 hours before or after phenytoin.
- Phenytoin can interact with many other drugs, including but not limited to acetaminophen, aspirin, cyclosporine, insulin, lidocaine, lithium, mebendazole, meperidine, tricyclic antidepressants, and warfarin.
- Avoid use of herbs that have sedative effects, such as hops, kava, passionflower, and valerian.
- Do not take phenytoin within 1 to 2 hours of ingesting high-calcium foods, such as milk or cheese.

SYMPTOMS OF OVERDOSE

An overdose can be fatal. Symptoms include clumsiness, confusion, dizziness, double or blurry vision, loss of coordination, slurred speech, staggering, and unsteadiness. If overdose occurs, seek immediate medical attention and bring the drug container(s) with you.

THINGS TO TELL YOUR DOCTOR

- Tell your doctor if your child has had allergic reactions to any medications in the past or if he or she is taking any medications, herbal remedies, or supplements now.
- Let your doctor know if your child has any of the following medical conditions: blood diseases, diabetes, heart disease, low blood pressure, kidney or liver disease, lupus, porphyria, slow heart rate, or thyroid disease.
- Consult your doctor if your child is pregnant or becomes pregnant during treatment. Phenytoin, like other anticonvulsants, is associated with an increased risk of birth defects.

IMPORTANT PRECAUTIONS

- Do not stop phenytoin suddenly or switch brands without first consulting your doctor.
- Because phenytoin can cause dizziness and drowsiness, make sure you know how your child reacts to this drug before he or she participates in potentially hazardous activities, such as riding a bike, driving a car, or operating machinery.
- Phenytoin increases sensitivity to sunlight, so make sure your child is adequately protected from the sun (e.g., sunscreen, appropriate clothing).
- Phenytoin can affect the gums, so be sure your child has regular dental checkups.
- Regular blood tests are necessary to monitor how your child's body is absorbing phenytoin, especially during the first few months of treatment.
- Store phenytoin in a tightly closed container and keep away from excess heat and moisture (e.g., the bathroom, near a stove or sink). Do not refrigerate the oral suspension.

PIMECROLIMUS

BRAND NAME
Elidel
Generic Not Available

ABOUT THIS DRUG
Pimecrolimus is a topical medication used to treat symptoms of atopic dermatitis, also known as eczema. It relieves itching, inflammation, and redness associated with this skin disorder.

SIDE EFFECTS
Contact your doctor if your child experiences any side effects that are persistent or troubling, including any that are not listed here.

- *Most common:* coldlike symptoms (e.g., sore throat, cough), feeling of warmth where applied, headache
- *Less common/rare:* viral skin infection

HOW TO USE THIS DRUG

Pimecrolimus is available as a cream. The dosages given here are ones that are usually recommended for children. However, your doctor will determine the most appropriate dose and schedule for your child.

- Children younger than 2 years: not recommended
- Children 2 years and older: apply a thin layer to the affected areas twice daily

Pimecrolimus can be applied to all areas of the skin, including the face and neck, but avoid contact with the eyes. If your child misses a dose, apply the cream as soon as you remember. If it is nearly time for the next dose, skip the missed dose and continue with the regular schedule.

TIME UNTIL IT TAKES EFFECT

Usually 8 to 15 days

POSSIBLE DRUG, FOOD, AND/OR SUPPLEMENT INTERACTIONS

Tell your doctor if your child is taking any prescription or over-the-counter medications or any vitamins, herbs, or other supplements. Possible interactions with pimecrolimus may include the following:

- Other topical medications may react with pimecrolimus. Consult with your doctor before using pimecrolimus with another topical drug.
- Caution should be used if using pimecrolimus along with drugs that inhibit liver enzymes, such as ketoconazole, itraconazole, erythromycin, or fluconazole.

SYMPTOMS OF OVERDOSE
Overdose is unlikely. If your child accidentally ingests pimecrolimus, seek immediate medical attention and bring the drug container(s) with you.

THINGS TO TELL YOUR DOCTOR
- Tell your doctor if your child has had allergic reactions to any medications in the past or if he or she is taking any medications, herbal remedies, or supplements now.
- Let your doctor know if your child has Netherton's syndrome or any other skin condition or a weakened immune system.

IMPORTANT PRECAUTIONS
- Pimecrolimus can increase your child's sensitivity to sunlight; therefore, be sure he or she uses sunscreen, sunglasses, protective clothing, and a hat to avoid excessive exposure to the sun.
- The potential risk of cancer associated with pimecrolimus is not clear; thus, this drug should not be the first drug used for your child's condition.
- Store pimecrolimus in a tightly closed container and keep away from excess heat and moisture (e.g., the bathroom, near a stove or sink).

PREDNICARBATE—
see *Corticosteroids, Topical*

PREDNISOLONE—see *Corticosteroids, Oral*

PREDNISONE—see *Corticosteroids, Oral*

PRIMIDONE

BRAND NAMES
Myidone, Mysoline
Generic Available

ABOUT THIS DRUG
Primidone is an anticonvulsant used to manage certain types of seizures associated with epilepsy. It appears to suppress the activity of specific areas of the brain and especially the abnormal firing of neurons that cause seizures.

SIDE EFFECTS
Contact your doctor if your child experiences any side effects that are persistent or troubling, including any that are not listed here.

- *Most common:* dizziness, drowsiness, double vision, hyperactivity, loss of coordination
- *Less common/rare:* lethargy followed by insomnia, loss of appetite, mental or mood changes, nausea, rash, vomiting

HOW TO USE THIS DRUG
Primidone is available in tablets and as a liquid suspension. The dosages given here are ones that are usually recommended for children. However, your doctor will determine the most appropriate dose and schedule for your child.

- Children younger than 8 years who have not been treated previously: 50 mg at bedtime on days 1 to 3, 50 mg twice daily days 4 to 6, 100 mg twice daily days 7 to 9, thereafter as maintenance 125 to 250 mg 3 times daily; alternatively, maintenance dosage can be 10 to 25 mg per 2.2 lb of body weight per day divided into smaller doses
- Children 8 years and older who have not been treated previously: 100 to 125 mg at bedtime on days 1 to 3, 100 to 125 mg twice daily days 4 to 6, 100 to 125 mg 3 times daily days 7 to 9; thereafter as maintenance 250 mg 3 times daily

- If your child is already receiving an anticonvulsant, the usual starting dose is 100 to 125 mg at bedtime. Your doctor may gradually increase this dose while decreasing the other drug's dose until a balance is reached with both drugs or primidone is the sole drug used.

Primidone can be taken with food to prevent stomach irritation. If your child misses a dose, give it as soon as you remember. If it is nearly time for the next dose, skip the missed dose and continue the regular dosing schedule. Do not give a double dose.

TIME UNTIL IT TAKES EFFECT
Several hours

POSSIBLE DRUG, FOOD, AND/OR SUPPLEMENT INTERACTIONS
Tell your doctor if your child is taking any prescription or over-the-counter medications or any vitamins, herbs, or other supplements. Possible interactions with primidone may include the following:

- Primidone may cause oral contraceptives to fail. A backup method of birth control is recommended if your child is taking primidone.
- Interactions may occur with the following drugs: other anticonvulsants (e.g., phenytoin), benzodiazepines, caffeine, calcium channel blockers, corticosteroids, corticotropin, cyclophosphamide, cyclosporine, digitoxin, disopyramide, doxycycline, general anesthetics, griseofulvin, haloperidol, isoniazid, loxapine, maprotiline, metoprolol, propranolol, quinidine, theophylline, tricyclic antidepressants, vitamin D, warfarin.

SYMPTOMS OF OVERDOSE
Symptoms include difficulty breathing, drowsiness, and loss of consciousness. If overdose occurs, seek immediate medical attention and bring the drug container(s) with you.

THINGS TO TELL YOUR DOCTOR

- Tell your doctor if your child has had allergic reactions to any medications in the past or if he or she is taking any medications, herbal remedies, or supplements now.
- Let your doctor know if your child has any of the following medical conditions: asthma, chronic lung disease, hyperactivity, kidney or liver disease, porphyria.
- Consult your doctor if your child is pregnant or becomes pregnant during treatment. Like other anticonvulsants, primidone is associated with birth defects and bleeding problems.

IMPORTANT PRECAUTIONS

- Primidone is often given as long-term therapy. If your child requires long-term treatment, your doctor will likely check his or her blood levels regularly.
- Your child should carry an identification card or bracelet saying that he or she is taking primidone and has a seizure disorder.
- Store primidone in a tightly closed container and keep away from excess heat and moisture (e.g., the bathroom, near a stove or sink). Do not freeze the liquid form.

PROMETHAZINE

BRAND NAMES

Anergan, Phenazine, Phencen, Phenergan, Prometh, Prorex, V-Gan
Generic Available

ABOUT THIS DRUG

Promethazine is an antihistamine that is prescribed to relieve the symptoms of hay fever and other allergies. It is also effective in preventing motion sickness and in the treatment of nausea and vomiting. It works by interfering with the release and activity of histamine, a naturally occurring agent that causes sneezing, watery eyes, itching, and other allergy symptoms. Promethazine also relaxes smooth muscle that controls the stomach, intestines, lungs, and other organs, which helps relieve symptoms of motion sickness and gastrointestinal irritation.

SIDE EFFECTS
Contact your doctor if your child experiences any side effects that are persistent or troubling, including any that are not listed here.

- *Most common:* drowsiness, thickened mucus
- *Less common/rare:* blurry vision, confusion, difficult urination, dizziness, dry mouth or nose, faintness, increased sweating, loss of appetite, rapid heartbeat, rash, ringing in ears, unusual irritability

HOW TO USE THIS DRUG
Promethazine is available in tablets, syrup, and suppositories and via injection. (Information on the injectable form is not provided here.) The dosages given here are ones that are usually recommended for children. However, your doctor will determine the most appropriate dose and schedule for your child.

For Allergies
- Children 2 to 12 years: Tablets or syrup—5 to 12.5 mg 3 times daily or 25 mg at bedtime; suppositories—6.25 to 12.5 mg 3 times daily or 25 mg at bedtime
- Children 13 years and older: Tablets or syrup—10 to 12.5 mg 4 times daily before meals and at bedtime, or 25 mg at bedtime; suppositories—25 mg at first, 25 mg 2 hours later, if needed

For Nausea and Vomiting
- Children 2 to 12 years: Tablets or syrup—10 to 25 mg every 4 to 6 hours; suppositories—25 mg at first, then 12.5 to 25 mg every 4 to 6 hours, if needed
- Children 13 years and older: Tablets or syrup—25 mg at first, then 10 to 25 mg every 4 to 6 hours as needed

Motion Sickness
- Children 2 to 12 years: Tablets or syrup—10 to 25 mg taken 30 to 60 minutes before traveling
- Children 13 years and older: 25 mg taken 30 to 60 minutes before traveling

Promethazine can be taken with food to prevent stomach irritation. If your child misses a dose, give it as soon as you remember. If it is nearly time for the next dose, skip the missed dose and continue with the regular dosing schedule. Never give a double dose.

TIME UNTIL IT TAKES EFFECT
15 to 60 minutes for oral forms

POSSIBLE DRUG, FOOD, AND/OR SUPPLEMENT INTERACTIONS
Tell your doctor if your child is taking any prescription or over-the-counter medications or any vitamins, herbs, or other supplements. Possible interactions with promethazine may include the following:

- Interactions may occur with the following drugs: amoxapine, anticholinergics, antihistamines, antipsychotic drugs, barbiturates, central nervous system depressants, monoamine oxidase (MAO) inhibitors, methyldopa, metoclopramide, metrizamide, pimozide, tricyclic antidepressants, and others.
- Avoid use of alcohol.

SYMPTOMS OF OVERDOSE
Symptoms include difficulty breathing; clumsiness; dizziness; dry mouth, nose, or throat; hallucinations; insomnia; jerky movements of the head and face; muscle spasms; seizures; and trembling hands. If overdose occurs, seek immediate medical attention and bring the drug container(s) with you.

THINGS TO TELL YOUR DOCTOR
- Tell your doctor if your child has had allergic reactions to any medications in the past or if he or she is taking any medications, herbal remedies, or supplements now.
- Let your doctor know if your child has any of the following medical conditions: blood disease, emphysema, epilepsy, glaucoma, heart disease, jaundice, liver disease, peptic ulcer, Reye's syndrome, sleep apnea, urinary tract blockage.
- Consult your doctor if your child is pregnant or becomes pregnant during treatment. Use of promethazine within 2 weeks of delivery may result in a newborn who has jaundice or blood clotting problems.

IMPORTANT PRECAUTIONS
- Prolonged use of promethazine can cause a decrease in salivary flow, which can result in thrush, periodontal disease, dental caries, and gingivitis. Therefore, make sure your child drinks plenty of fluids and brushes after every meal.
- Store promethazine in a tightly closed container and keep away from excess heat and moisture (e.g., the bathroom, near a stove or sink). Do not allow the syrup to freeze.

PSEUDOEPHEDRINE

BRAND NAMES
Afrinol, Decofed Syrup, Drixoral Non-Drowsy, Neofed, Novafed, PediaCare Oral, Sudafed, Sudafed 12 Hour, Sufedrin, Triaminic AM Decongestant Formula
Generic Available/Over-the-Counter Available

ABOUT THIS DRUG
Pseudoephedrine is a decongestant and cough medication used to relieve nasal and sinus congestion associated with hay fever and other respiratory allergies, sinus infections, and colds. This drug constricts blood vessels, which in turn

reduces the flow of blood to swollen nasal passages and thus improves air flow in the nasal passages.

SIDE EFFECTS

Contact your doctor if your child experiences any side effects that are persistent or troubling, including any that are not listed here.

- *Most common:* insomnia, nervousness, restlessness
- *Less common/rare:* dizziness, difficult or painful urination, increased sweating, nausea, paleness, rapid or pounding heartbeat, trembling, vomiting, weakness

HOW TO USE THIS DRUG

Pseudoephedrine is available in tablets, extended-release capsules, oral solution, and syrup. The dosages given here are ones that are usually recommended for children. However, your doctor will determine the most appropriate dose and schedule for your child.

- Children 2 to 6 years: 15 mg every 4 hours, not to exceed 60 mg in 24 hours
- Children 7 to 12 years: 30 mg every 4 to 6 hours, not to exceed 120 mg in 24 hours
- Children 13 years and older: 60 mg every 4 to 6 hours, not to exceed 240 mg in 24 hours. If taking extended-release capsules, 120 mg every 12 hours or 240 mg every 24 hours. Neither form should exceed 240 mg in 24 hours.

TIME UNTIL IT TAKES EFFECT

15 to 30 minutes

POSSIBLE DRUG, FOOD, AND/OR SUPPLEMENT INTERACTIONS

Tell your doctor if your child is taking any prescription or over-the-counter medications or any vitamins, herbs, or other supplements. Possible interactions with pseudoephedrine may include the following:

- Monoamine oxidase (MAO) inhibitors should not be taken with or within 2 weeks of pseudoephedrine, as serious side effects may occur.
- Talk to your doctor if your child is taking beta-blockers.

SYMPTOMS OF OVERDOSE
Symptoms include changes in mental state, dizziness, drowsiness, hallucinations, loss of consciousness, low blood pressure, profuse sweating, reduced urine output, and seizures. If overdose occurs, seek immediate medical attention and bring the drug container(s) with you.

THINGS TO TELL YOUR DOCTOR
- Tell your doctor if your child has had allergic reactions to any medications in the past or if he or she is taking any medications, herbal remedies, or supplements now.
- Let your doctor know if your child has blood vessel disease, diabetes, heart disease, high blood pressure, or hypothyroidism.
- Consult your doctor if your child is pregnant or becomes pregnant during treatment.

IMPORTANT PRECAUTIONS
- To help prevent insomnia, the last dose of the day should be taken at least 2 hours before bedtime.
- If your child's symptoms don't improve within 7 days, contact your doctor.
- Store pseudoephedrine in a tightly closed container and keep away from excess heat and moisture (e.g., the bathroom, near a stove or sink). Do not allow the liquid form to freeze.

PSYLLIUM

BRAND NAMES
Fiberall Powder, Fiberall Wafer, Konsyl, Metamucil, Modane Bulk, Natural Vegetable, Perdiem Fiber, Reguloid, Serutan, Syllact
Generic Available/Over-the-Counter Available

ABOUT THIS DRUG
Psyllium is a bulk-forming laxative that is used to relieve constipation, although it can also be used to treat diarrhea. It is a natural fiber that absorbs liquid in the intestines and swells to produce bulky stool, which in turn stimulates bowel activity and defecation.

SIDE EFFECTS
Contact your doctor if your child experiences any side effects that are persistent or troubling, including any that are not listed here.

- *Most common:* none
- *Less common/rare:* abdominal pain or cramps, nausea, partial intestinal obstruction, vomiting

HOW TO USE THIS DRUG
Psyllium is available as granules, powder, wafers, and caramels. The dosages given here are ones that are usually recommended for children. However, your doctor will determine the most appropriate dose and schedule for your child.

- Children younger than 6 years: not recommended
- Children 6 years and older: 1 level teaspoon of granules or powder in 4 to 8 ounces of water 1 to 3 times per day, as needed

Each dose of psyllium should be followed by a full (8-ounce) glass of water or juice. If your child misses a dose, give it as soon as you remember. If it is nearly time for the next dose, skip the missed dose and continue with the regular dosing schedule. Never give a double dose.

TIME UNTIL IT TAKES EFFECT
Usually 12 to 24 hours, but may be as long as 3 days

POSSIBLE DRUG, FOOD, AND/OR SUPPLEMENT INTERACTIONS
Tell your doctor if your child is taking any prescription or over-the-counter medications or any vitamins, herbs, or other supplements. Possible interactions with psyllium may include the following:

- Talk to your doctor if your child is taking oral tetracycline antibiotics.
- Concomitant use of lithium, carbamazepine, digoxin, or warfarin may reduce the absorption of these drugs.
- Psyllium may increase the cholesterol-reducing abilities of cholestyramine.
- Psyllium may reduce the body's absorption of minerals such as calcium, copper, iron, magnesium, and zinc.

SYMPTOMS OF OVERDOSE
An overdose could result in intestinal blockage. If overdose occurs, seek immediate medical attention and bring the drug container(s) with you.

THINGS TO TELL YOUR DOCTOR
- Tell your doctor if your child has had allergic reactions to any medications in the past or if he or she is taking any medications, herbal remedies, or supplements now.
- Let your doctor know if your child has any type of fecal impaction, intestinal obstruction, difficulty swallowing, or esophageal narrowing or if he or she has a colostomy or ileostomy, diabetes, heart disease, high blood pressure, kidney disease, or unexplained rectal bleeding.
- Consult your doctor if your child is pregnant or becomes pregnant during treatment.

IMPORTANT PRECAUTIONS

- Store psyllium in a tightly closed container and keep away from excess heat and moisture (e.g., the bathroom, near a stove or sink).

PYRETHRIN PLUS PIPERONYL BUTOXIDE

BRAND NAMES

A-200 Gel Concentrate, A-200 Shampoo Concentrate, Barc, Blue, Licetrol, Pronto Lice Killing Shampoo Kit, Pyrinyl, R&C, Rid, Tisit, Triple X
Generic Available/Over-the-Counter Available

ABOUT THIS DRUG

Pyrethrin + piperonyl butoxide is a combination topical antiparasitic medication used to treat lice infestations. The medication is absorbed into the bodies of lice, where it damages the nervous system, causing paralysis and death. The drug does not have this effect on humans.

SIDE EFFECTS

Contact your doctor if your child experiences any side effects that are persistent or troubling, including any that are not listed here.

- *Most common:* none
- *Less common/rare:* skin irritation, rash

HOW TO USE THIS DRUG

Pyrethrin + piperonyl butoxide is available as gel, shampoo, and topical solution. The use instructions given here are ones that are usually recommended for children. However, your doctor will determine the most appropriate dose and schedule for your child.

- Gel or solution: apply enough of the medication to thoroughly wet your infant's or child's hair, scalp, or skin. Allow the medication to remain on the treated areas for 10 minutes, then wash it off with warm water and soap or regular shampoo. Dry the skin or hair with a clean towel.

• Shampoo: Apply enough of the medicated shampoo to wet your infant's or child's hair, scalp, or skin. Allow the medication to remain on the treated areas for 10 minutes, then use a small amount of water to work the shampoo more thoroughly into the treated areas. Rinse thoroughly and dry with a clean towel.

You should use a nit-removal comb to remove dead lice and eggs from your child's hair. This entire process should be repeated one more time 7 to 10 days after the first treatment. If you forget to do the second treatment within that time, do it as soon as you remember.

TIME UNTIL IT TAKES EFFECT
Within 10 minutes

POSSIBLE DRUG, FOOD, AND/OR SUPPLEMENT INTERACTIONS
Tell your doctor if your child is taking any prescription or over-the-counter medications or any vitamins, herbs, or other supplements. There are no significant interactions to note.

SYMPTOMS OF OVERDOSE
If your child accidentally ingests pyrethrin + piperonyl butoxide, he or she may experience the following symptoms: central nervous system depression, muscle paralysis, nausea, and vomiting. If accidental ingestion does occur, seek immediate medical attention and bring the drug container(s) with you.

THINGS TO TELL YOUR DOCTOR
• Tell your doctor if your child has had allergic reactions to any medications in the past or if he or she is taking any medications, herbal remedies, or supplements now. Also tell your doctor about any history of negative re-

actions to ragweed, chrysanthemum plants, kerosene, or other petroleum products.
- Let your doctor know if your child has any severe skin inflammations.
- Consult your doctor if your child is pregnant.

IMPORTANT PRECAUTIONS
- Store pyrethrin + piperonyl butoxide in a tightly closed container and keep at room temperature away from excess heat and moisture (e.g., the bathroom, near a stove or sink).

RIMANTADINE

BRAND NAME
Flumadine
Generic Not Available

ABOUT THIS DRUG
Rimantadine is an antiviral medication used to prevent or treat influenza type A. This drug hinders the activity of the virus's genetic material by blocking a process that allows it to reproduce. Rimantadine is effective against only certain strains of the influenza type A virus.

SIDE EFFECTS
Contact your doctor if your child experiences any side effects that are persistent or troubling, including any that are not listed here.

- *Most common:* diarrhea (mild), nausea, vomiting
- *Less common/rare:* dizziness, dry mouth, fatigue, insomnia, loss of appetite, nervousness, stomach pain, trouble with concentration

HOW TO USE THIS DRUG
Rimantadine is available as tablets and syrup. The dosages given here are ones that are usually recommended for chil-

dren. However, your doctor will determine the most appropriate dose and schedule for your child.

- Children younger than 10 years: 2.3 mg per lb of body weight once daily, not to exceed 150 mg daily
- Children 10 years and older: 100 mg twice daily

Rimantadine should be taken for about 7 days. It is best taken on an empty stomach at least 1 hour before or 2 hours after a meal. If your child misses a dose, give it as soon as you remember. If it is nearly time for the next dose, skip the missed dose and continue with the regular dosing schedule. Never give a double dose.

TIME UNTIL IT TAKES EFFECT
Unknown. To prevent the flu, give rimantadine to your child prior to or immediately after your child is exposed to the flu.

POSSIBLE DRUG, FOOD, AND/OR SUPPLEMENT INTERACTIONS
Tell your doctor if your child is taking any prescription or over-the-counter medications or any vitamins, herbs, or other supplements. Possible interactions with rimantadine may include the following:

- Medications that stimulate the central nervous system (e.g., caffeine, decongestants, diet pills) may increase the side effects of rimantadine.
- Acetaminophen and aspirin may decrease the level of rimantadine in the blood.
- Cimetidine may increase the level of rimantadine in the blood and lead to toxic effects. Your child should not take cimetidine while using rimantadine without your doctor's approval.

SYMPTOMS OF OVERDOSE
Symptoms include agitation and heart rhythm abnormalities. If overdose occurs, seek immediate medical attention and bring the drug container(s) with you.

THINGS TO TELL YOUR DOCTOR

- Tell your doctor if your child has had allergic reactions to any medications in the past or if he or she is taking any medications, herbal remedies, or supplements now.
- Let your doctor know if your child has epilepsy or a history of any type of seizure disorder or kidney or liver disease.
- Consult your doctor if your child is pregnant or becomes pregnant while taking rimantadine. This drug causes birth defects in animals, but its effect in humans is not known.

IMPORTANT PRECAUTIONS

- Store rimantadine in a tightly closed container and keep away from excess heat and moisture (e.g., the bathroom, near a stove or sink). Do not allow the syrup to freeze.

RISPERIDONE

BRAND NAME
Risperdal
Generic Not Available

ABOUT THIS DRUG
Risperidone is used to treat severe mental illnesses such as schizophrenia and bipolar disease, and irritability in autistic children. Specifically, it reduces symptoms such as delusions, hostility, and hallucinations.

This drug works by blocking the action of dopamine and serotonin, two nerve transmitters in the brain, which correct an imbalance that is believed to cause or contribute to various mental disorders.

SIDE EFFECTS
Contact your doctor if your child experiences any side effects that are persistent or troubling, including any that are not listed here.

- *Common:* agitation, anxiety, headache, sleepiness, sleeplessness, runny nose
- *Less common/rare:* abdominal pain, difficulty breathing, chest pain, constipation, dandruff, dizziness, dizziness or fainting upon rising, dry skin, fever, joint or back pain, nausea, rapid heart rate, sinus infection, sore throat, sun sensitivity, difficulty swallowing, toothache, visual disturbances, vomiting, urinary infection

On rare occasions, Parkinson's disease–like reactions (e.g., uncontrollable jerking movements), symptoms of tardive dyskinesia (e.g., lip smacking, wormlike movements of the tongue, and slow, rhythmical, involuntary movements), or seizures occur. Seek immediate medical attention if your child experiences any of these symptoms.

HOW TO USE THIS DRUG
Risperidone is available in tablets and liquid. The dosages given here are ones that are usually recommended for children. However, your doctor will determine the most appropriate dose and schedule for your child.

- Children younger than 6 years: not recommended
- Children 6 years and older: starting dose 0.11 to 0.34 mg per lb of body weight daily, with total doses ranging from 0.5 to 3.5 g per day

Risperidone can be taken with or without food. The liquid form can be taken with water, orange juice, coffee, or low-fat milk, but not with colas or tea. If your child misses a dose, give it as soon as you remember. If it is nearly time for the next dose, do not give the missed dose. Continue with the regular dosing schedule and never give a double dose.

TIME UNTIL IT TAKES EFFECT
Sedation takes 1 to 5 hours; the antipsychotic effect takes a few weeks

POSSIBLE DRUG, FOOD, AND/OR SUPPLEMENT INTERACTIONS

Tell your doctor if your child is taking any prescription or over-the-counter medications or any vitamins, herbs, or other supplements. Possible interactions with risperidone may include the following:

- Use of high blood pressure medications (e.g., antihypertensives, beta-blockers) may result in very low blood pressure.
- Use of central nervous system depressants (e.g., sedatives, narcotics, tranquilizers) may cause increased drowsiness.
- Clozapine and carbamazepine reduce the amount of risperidone that the body absorbs.
- Alcohol should be avoided when using risperidone.
- Herbs that produce sedation, such as catnip, goldenseal, gotu kola, hops, kava, lemon balm, skullcap, St. John's wort, and valerian, should not be used along with risperidone.
- Stimulating herbs, such as ginseng or ephedra, should not be used with risperidone.

SYMPTOMS OF OVERDOSE

Symptoms of overdose include drowsiness, rapid heartbeat, low blood pressure, and sedation. If overdose occurs, seek immediate medical attention and bring the prescription container(s) with you.

THINGS TO TELL YOUR DOCTOR

- Tell your doctor if your child has had allergic reactions to any medications in the past or if he or she is taking any medications, herbal remedies, or supplements now.
- Let your doctor know if your child has any of the following medical conditions: kidney or liver disease, a seizure disorder, thyroid disorders, dehydration, or history of stroke.
- If your child is scheduled for surgery (including dental surgery), tell your doctor or dentist that your child is taking risperidone.

IMPORTANT PRECAUTIONS

- Use of risperidone increases the level of prolactin in the body. High levels of this hormone are associated with an increased risk of pancreatic, pituitary, and breast tumors.
- Because risperidone can cause drowsiness and dizziness, make sure you know how your child reacts to it before he or she participates in potentially hazardous activities, such as riding a bike, driving a car, or operating machinery.
- Risperidone may cause increased sensitivity to the sun. Your child should wear protective clothing and sunscreen when using this drug.
- Your child should drink lots of fluids and avoid extreme heat, as excessive sweating can cause dizziness, lightheadedness, fainting, vomiting, and dehydration.
- Store risperidone in a tightly closed container and keep away from excess heat and moisture (e.g., the bathroom, near a stove or sink). Do not allow the liquid to freeze.

SALMETEROL

BRAND NAME
Serevent
Generic Not Available

ABOUT THIS DRUG
Salmeterol is a bronchodilator that is used to dilate narrowed air passages in the lungs, which is usually the result of asthma or chronic obstructive pulmonary disease (COPD). It is also used to prevent exercise-induced asthma, but it is not meant to be used to treat acute asthma attacks. This drug widens the air passages by relaxing the smooth muscles that surround them.

SIDE EFFECTS
Contact your doctor if your child experiences any side effects that are persistent or troubling, including any that are not listed here.

- *Most common:* headache, runny or stuffy nose, sore throat
- *Less common/rare:* abdominal pain, cough, diarrhea, muscle aches, nausea

HOW TO USE THIS DRUG

Salmeterol is available as inhalation aerosol and inhalation powder. The dosages given here are ones that are usually recommended for children. However, your doctor will determine the most appropriate dose and schedule for your child.

- Children younger than 12 years: not recommended
- Children 12 years and older: for aerosol—2 inhalations twice daily, about 12 hours apart; for inhalation powder, 1 inhalation twice daily, about 12 hours apart

If your child misses a dose, give it as soon as you remember. However, if it is nearly time for the next dose, skip the missed dose and continue with the regular dosing schedule. Never give a double dose.

TIME UNTIL IT TAKES EFFECT

Within 15 minutes

POSSIBLE DRUG, FOOD, AND/OR SUPPLEMENT INTERACTIONS

Tell your doctor if your child is taking any prescription or over-the-counter medications or any vitamins, herbs, or other supplements. Possible interactions with salmeterol may include the following:

- Beta-blockers may result in a negative response; talk to your doctor.
- Tricyclic antidepressants should not be used along with salmeterol.

SYMPTOMS OF OVERDOSE

Symptoms include chest pain; dizziness; fainting; irregular, racing, or pounding heartbeat; lightheadedness; and severe headache. If overdose occurs, seek immediate medical attention and bring the drug container(s) with you.

THINGS TO TELL YOUR DOCTOR
- Tell your doctor if your child has had allergic reactions to any medications in the past or if he or she is taking any medications, herbal remedies, or supplements now.
- Let your doctor know if your child has any of the following medical conditions: liver disease, coronary heart disease, high blood pressure.
- Consult your doctor if your child is pregnant or becomes pregnant while taking salmeterol.

IMPORTANT PRECAUTIONS
- Do not use this drug for acute or sudden asthma attacks.
- Store salmeterol in a tightly closed container and keep at room temperature away from excess heat and moisture (e.g., the bathroom, near a stove or sink).

SERTRALINE

BRAND NAME
Zoloft
Generic Available

ABOUT THIS DRUG
Sertraline is a selective serotonin reuptake inhibitor (SSRI) antidepressant that is prescribed to treat symptoms of major depression, panic disorder, and obsessive-compulsive disorder. This drug affects serotonin, a brain chemical that has an impact on mood, mental state, and emotions.

SIDE EFFECTS
Contact your doctor if your child experiences any side effects that are persistent or troubling, including any that are not listed here.

- *Most common:* abdominal pain, decreased appetite, diarrhea, dizziness, drowsiness, dry mouth, fatigue, increased sweating, insomnia, loss of initiative, stomach cramps, weight loss
- *Less common/rare:* anxiety, agitation, blurry vision, constipation, flushing, increased appetite, irregular heartbeat, sensitivity to light, taste alterations, vomiting

HOW TO USE THIS DRUG

Sertraline is available in capsules and tablets. The dosages given here are ones that are usually recommended for children. However, your doctor will determine the most appropriate dose and schedule for your child.

- Children 6 to 12 years: to start, 25 mg once daily; your doctor may increase the dose gradually
- Children 13 years and older: to start, 50 mg once daily; your doctor may increase the dose gradually

If your child misses a dose, give it as soon as you remember. If it is nearly time for the next dose, skip the missed dose and continue with the regular dosing schedule.

TIME UNTIL IT TAKES EFFECT

1 to 4 weeks

POSSIBLE DRUG, FOOD, AND/OR SUPPLEMENT INTERACTIONS

Tell your doctor if your child is taking any prescription or over-the-counter medications or any vitamins, herbs, or other supplements. Possible interactions with sertraline may include the following:

- Monoamine oxidase (MAO) inhibitors should not be used within 14 days of sertraline. The combination of MAO inhibitors and sertraline can cause potentially fatal serotonin syndrome, characterized by diarrhea, fever, increased sweating, mood or behavior changes, overactive reflexes, racing heartbeat, and shivering.

- Cimetidine may increase the effects of sertraline.
- The following drugs may interact with sertraline: anti-histamines, buspirone, cough medicines, digitoxin, lithium, meperidine, naratriptan, oral antidiabetic drugs, sedatives, sumatriptan, tricyclic antidepressants, and venlafaxine.
- Warfarin may result in increased bleeding.
- Avoid alcohol when using sertraline.

SYMPTOMS OF OVERDOSE
Symptoms include anxiety, dilated pupils, nausea, rapid heartbeat, sleepiness, and vomiting. If overdose occurs, seek immediate medical attention and bring the drug container(s) with you.

THINGS TO TELL YOUR DOCTOR
- Tell your doctor if your child has had allergic reactions to any medications in the past or if he or she is taking any medications, herbal remedies, or supplements now.
- Let your doctor know if your child has brain disease, mental retardation, liver or kidney disease, or a history of seizures or convulsions.
- If your child needs to undergo surgery or a dental procedure, tell your physician or dentist that he or she is taking sertraline.
- Consult your doctor if your child is pregnant or becomes pregnant while taking sertraline.

IMPORTANT PRECAUTIONS
- Sertraline is one of the antidepressants for which the U.S. Food and Drug Administration (FDA) ordered manufacturers to place a "black box warning" on the label, alerting patients to the possibility of clinical worsening of depression or the emergence of suicidality when using this drug (see "Psychiatric Drugs" in the introductory material section of this book). These risks are especially relevant when beginning the drug or when the dose changes (either increased or decreased).
- Because sertraline can cause drowsiness and dizziness,

make sure you know how your child reacts to it before he or she participates in potentially hazardous activities, such as riding a bike, driving a car, or operating machinery.

- Store sertraline in a tightly closed container and keep away from excess heat and moisture (e.g., the bathroom, near a stove or sink).

SODIUM PHOSPHATE

BRAND NAMES
Fleet Enema, Fleet Enema for Children, Fleet Phospho-soda
Generic Available/Over-the-Counter Available

ABOUT THIS DRUG
Sodium phosphate and sodium biphosphate are laxatives used to treat short-term constipation or to empty the colon before surgery or a rectal examination. This medication rapidly attracts and retains water in the intestines and then increases bowel activity, resulting in an urge to defecate.

SIDE EFFECTS
Contact your doctor if your child experiences any side effects that are persistent or troubling, including any that are not listed here.

- *Most common:* cramps, diarrhea, gas, increased thirst
- *Less common/rare:* none

HOW TO USE THIS DRUG
Sodium phosphate is available as oral solution and enema. The dosages given here are ones that are usually recommended for children. However, your doctor will determine the most appropriate dose and schedule for your child.

Oral Form
- Children younger than 5 years: not recommended
- Children 5 to 9 years: 5 mL (1 teaspoon) mixed with 4 ounces cool water

- Children 10 to 12 years: 10 mL (2 teaspoons) mixed with 4 ounces cool water
- Children 13 years and older: 20 to 30 mL (4 to 6 teaspoons) mixed with 4 ounces cool water

Enema
- Children younger than 2 years: do not use
- Children 2 to 4 years: half the contents of 1 disposable pediatric enema given rectally (50% of 2.25 fl oz = 1.12 oz)
- Children 5 to 12 years: the contents of 1 disposable pediatric enema (2.25 oz) given rectally
- Children 13 years and older: the contents of 1 disposable adult enema (4.5 fl oz) given rectally

The oral form should be taken when your child gets up in the morning, 30 minutes before a meal, or before bedtime. Never give more than the recommended dose of either form within a 24-hour period, and do not give sodium phosphate or biphosphate for longer than 1 week.

TIME UNTIL IT TAKES EFFECT
Oral form, 30 minutes to 3 hours; enema, 3 to 5 minutes

POSSIBLE DRUG, FOOD, AND/OR SUPPLEMENT INTERACTIONS
Tell your doctor if your child is taking any prescription or over-the-counter medications or any vitamins, herbs, or other supplements. Possible interactions with sodium phosphate or biphosphate may include the following:

- Anticoagulants (e.g., warfarin), ciprofloxacin, digitalis drugs, etidronate, oral tetracyclines, and sodium polystyrene sulfonate may result in negative reactions. Talk to your doctor if your child is using any of these medications.
- Alcohol use should be avoided.
- Use of other laxatives should be avoided unless prescribed by your doctor.

SYMPTOMS OF OVERDOSE

Symptoms include abnormal heartbeat, blood chemistry abnormalities, dehydration, excessive bowel activity, low blood pressure, and metabolic acidosis. If overdose occurs, seek immediate medical attention and bring the drug container(s) with you.

THINGS TO TELL YOUR DOCTOR

- Tell your doctor if your child has had allergic reactions to any medications in the past or if he or she is taking any medications, herbal remedies, or supplements now.
- Let your doctor know if your child has a history of appendicitis, rectal bleeding of unknown cause, colostomy, intestinal blockage, or ileostomy or diabetes, heart disease, high blood pressure, kidney disease, or any difficulty swallowing.
- If you administer the enema and no stools are released, contact your doctor immediately, as dehydration could occur.
- Consult your doctor if your child is pregnant. This laxative contains a large amount of sodium, which may cause negative effects during pregnancy.

IMPORTANT PRECAUTIONS

- Store sodium phosphate or biphosphate in a tightly closed container and keep at room temperature away from excess heat and direct light.

SUCCIMER

BRAND NAME

Chemet
Generic Available

ABOUT THIS DRUG

Succimer is a chelating agent used to treat acute lead poisoning, especially in small children. It works by attaching itself to lead in the blood stream and the combination is then removed from the body by the kidneys through urination;

thus, succimer helps reduce the damage to organs and other tissues caused by excess lead in the body.

SIDE EFFECTS
Contact your doctor if your child experiences any side effects that are persistent or troubling, including any that are not listed here.

- *Most common:* diarrhea, loss of appetite, nausea, rash, vomiting
- *Less common/rare:* chills, fever

HOW TO USE THIS DRUG
Succimer is available in capsules. The dosages given here are ones that are usually recommended for children. However, your doctor will determine the most appropriate dose and schedule for your child.

- Children younger than 1 year: dose to be determined by your doctor
- Children 1 to 11 years (dose based on body weight): the usual dose is 4.5 mg per lb of body weight every 8 hours for 5 days; the same dose is then given every 12 hours for 14 days, for a total of 19 days of treatment
- Children 12 years and older (dose based on body weight): the usual dose is 4.5 mg per lb of body weight every 8 hours for 5 days

If your child cannot swallow the capsules, the contents of the capsules can be sprinkled on soft food, which should be consumed immediately. The contents can also be taken from a spoon and followed by a fruit drink.

If your child misses a dose, give it as soon as you remember. If it is nearly time for the next dose, skip the missed dose and continue with the regular dosing schedule. Never give a double dose.

TIME UNTIL IT TAKES EFFECT
Unknown

POSSIBLE DRUG, FOOD, AND/OR SUPPLEMENT INTERACTIONS

Tell your doctor if your child is taking any prescription or over-the-counter medications or any vitamins, herbs, or other supplements. Succimer is not known to interact with other drugs, foods, or supplements. However, other chelating agents should not be used along with succimer.

SYMPTOMS OF OVERDOSE

No cases of overdose have been reported. Symptoms are believed to include difficulty breathing, poor coordination, weakness, and seizures. If you believe an overdose has occurred, seek medical attention immediately and bring the prescription container with you.

THINGS TO TELL YOUR DOCTOR

- Tell your doctor if your child has had allergic reactions to any medications in the past or if he or she is taking any medications now.
- Let your doctor know if your child has liver or kidney disease or any blood disease.
- Consult your doctor if your child is pregnant or becomes pregnant while taking succimer.

IMPORTANT PRECAUTIONS

- Use of succimer can lower your child's resistance to infection. Try to avoid exposure to individuals who have an infectious disease.
- Your doctor may conduct blood tests during treatment to monitor blood levels of the drug.
- Store succimer in a tightly sealed container away from heat and moisture (e.g., the bathroom, near a stove or sink).

CLASS: SULFA DRUGS (SULFONAMIDES)

GENERICS
(1) sulfadiazine; (2) sulfamethoxazole + phenazopyridine;
(3) sulfamethoxazole + trimethoprim; (4) sulfasalazine; (5)
sulfisoxazole

BRAND NAMES
(1) Microsulfon; (2) Azo Gantanol, Azo-sulfamethoxazole;
(3) Bactrim, Bactrim DS, Bactrim Pediatric, Cotrim, Cotrim
DS, Cotrim Pediatric, Septra, Septra DS, Septra Pediatric,
Sulfatrim, Sulfatrim Pediatric; (4) Azaline, Azulfidine,
Azulfidine EN-Tabs; (5) Gantrisin
Generics Available

ABOUT THESE DRUGS
Sulfa drugs, also known as sulfonamides, are used to treat a
variety of bacterial and protozoal infections, including urinary tract infections, inflammatory bowel disease, and ulcerative colitis. Each drug in the sulfa family kills certain
bacteria or protozoa, so these drugs are prescribed to meet
an individual's specific needs.

SIDE EFFECTS
Contact your doctor if your child experiences any side effects that are persistent or troubling, including any that are
not listed here.

- *Most common:* diarrhea, dizziness, headache, increased sensitivity to sunlight, itching, loss of appetite,
  nausea, rash, tiredness, vomiting
- *Less common/rare:* blood diseases, blood in urine,
  bloody diarrhea, extreme weakness or fatigue, jaundice, joint and muscle aches, pallor, peeling skin, severe abdominal pain, sore throat, difficulty swallowing

HOW TO USE THESE DRUGS
Sulfa drugs are available in various forms, including tablets,
capsules, suspension, and syrup. The dosages given here are

ones that are usually recommended for children. However, your doctor will determine the most appropriate dose and schedule for your child.

Sulfadiazine
- Children 2 months to 12 years (dose based on body weight): the usual dose is 34 mg per lb of body weight for first dose, then 17 mg per lb of body weight every 6 hours; or 11.4 mg per lb of body weight every 4 hours
- Children 13 years and older: 2 to 4 g for the first dose, then 1 g every 4 to 6 hours

Sulfamethoxazole + Phenazopyridine
- Children younger than 12 years: not recommended
- Children 12 years and older: 2 g sulfamethoxazole and 400 mg phenazopyridine as the initial dose, then 1 g sulfamethoxazole and 200 mg phenazopyridine every 12 hours for up to 2 days

Sulfamethoxazole + Trimethoprim
- Infants 2 months and older and children weighing less than 88 lbs: for bacterial infection (dose based on body weight)—the usual dose is 9.1 to 13.6 mg of sulfamethoxazole and 1.8 to 2.7 mg trimethoprim per lb of body weight every 12 hours
- Children weighing 88 lbs or more: for bacterial infection—800 mg sulfamethoxazole and 160 mg trimethoprim every 12 hours
- Children 2 months and older: for treatment of *Pneumocystis carinii* pneumonia (dose based on body weight)—the usual dose is 8.5 to 11.4 mg sulfamethoxazole and 1.7 to 2.3 mg trimethoprim per lb of body weight every 6 hours

Sulfasalazine

For Prevention or Treatment of Inflammatory Bowel Disease
- Children 2 years to 12 years (dose based on body weight): to start, usual dose is 3.05 to 4.55 mg per lb

of body weight every 4 hours or 4.55 to 6.82 mg per lb of body weight every 6 hours; or 6.05 to 9.09 mg per lb of body weight every 8 hours, then dose is usually 3.41 mg per lb of body weight every 6 hours
- Children 13 years and older: to start, 500 to 1,000 mg every 6 to 8 hours; your doctor may change the dose as needed

For Treatment of Rheumatoid Arthritis
- Children 6 to 12 years: 13.6 to 22.7 mg per lb of body weight daily, divided into 2 doses; the exact dose will be determined by your doctor
- Children 13 years and older: to start, 500 to 1,000 mg daily; your doctor may increase the dose as needed.

Sulfisoxazole

For Bacterial or Protozoal Infections
- Children 2 months to 12 years (dose based on body weight): the usual dose is 34 mg per lb of body weight for the first dose, then 11.4 mg per lb of body weight every 4 hours; or 17 mg per lb of body weight every 6 hours
- Children 13 years and older: 2 to 4 g for the first dose, then 750 mg to 1.5 g every 4 hours; or 1 to 2 g every 6 hours

Sulfa drugs should be taken with a full glass (8 ounces) of water. If your child experiences stomach irritation, the drugs can be taken with food or milk. If your child misses a dose, give it as soon as you remember. If it is nearly time for the next dose, skip the missed dose and continue with the regular dosing schedule. Never give a double dose.

TIME UNTIL THEY TAKE EFFECT
Unknown

POSSIBLE DRUG, FOOD, AND/OR SUPPLEMENT INTERACTIONS

Tell your doctor if your child is taking any prescription or over-the-counter medications or any vitamins, herbs, or other supplements. Possible interactions with sulfa drugs may include the following:

- Taking vitamin K, dapsone, methyldopa, nitrofurantoin, procainamide, quinidine, or quinine with sulfa drugs increases the risk of blood-related side effects.
- Sulfa drugs may increase the side effects of aspirin, indomethacin, methotrexate, warfarin, sulfonylurea drugs, and hydantoin anticonvulsive drugs such as phenytoin.
- Use of disulfiram, divalproex, methyldopa, naltrexone, oral contraceptives, phenothiazines, valproic acid, or other anti-infective drugs along with sulfa drugs increases the risk of liver side effects.

SYMPTOMS OF OVERDOSE

Symptoms include colic, dizziness, drowsiness, high fever, loss of appetite, nausea, and vomiting. If overdose occurs, seek immediate medical attention and bring the drug container(s) with you.

THINGS TO TELL YOUR DOCTOR

- Tell your doctor if your child has had allergic reactions to any medications in the past, including aspirin, anesthetics, diuretics, and sulfonylurea drugs, or if he or she is taking any medications, herbal remedies, or supplements now.
- Before surgery or a dental procedure, tell the doctor or dentist that your child is taking a sulfa drug.
- Let your doctor know if your child has anemia, G6PD (glucose-6-phosphate dehydrogenase) deficiency, porphyria, or liver or kidney disease.
- Consult your doctor if your child is pregnant or becomes pregnant while taking sulfa drugs. Sulfa drugs have caused birth defects in animals.

IMPORTANT PRECAUTIONS

- Because sulfa drugs can cause dizziness, make sure you know how your child reacts to them before he or she participates in potentially hazardous activities, such as riding a bike, driving a car, or operating machinery.
- Sulfa drugs can increase your child's sensitivity to sunlight, so make sure he or she takes precautions when outside, such as wearing sunscreen and protective clothing.
- Store sulfa drugs in a tightly closed container and keep away from excess heat and moisture (e.g., the bathroom, near a stove or sink). Do not allow the liquid forms to freeze.

SULFADIAZINE—see *Sulfa Drugs*

SULFAMETHOXAZOLE—see *Sulfa Drugs*

SULFASALAZINE—see *Sulfa Drugs*

SULFISOXAZOLE—see *Sulfa Drugs*

TERBUTALINE

BRAND NAMES
Brethaire, Brethine, Bricanyl
Generic Not Available

ABOUT THIS DRUG
Terbutaline is a bronchodilator used to prevent and treat shortness of breath, wheezing, and other breathing difficulties associated with asthma, chronic bronchitis, emphysema, and other lung diseases. It works by relaxing and opening the air passages in the lungs and dilating bronchial tubes when they be-

come constricted. Terbutaline has a less aggressive effect on the heart and blood vessels than other bronchodilators, which makes it a better choice for individuals who have heart disease.

SIDE EFFECTS

Contact your doctor if your child experiences any side effects that are persistent or troubling, including any that are not listed here.

- *Most common:* difficulty breathing, chest discomfort, dizziness, drowsiness, fast heartbeat, flushing, headache, heart palpitations, increased heart rate, nausea, nervousness, trembling, weakness
- *Less common/rare:* anxiety, changes in taste and smell, dry mouth, inflamed blood vessels, muscle cramps, sleeplessness, sore throat, sweating

HOW TO USE THIS DRUG

Terbutaline is available in tablets and as an inhalation aerosol. The tablets are used to prevent symptoms, whereas the aerosol helps prevent or relieve symptoms. The dosages given here are ones that are usually recommended for children. However, your doctor will determine the most appropriate dose and schedule for your child.

Aerosol

- Children younger than 12 years: not recommended
- Children 12 years and older: 1 or 2 puffs every 4 to 6 hours

Tablets

- Children younger than 12 years: not recommended
- Children 12 to 14 years: 2.5 mg 3 times daily
- Children 15 years and older: 2.5 to 5 mg 3 times daily

Terbutaline should not be taken more than prescribed, as it can cause increased difficulty breathing and heart rhythm disturbances. The oral form is most effective when taken on an empty stomach.

If your child misses a dose, give it as soon as you remember. If it is nearly time for the next dose, skip the missed dose and continue with the regular dosing schedule. Never give a double dose.

TIME UNTIL IT TAKES EFFECT
Aerosol, within 5 minutes; tablets, 1 to 2 hours

POSSIBLE DRUG, FOOD, AND/OR SUPPLEMENT INTERACTIONS
Tell your doctor if your child is taking any prescription or over-the-counter medications or any vitamins, herbs, or other supplements. Possible interactions with terbutaline may include the following:

- Monoamine oxidase (MAO) inhibitors should not be taken along with or within 14 days of terbutaline, as dangerously high blood pressure can result.
- Terbutaline should not be taken along with theophylline.
- Over-the-counter cold, cough, sinus, allergy, and weight loss medications can raise blood pressure and should not be used along with terbutaline without first consulting your physician.
- Other inhaled medications should not be used along with terbutaline without first consulting your physician.
- Tricyclic antidepressants should be used with caution.
- Beta-blockers may reduce the effects of terbutaline.

SYMPTOMS OF OVERDOSE
Symptoms include chest pain, headache, heart palpitations, nervousness, rapid heart rate, sweating, tremor, and vomiting. If overdose occurs, seek medical attention immediately and bring the prescription container with you.

THINGS TO TELL YOUR DOCTOR
- Tell your doctor if your child has had allergic reactions to any medications in the past or if he or she is taking any medications now.
- Let your doctor know if your child has any of the fol-

lowing medical conditions: anxiety disorder, diabetes, glaucoma, heart disease, high blood pressure, hyperthyroidism, seizures.
- Consult your doctor if your child is pregnant or becomes pregnant while taking terbutaline. Generally, terbutaline should be avoided during the first trimester of pregnancy.

IMPORTANT PRECAUTIONS
- Because terbutaline can cause dizziness and drowsiness, make sure you know how your child reacts to it before he or she participates in potentially hazardous activities, such as riding a bike, driving a car, or operating machinery.
- Store terbutaline in a tightly closed container and keep away from excess heat and moisture (e.g., the bathroom, near a stove or sink). Do not refrigerate the aerosol.

TETRACYCLINE–
see *Tetracycline Antibiotics*

CLASS: **TETRACYCLINE ANTIBIOTICS**

GENERICS
(1) demeclocycline; (2) doxycycline; (3) minocycline; (4) oxytetracycline; (5) tetracycline

BRAND NAMES
(1) Declomycin; (2) Doryx, DoxyCaps, Monodox, Periostat, Vibramycin, Vibra-Tabs; (3) Dynacin, Minocin, Vectrin; (4) Terramycin; (5) Achromycin, Sumycin, Tetracyn
Generics Available for all except demeclocycline

ABOUT THESE DRUGS
Tetracycline antibiotics are broad-spectrum antibiotics that are used to treat bacterial or protozoan infections, including but not limited to acne, amebic dysentery, anthrax, cholera,

Lyme disease, respiratory infections (e.g., pneumonia), Rocky Mountain spotted fever, and urinary tract infections. In cases when penicillin cannot be given, tetracycline antibiotics are prescribed for treatment of gonorrhea and syphilis.

Tetracycline antibiotics work by preventing the disease-causing bacteria and protozoa from manufacturing the proteins they need to survive. These drugs are not effective against other types of microorganisms, such as fungi, parasites, and viruses. Many bacteria are also resistant to tetracycline antibiotics.

SIDE EFFECTS
Contact your doctor if your child experiences any side effects that are persistent or troubling, including any that are not listed here.

- *Most common:* diarrhea, discolored teeth (in infants and children), increased sensitivity to sunlight, increased skin pigmentation, nausea, stomach upset, thrush, vaginal yeast infection
- *Less common/rare:* colitis, loss of appetite, inflamed genitals or anus, pain and swelling of legs, sore throat, tongue irritation

HOW TO USE THESE DRUGS
Demeclocycline is available in tablets; doxycycline is available in capsules, delayed-release capsules, oral suspension, and tablets; minocycline is available in capsules and suspension; and oxytetracycline, and tetracycline are available in capsules. The dosages given here are ones that are usually recommended for children. However, your doctor will determine the most appropriate dose and schedule for your child.

Demeclocycline
- Children 9 to 12 years (dose based on body weight): the usual dose is 0.8 to 1.5 mg per lb of body weight every 6 hours; or 1.5 to 3 mg per lb of body weight every 12 hours
- Children 13 years and older: 150 mg every 6 hours, or 300 mg every 12 hours

Doxycycline

For Bacterial and Protozoan Infections
- Children older than 8 years weighing 99 lbs or less: 1 mg per lb of body weight in 2 doses on first day, followed by 1 to 2 mg per lb per day in 1 or 2 divided doses
- Children weighing 100 lbs or more: 100 mg every 12 hours (twice daily) on the first day, followed by 100 to 200 mg daily

For Gonorrhea
- Children weighing 100 lbs or more: 200 mg to start, then 100 mg twice daily for 3 days

Minocycline
- Children 9 to 12 years (dose based on body weight): the usual dose is 1.8 mg per lb of body weight at first, then 0.9 mg per lb of body weight every 12 hours
- Children 13 years and older: 200 mg at first, then 100 mg every 12 hours; or 100 to 200 mg at first, then 50 mg every 6 hours

Oxytetracycline
- Children 9 to 12 years (dose is based on body weight): the usual dose is 2.8 to 5.7 mg per lb of body weight every 6 hours
- Children 13 years and older: 250 to 500 mg every 6 hours

Tetracycline
- Children 9 to 12 years (dose is based on body weight): the usual dose is 2.8 to 5.7 mg per lb of body weight every 6 hours; or 5.7 to 11.4 mg per lb of body weight every 12 hours
- Children 13 years and older: 250 to 500 mg every 6 hours, or 500 mg to 1 g every 12 hours

Tetracycline antibiotics should be taken with a full glass (8 ounces) of water to help prevent irritation of the esophagus and stomach. Demeclocycline, oxytetracycline, and tetracycline are best taken on an empty stomach, either 1 hour before or 2 hours after meals. However, if your child experiences irritation, he or she can take these medications with food, except milk or other dairy products, which may prevent the antibiotic from working properly.

If your child misses a dose, give it as soon as you remember. If it is nearly time for the next dose, skip the missed dose and resume your regular dosing schedule. Never give a double dose.

TIME UNTIL THEY TAKE EFFECT
Up to 5 days

POSSIBLE DRUG, FOOD, AND/OR SUPPLEMENT INTERACTIONS
Tell your doctor if your child is taking any prescription or over-the-counter medications or any vitamins, herbs, or other supplements. Possible interactions with tetracycline antibiotics may include the following:

- Antacids and supplements that contain calcium, iron, magnesium, or sodium bicarbonate should be taken more than 2 hours after taking tetracycline antibiotics, as these substances can decrease the effectiveness of the antibiotics.
- Dairy products can decrease absorption of tetracycline antibiotics. Have your child take his or her medication 2 hours after or 1 hour before consuming milk or other dairy products.
- Do not allow your child to eat meat or iron-fortified foods for 2 hours before and after taking tetracycline antibiotics.
- Birth control pills may not be effective during treatment with tetracycline antibiotics. Use a backup form of birth control while taking these drugs.

SYMPTOMS OF OVERDOSE
Symptoms include diarrhea, difficulty swallowing, nausea, vomiting. If overdose occurs, seek immediate medical attention and bring the drug container(s) with you.

THINGS TO TELL YOUR DOCTOR

- Tell your doctor if your child has had allergic reactions to any medications in the past or if he or she is taking any medications now.
- Let your doctor know if your child has any of the following medical conditions: kidney or liver disease, lupus, myasthenia gravis.
- Consult your doctor if your child is pregnant or becomes pregnant during treatment with these antibiotics. Tetracycline antibiotics should not be used during pregnancy, as they can hinder the development of the infant's bones and teeth.

IMPORTANT PRECAUTIONS

- Tetracycline antibiotics should be taken for the entire course of treatment prescribed by your doctor. Stopping treatment before the scheduled time can result in a more serious drug-resistant infection.
- Store doxycycline in a tightly closed container and keep at room temperature away from excess heat and moisture (e.g., the bathroom, near stoves or sinks).
- Tetracycline antibiotics should not be given to children younger than 8 years of age because they can cause permanent tooth staining.

THEOPHYLLINE—
see *Xanthine Bronchodilators*

THIABENDAZOLE

BRAND NAME
Mintezol
Generic Not Available

ABOUT THIS DRUG
Thiabendazole is an anthelmintic that is prescribed to treat infections caused by worms, including strongyloidiasis

(threadworms), cutaneous larva migrans, visceral larva migrans, and trichinosis. The drug appears to work by interfering with the metabolism of the worms, which eventually leads to their death.

SIDE EFFECTS
Contact your doctor if your child experiences any side effects that are persistent or troubling, including any that are not listed here.

- *Most common:* buzzing or ringing in the ears, dizziness, drowsiness, dry eyes or mouth, headache
- *Less common/rare:* fever, flushing of the face, swelling

HOW TO USE THIS DRUG
Thiabendazole is available as chewable tablets and oral suspension. The dosages given here are ones that are usually recommended for children. However, your doctor will determine the most appropriate dose and schedule for your child.

- Children weighing less than 30 lbs: dose is based on body weight and is determined by your physician.
- Children weighing 30 lbs or more: dose is usually determined by your physician. Generally, the dose is 11.4 mg per lb of body weight twice daily, up to a maximum of 3,000 mg per day for 2 to 5 days. For cutaneous larva migrans and strongyloidiasis—treatment is for 2 days; for trichinosis—2 to 4 days; and for visceral larva migrans—7 days

Thiabendazole can be taken after meals to reduce stomach irritation and some of the common side effects. If your child misses a dose, give it as soon as you remember. If it is nearly time for the next dose, skip the missed dose and continue with the regular dosing schedule. Never give a double dose.

TIME UNTIL IT TAKES EFFECT
Unknown

POSSIBLE DRUG, FOOD, AND/OR SUPPLEMENT INTERACTIONS

Tell your doctor if your child is taking any prescription or over-the-counter medications or any vitamins, herbs, or other supplements. Possible interactions with thiabendazole may include the following:

- Toxic levels of theophylline may result if theophylline is taken along with thiabendazole.
- If your child has trichinosis, your doctor may prescribe a corticosteroid along with thiabendazole, and it is important that your child take these two drugs together.

SYMPTOMS OF OVERDOSE

Symptoms include changes in behavior and personality and vision problems. If overdose occurs, seek medical attention immediately and bring the prescription container with you.

THINGS TO TELL YOUR DOCTOR

- Tell your doctor if your child has had allergic reactions to any medications in the past or if he or she is taking any medications now.
- Let your doctor know if your child has liver or kidney disease.
- Consult your doctor if your child is pregnant. Thiabendazole should not be used during pregnancy.

IMPORTANT PRECAUTIONS

- Because thiabendazole can cause dizziness and drowsiness, make sure you know how your child reacts to it before he or she participates in potentially hazardous activities, such as riding a bike, driving a car, or operating machinery.
- Store thiabendazole in a tightly sealed container away from heat and moisture (e.g., in the bathroom, near a stove or sink). Do not allow the oral suspension to freeze.

THYROID HORMONE—
see *Thyroid Hormone Replacements*

CLASS: THYROID HORMONE REPLACEMENTS

GENERICS
(1) levothyroxine sodium; (2) liothyronine sodium; (3) liotrix; (4) thyroid hormone

BRAND NAMES
(1) Euthyrox, Levothroid, Novothyrox, Synthroid; (2) Cytomel; (3) Thyrolar; (4) Armour Thyroid, S-P-T, Thyrar, Thyroid Strong, Westhroid
Generic Available

ABOUT THESE DRUGS
Thyroid hormone replacements are hypothyroid agents used to treat an underactive thyroid gland, or hypothyroidism. Symptoms of hypothyroidism include fatigue, weight gain, and sluggishness. These hormone replacements speed up metabolism and help promote normal growth and development.

The main differences among thyroid hormone replacements are their source and hormone content. Thyroid hormone is manufactured from cow thyroid; the other forms, including the most commonly prescribed thyroid hormone replacement, levothyroxine sodium, are synthetically produced.

SIDE EFFECTS
Side effects rarely occur if the dosage has been adjusted correctly. However, contact your doctor if your child experiences any side effects that are persistent or troubling, including any that are not listed here.

- *Most common:* changes in appetite, diarrhea, fever, hand tremor, headache, increased sensitivity to heat, ir-

ritability, leg cramps, nervousness, sweating, trouble
sleeping, vomiting, weight loss
- *Less common/rare:* severe headache, hives, rash

HOW TO USE THESE DRUGS

Thyroid hormone replacements are available mainly in
tablet form; however, injections are available. (Information
on injectable forms is not provided here.) The dosages given
here are ones that are usually recommended for children.
However, your doctor will determine the most appropriate
dose and schedule for your child.

Levothyroxine
- Children younger than 6 months: 0.025 to 0.05 mg
  once daily
- Children 6 to 12 months: 0.05 to 0.075 mg once daily
- Children 1 to 5 years: 0.075 to 0.1 mg once daily
- Children 6 to 10 years: 0.1 to 0.15 mg once daily
- Children 11 to 13 years: 0.15 to 0.2 mg once daily.
- Children 14 years and older: 0.0125 to 0.05 mg once
  daily to start, then your doctor may increase the dose
  gradually to 0.075 to 0.125 mg daily. The dose usually
  does not exceed 0.15 mg once daily.

Liothyronine
- Dosing is highly individualized. Starting dose is usually 25 µg daily, but children who have a serious condition may begin at 2.5 to 5 µg. Your doctor may
  increase the dose up to 50 µg daily if needed and/or divide the dose into smaller amounts to be taken twice or
  more daily.

Liotrix (Levothyroxine and Liothyronine Combination)
- Dosing is highly individualized. Starting dose is usually 50 µg of levothyroxine and 12.5 µg of liothyronine once daily, but children who have a serious
  condition may begin at 12.5 µg levothyroxine and 3.1
  µg liothyronine once daily. Your doctor may increase

the dose up to 100 µg levothyroxine and 25 µg liothyronine daily.

Thyroid Hormone
- Dosing is highly individualized. Starting dose is usually 60 mg daily, but children who have a serious condition may begin at 15 mg once daily. Your doctor may increase the dose up to 60 to 120 mg daily, if needed.

Thyroid hormone replacements should be taken at the same time each day, preferably before breakfast on an empty stomach. If your child misses a dose, give it as soon as you remember. If it is nearly time for the next dose, skip the missed dose and continue with the regular dosing schedule. If your child misses two or more doses in a row, call your doctor.

TIME UNTIL THEY TAKE EFFECT
24 hours (levothyroxine); 48 to 72 hours (liothyronine)

POSSIBLE DRUG, FOOD, AND/OR SUPPLEMENT INTERACTIONS
Tell your doctor if your child is taking any prescription or over-the-counter medications or any vitamins, herbs, or other supplements. Possible interactions with thyroid hormone replacements may include the following:

- Amphetamines, anticoagulants, appetite suppressants, asthma medications, cholestyramine, colestipol, and medications for colds, sinus conditions, or allergies may cause adverse effects. Consult your doctor for advice before giving your child any of these drugs.
- Thyroid hormone replacements should be taken at least 4 hours before or after iron supplements or calcium supplements.

SYMPTOMS OF OVERDOSE
Symptoms include fever, headache, heartbeat irregularity, increased bowel movements, irritability, nervousness, rapid

heartbeat, seizures, sweating, and vomiting. If overdose occurs, seek immediate medical attention and bring the drug container(s) with you.

THINGS TO TELL YOUR DOCTOR
- Tell your doctor if your child has had allergic reactions to any medications in the past or if he or she is taking any medications, herbal remedies, or supplements now.
- Let your doctor know if your child has any of the following medical conditions: diabetes, heart problems, high blood pressure, history of overactive thyroid, underactive adrenal or pituitary glands.

IMPORTANT PRECAUTIONS
- Before undergoing any medical or dental procedure, tell your doctor or dentist that your child is taking a thyroid hormone replacement.
- Store thyroid hormone replacements in a tightly closed container and keep away from excess heat and moisture (e.g., the bathroom, near a stove or sink).

TOBRAMYCIN

BRAND NAMES
AK-Tob, Tobrex
Generic Available

ABOUT THIS DRUG
Tobramycin is an aminoglycoside antibiotic used to treat various bacterial infections, including those that affect the bones and joints, abdominal cavity, lungs, skin, urinary tract, blood, and eyes. It is given via injection for most of these infections, except of the eyes. Tobramycin is also used to manage lung infections in individuals who have cystic fibrosis.

This drug interferes with the genetic material of the bacteria and prevents them from manufacturing the proteins they need to survive.

SIDE EFFECTS

Contact your doctor if your child experiences any side effects that are persistent or troubling, including any that are not listed here.

- *Most common:* for ophthalmic ointment—temporary blurry vision; for inhalation—hoarseness
- *Less common/rare:* for ophthalmic forms—burning or stinging of the eyes; for inhalation—dizziness, ringing in the ears

HOW TO USE THIS DRUG

Tobramycin is available as ophthalmic solution and ointment, for inhalation via nebulizer, and via injection. (Information on the injectable form is not provided here.) The dosages given here are ones that are usually recommended for children. However, your doctor will determine the most appropriate dose and schedule for your child.

Ophthalmic Forms

- Ointment, for all ages: apply ½ inch to affected eye(s) every 8 to 12 hours. For severe infections, use every 3 to 4 hours until improvement is noted.
- Eye drops, for all ages: 1 drop every 4 hours. For severe infections, 1 drop every hour until improvement is noted.

Inhalation

- 300 mg (1 ampoule) twice daily for 28 days, stop therapy for 28 days, then resume for 28 days. Inhalations should be taken as close to 12 hours apart as possible, and never less than 6 hours apart.

If your child misses a dose, give it as soon as you remember. If it is nearly time for the next dose, skip the missed dose and continue with the regular dosing schedule. Never give a double dose.

TIME UNTIL IT TAKES EFFECT

Variable

POSSIBLE DRUG, FOOD, AND/OR SUPPLEMENT INTERACTIONS

Tell your doctor if your child is taking any prescription or over-the-counter medications or any vitamins, herbs, or other supplements. Possible interactions with tobramycin may include the following:

- Other aminoglycosides, methoxyflurane, cyclosporine, dornase alfa, and vancomycin may cause reactions.
- Use of alcohol should be avoided

SYMPTOMS OF OVERDOSE

Symptoms related to the ophthalmic forms include eye pain and redness, increased tear production, itchy eyes or eyelids, and swelling. No symptoms have been reported for the inhalation form. If overdose occurs, seek medical attention immediately and bring the prescription container with you.

THINGS TO TELL YOUR DOCTOR

- Tell your doctor if your child has had allergic reactions to any medications in the past or if he or she is taking any medications now.
- Let your doctor know if your child has a hearing or balance disorder, kidney disease, asthma, or muscle disease.
- Contact your doctor if your child's eye condition does not improve within 3 days of starting treatment.

IMPORTANT PRECAUTIONS

- Your child should drink plenty of fluids while taking this medication.
- Store tobramycin in a tightly sealed container away from heat and direct light. The inhalation form should be refrigerated, but do not allow it to freeze.

TRIAMCINOLONE—see *Corticosteroids, Nasal Inhalants; Corticosteroids, Oral; Corticosteroids, Oral Inhalants; Corticosteroids, Topical*

CLASS: TRICYCLIC ANTIDEPRESSANTS

GENERICS
(1) amitriptyline; (2) clomipramine; (3) desipramine; (4) doxepin; (5) imipramine; (6) nortriptyline; (7) trimipramine

BRAND NAMES
(1) Endep; (2) Anafranil; (3) Norpramin; (4) Sinequan; (5) Tofranil, Tofranil-PM; (6) Aventyl, Pamelor; (7) Surmontil
Generics Available

ABOUT THESE DRUGS
Tricyclic antidepressants are used to treat mental depression. Symptoms of depression include sadness, feelings of guilt and shame, sleep and appetite changes, anxiety, fatigue, and low self-esteem. Imipramine is also prescribed for bed-wetting in children, and clomipramine is used to treat obsessive-compulsive disorders. Amitriptyline is prescribed for anxiety and depression.

Tricyclic antidepressants work by making more of the neurotransmitters serotonin and norepinephrine available to the brain, which in turn helps improve mood.

SIDE EFFECTS
Contact your doctor if your child experiences any side effects that are persistent or troubling, including any that are not listed here.

- *Most common:* blurry vision, constipation, dizziness, drowsiness, dry mouth, headache, impaired urination, increased appetite, lightheadedness, nausea, tiredness, weight gain

- *Less common/rare:* abnormal heart rate, anxiety, confusion, delirium, diarrhea, disorientation, fainting, fever, fluid retention, heartburn, nervousness, numbness and tingling, poor coordination, photosensitivity, restlessness, sleep disturbances, tremors, vivid dreams, vomiting

A rare but life-threatening condition known as neuroleptic malignant syndrome may occur when taking tricyclic antidepressants. Symptoms include difficulty breathing, fever, rapid heartbeat, rigid muscles, increased sweating, irregular blood pressure, and convulsions. Seek immediate medical attention if these occur in your child.

HOW TO USE THESE DRUGS
Tricyclic antidepressants are available in various forms, depending on the brand, and include capsules, tablets, oral solution, and syrup. The dosages given here are ones that are usually recommended for children. However, your doctor will determine the most appropriate dose and schedule for your child.

Amitriptyline (Tablets and Syrup) for Depression
- Children younger than 6 years: your doctor will determine the dose
- Children 6 to 12 years: 10 to 30 mg daily
- Children 13 years and older: starting dose is 10 mg 3 times daily, with 20 mg at bedtime; your doctor may increase the dose as needed, but dosage usually should not exceed 100 mg daily

Clomipramine (Tablets and Capsules) for Obsessive-Compulsive Disorders
- Children up to 10 years: your doctor will determine the dose
- Children 11 years and older: starting dose is 25 mg once daily, but your doctor may increase the dose as needed; dosage should not exceed 200 mg daily

Desipramine (Tablets) for Depression
- Children 6 to 12 years: 10 to 30 mg daily
- Children 13 years and older: 25 to 50 mg daily; your doctor may increase the dose as needed, but maximum dose usually does not exceed 150 mg daily

Doxepin (Capsules and Solution) for Depression
- Children up to 12 years: your doctor will determine the dose
- Children 13 years and older: starting dose is 25 mg 3 times daily; your doctor may increase the dose as needed, but maximum dose usually does not exceed 150 mg daily

Imipramine (Tablets) for Depression
- Children up to 6 years: your doctor will determine the dose
- Children 7 to 12 years: 10 to 30 mg daily
- Children 13 years and older: 25 to 50 mg daily; your doctor may increase the dose as needed, but maximum dose usually does not exceed 100 mg daily

Imipramine (Tablets) for Bed-wetting
- Children 5 years and older: 25 mg once daily, taken 1 hour before bedtime; your doctor may increase the dose if needed

Imipramine (Capsules) for Depression
- Children up to 12 years: your doctor will determine the dose
- Children 13 years and older: starting dose is 75 mg daily taken at bedtime; your doctor may increase the dose, but maximum dose usually does not exceed 200 mg daily

Nortriptyline (Capsules and Solution) for Depression
- Children 6 to 12 years: 10 to 20 mg daily
- Children 13 years and older: 25 to 50 mg daily; your doctor may increase the dose

Trimipramine (Capsules and Tablets) for Depression

- Children up to 12 years: your doctor will determine the dose
- Children 13 years and older: starting dose is 50 mg daily; your doctor may increase the dose, but maximum dose usually does not exceed 100 mg daily

If any of these tricyclic antidepressants cause stomach irritation, your child can take them with food. If your child misses a dose, give it as soon as you remember. If it is nearly time for the next dose, skip the missed dose and continue with the normal schedule. Never give a double dose.

TIME UNTIL THEY TAKE EFFECT
Some effects are seen within 7 to 21 days, but full benefits may take 3 to 6 weeks.

POSSIBLE DRUG, FOOD, OR SUPPLEMENT INTERACTIONS
Tell your doctor if your child is taking any prescription or over-the-counter medications or any vitamins, herbs, or other supplements. Possible interactions with tricyclic antidepressants may include the following:

- Monoamine oxidase (MAO) inhibitor antidepressants should not be taken at the same time or within 14 days of a tricyclic antidepressant. This combination can cause potentially fatal reactions.
- Central nervous system depressants such as tranquilizers and sleep aids can increase the effects of tricyclic antidepressants.
- Allergy and asthma medications, amphetamines, appetite suppressants, cold and cough remedies, ephedrine, isoproterenol, and phenylephrine may increase the risk of serious effects on the heart.
- Use of cimetidine, methylphenidate, or phenothiazine drugs may lead to severe side effects.
- Tricyclic antidepressants may reduce the effects of guanethidine.

- Caution should be exercised if using antihypertensive drugs along with tricyclic antidepressants, as the latter can also reduce blood pressure.
- Alcohol should be avoided when taking tricyclic antidepressants.
- Consult your physician before your child takes any of these antidepressants with grapefruit juice.
- Do not combine tricyclic antidepressants with supplements such as dong quai, hops, passionflower, St. John's wort, valerian, 5-HTP (5-hydroxytryptophan), or SAMe (S-adenosylmethionine).

SYMPTOMS OF OVERDOSE

Symptoms include difficulty breathing, confusion, dilated pupils, fever, hallucinations, irregular heartbeat, seizures, and severe fatigue. If overdose occurs, seek medical attention immediately and bring the prescription container with you to the hospital.

THINGS TO TELL YOUR DOCTOR

- Tell your doctor if your child has had allergic reactions to any medications in the past, especially to other tricyclic antidepressants, or if he or she is taking any medications now.
- Let your doctor know if your child has asthma, bipolar disorder, blood disorders, convulsions, difficult urination, glaucoma, heart disease, high blood pressure, hypothyroidism, kidney or liver disease, schizophrenia, or stomach or intestinal problems.
- Before undergoing any surgery or dental procedure, tell our doctor or dentist that your child is taking a tricyclic antidepressant.
- Consult your doctor if your child is pregnant or becomes pregnant while taking tricyclic antidepressants. Although adequate studies of the impact of these drugs on pregnant women have not been done, the newborns of mothers who take these drugs have experienced breathing, urinary, and heart problems.

IMPORTANT PRECAUTIONS

- The U.S. Food and Drug Administration (FDA) ordered manufacturers of tricyclic antidepressants to place a "black box warning" on their labels, alerting patients to the possibility of clinical worsening of depression or the emergence of suicidality when using these drugs (see "Psychiatric Drugs" in the introductory section of this book). These risks are especially relevant when beginning the drug or when the dose changes (either increased or decreased).
- Tricyclic antidepressants, especially desipramine, can cause changes in cardiac conduction; children are more susceptible to this reaction than are adults. Children who are taking tricyclics need to be monitored regularly with blood tests and electrocardiography.
- Because tricyclic antidepressants increase sensitivity to the sun, your child should take precautions, such as wearing sunscreen and protective clothing when outside.
- Blurry vision, dizziness, and drowsiness are common side effects, so make sure you know how your child reacts to these drugs before he or she participates in potentially hazardous activities, such as riding a bike, driving a car, or operating machinery.
- Store tricyclic antidepressants in a tightly sealed container and keep away from excess heat and moisture (e.g., the bathroom, near a stove or sink). Do not allow the liquid forms to freeze.

TRIMETHOBENZAMIDE

BRAND NAMES
Arrestin, Tebamide, T-Gen, Tigan, Triban
Generic Available

ABOUT THIS DRUG
Trimethobenzamide is an antiemetic (antinauseant) used to treat nausea, vomiting, and motion sickness. The drug works by acting on the area of the brain that controls vomiting.

SIDE EFFECTS

Contact your doctor if your child experiences any side effects that are persistent or troubling, including any that are not listed here.

- *Most common:* drowsiness
- *Less common/rare:* blurry vision, diarrhea, dizziness, fainting, headache, lightheadedness, muscle cramps

HOW TO USE THIS DRUG

Trimethobenzamide is available in capsules and suppositories, and via injection. (Information on injectable forms is not provided here.) The dosages given here are ones that are usually recommended for children. However, your doctor will determine the most appropriate dose and schedule for your child.

Capsules

- Children weighing 30 to 90 lbs: 6.8 mg per lb of body weight, not to exceed 200 mg, 3 or 4 times daily
- Children 12 years and older: 250 mg 3 or 4 times daily as needed

Suppositories

- Children less than 30 lbs: ½ suppository (100 mg) 3 or 4 times daily
- Children 30 to 90 lbs: ½ to 1 suppository (100 to 200 mg) 3 or 4 times daily
- Children 12 years and older: 200 mg 3 or 4 times daily

If your child cannot tolerate swallowing the capsules, the capsules can be opened and the contents mixed with food. If your child misses a dose, give it as soon as you remember. If it is nearly time for the next dose, skip the missed dose and continue the regular dosage schedule. Never give a double dose.

TIME UNTIL IT TAKES EFFECT

Capsules, 3 to 4 hours; suppositories, variable

POSSIBLE DRUG, FOOD, AND/OR SUPPLEMENT INTERACTIONS

Tell your doctor if your child is taking any prescription or over-the-counter medications or any vitamins, herbs, or other supplements. Possible interactions with trimethobenzamide may include the following:

- Aspirin, phenobarbital, tricyclic antidepressants, or other central nervous system depressants (e.g., tranquilizers, sleeping pills, cold medications) may cause adverse reactions.
- Alcohol should be avoided.

SYMPTOMS OF OVERDOSE

Symptoms include blurry vision, difficulty breathing, drowsiness, seizures, unconsciousness, uncontrollable movements, and death. If overdose occurs, seek medical attention immediately and bring the prescription container with you.

THINGS TO TELL YOUR DOCTOR

- Tell your doctor if your child has had allergic reactions to any medications in the past or if he or she is taking any medications now.
- Let your doctor know if your child has any of the following medical conditions: kidney or liver disease, bladder problems, glaucoma, asthma, heart disease, difficulty urinating.
- Consult your doctor if your child is pregnant or becomes pregnant while taking trimethobenzamide.

IMPORTANT PRECAUTIONS

- Because trimethobenzamide can cause drowsiness, make sure you know how your child reacts to it before he or she participates in potentially hazardous activities, such as riding a bike, driving a car, or operating machinery.
- Store trimethobenzamide in a tightly closed container and keep it away from heat and moisture (e.g., in the

bathroom, near a stove or sink). The suppositories
should be refrigerated, but do not allow them to freeze.

TRIMIPRAMINE—
see *Tricyclic Antidepressants*

TRIPROLIDINE

BRAND NAMES
Actidil; Actifed (with pseudoephedrine)
Generic Available/Over-the-Counter Available

ABOUT THIS DRUG
Triprolidine is an antihistamine and triprolidine + pseudoephedrine is an antihistamine plus decongestant that are
prescribed to relieve symptoms of hay fever and other allergies. Triprolidine interferes with the activities of histamine,
a substance that occurs naturally in the body and causes
sneezing, itching, watery eyes, and other symptoms of an allergic reaction.

SIDE EFFECTS
Contact your doctor if your child experiences any side effects that are persistent or troubling, including any that are
not listed here.

- *Most common:* drowsiness, thickening of mucus
- *Less common/rare:* blurry vision; confusion; difficult
  or painful urination; dry mouth, nose, or throat; dizziness; irritability; loss of appetite; nervousness, ringing
  in the ears

HOW TO USE THIS DRUG
Triprolidine is available as a syrup and the triprolidine +
pseudoephedrine combination is available as tablets, capsules, extended-release capsules, and liquid. The dosages
given here are ones that are usually recommended for chil-

dren. However, your doctor will determine the most appropriate dose and schedule for your child.

TIME UNTIL IT TAKES EFFECT
15 to 60 minutes

POSSIBLE DRUG, FOOD, AND/OR SUPPLEMENT INTERACTIONS
Tell your doctor if your child is taking any prescription or over-the-counter medications or any vitamins, herbs, or other supplements. Possible interactions with triprolidine and the triprolidine + pseudoephedrine combination may include the following:

- Anticholinergics, clarithromycin, erythromycin, itraconazole, ketoconazole, bepridil, maprotiline, phenothiazines, procainamide, quinidine, tricyclic antidepressants, central nervous system depressants, and quinine may have a negative effect. Consult your doctor.

SYMPTOMS OF OVERDOSE
Symptoms include central nervous system depression, nervous system stimulation, difficulty breathing, seizures, loss of consciousness, and severe dryness of the mouth, nose, or throat. If overdose occurs, seek immediate medical attention and bring the drug container(s) with you.

THINGS TO TELL YOUR DOCTOR
- Tell your doctor if your child has had allergic reactions to any medications in the past or if he or she is taking any medications, herbal remedies, or supplements now.
- Let your doctor know if your child has difficulty urinating, urinary tract blockage, liver disease, or glaucoma.
- Consult your doctor if your child is pregnant or becomes pregnant while taking triprolidine.

IMPORTANT PRECAUTIONS
- Because drowsiness is a side effect of triprolidine, make sure you know how your child reacts to it before

you allow him or her to participate in potentially hazardous activities, such as riding a bike, driving a car, or operating machinery.

- Store triprolidine in a tightly closed container and keep away from excess heat and moisture (e.g., the bathroom, near a stove or sink). Do not allow the liquid forms to freeze.

VALPROIC ACID

BRAND NAMES
Depakene, Depakote, Myproic Acid
Generic Available

ABOUT THIS DRUG
Valproic acid is an anticonvulsant that is prescribed to control certain types of epileptic seizures, including absence seizures, tonic-clonic seizures, myoclonic seizures, and psychomotor seizures. It is also prescribed to treat acute mania associated with bipolar disorder. It works by depressing the abnormal firing of neurons in the brain that causes seizures.

SIDE EFFECTS
Contact your doctor if your child experiences any side effects that are persistent or troubling, including any that are not listed here.

- *Most common:* clumsiness or unsteadiness, confusion, cramps, diarrhea, dizziness, hair loss, heartburn, increased appetite and weight gain, loss of appetite and weight loss, nausea, sedation, vomiting
- *Less common/rare:* blurry or double vision, constipation, drowsiness, excitability, headache, irritability, rash, restlessness

HOW TO USE THIS DRUG
Valproic acid is available in capsules and syrup. The dosages given here are ones that are usually recommended for chil-

dren. However, your doctor will determine the most appropriate dose and schedule for your child.

- Children 1 to 12 years: usual starting dose is 6.9 to 20.7 mg per lb of body weight per day
- Children 13 years and older: starting dose is usually 2.3 to 6.9 mg per lb of body weight per day; your doctor may increase the dosage each week until an optimal response is achieved

If valproic acid irritates your child's stomach, it can be taken with food. The capsules should be swallowed whole, never chewed. The syrup can be taken with food or liquid, but not carbonated beverages.

If your child misses a dose, give it as soon as you remember. If it is nearly time for the next dose, skip the missed dose and continue with the regular dosing schedule. Never give a double dose.

TIME UNTIL IT TAKES EFFECT
Within several hours

POSSIBLE DRUG, FOOD, AND/OR SUPPLEMENT INTERACTIONS
Tell your doctor if your child is taking any prescription or over-the-counter medications or any vitamins, herbs, or other supplements. Possible interactions with valproic acid may include the following:

- Aspirin, cimetidine, chlorpromazine, erythromycin, and felbamate may increase the risk of side effects of valproic acid.
- Acyclovir, ritonavir, and antacids may reduce the effects of valproic acid.
- Valproic acid may increase the effects of antidepressants, benzodiazepines, and blood thinners.
- Avoid alcohol while using valproic acid.
- Use of other central nervous system depressants (e.g.,

sedatives, antidepressants, narcotics, tranquilizers)
with valproic acid can cause excessive sedation.

- Valproic acid may alter the absorption of other anticonvulsants, such as phenobarbital, phenytoin, and carbamazepine.

SYMPTOMS OF OVERDOSE
Symptoms include hallucinations, loss of consciousness,
restlessness, sleepiness, and trembling of the arms and
hands. If overdose occurs, seek immediate medical attention
and bring the drug container(s) with you.

THINGS TO TELL YOUR DOCTOR
- Tell your doctor if your child has had allergic reactions
to any medications in the past or if he or she is taking
any medications, herbal remedies, or supplements now.
- Let your doctor know if your child has any of the following medical conditions: bleeding disorder, liver disease, myasthenia gravis.
- Consult your doctor if your child is pregnant or becomes pregnant while taking valproic acid. Birth defects have been noted in animal studies.

IMPORTANT PRECAUTIONS
- Because valproic acid can affect vision and cause
drowsiness, make sure you know how your child reacts
to it before he or she participates in potentially hazardous activities, such as riding a bike, driving a car, or
operating machinery.
- Store valproic acid in a tightly closed container and
keep away from excess heat and moisture (e.g., the
bathroom, near a stove or sink).
- In rare cases, valproic acid has caused liver failure. Children younger than 2 years of age, those with mental retardation or organic brain disease, those taking several
seizure medications, or those with metabolic disease are at
greatest risk of liver failure. Contact your doctor immediately if your child develops loss of seizure control, fatigue,

facial swelling, vomiting, loss of appetite, and weakness, which may be early indications of liver damage.

- In rare cases, valproic acid has caused pancreatitis (inflamed pancreas), some cases of which have been fatal. Contact your doctor immediately if your child develops abdominal pain, nausea, vomiting, and loss of appetite, which may be early indications of pancreatitis.

CLASS: XANTHINE BRONCHODILATORS

GENERICS
(1) aminophylline; (2) oxtriphylline; (3) theophylline

BRAND NAMES
(1) Aminophyllin, Phyllocontin, Truphylline; (2) Choledyl, Choledyl SA; (3) Aerolate III, Aerolate JR, Aerolate SR, Aquaphyllin, Asmalix, Bronkodyl, Elixicon, Elixophyllin, Elixophyllin SR, Quibron-T, Quibron-T/SR, Respbid, Slobid, Slo-Phyllin, Sustaire, Theo-24, Theobid, Theochron, Theoclear LA, Theo-Dur, Theo-Dur Sprinkle, Theolair, Theospan SR, Theovent, Theo-X, Uniphyl
Generic Available

ABOUT THESE DRUGS
Xanthine bronchodilators are drugs that are used to prevent and treat symptoms associated with asthma, bronchitis, emphysema, and other lung diseases. They work by relaxing and opening constricted air passages in the lungs, which then make it easier to breathe.

SIDE EFFECTS
Contact your doctor if your child experiences any side effects that are persistent or troubling, including any that are not listed here.

- *Most common:* diarrhea, difficulty sleeping, headache, irritability, nausea, nervousness, restlessness, stomach pain, upset stomach, vomiting

- *Less common/rare:* dizziness, excitability, fever, heart palpitations, irregular heartbeat, muscle spasms, rash, seizures

HOW TO USE THESE DRUGS

Xanthine bronchodilators are available as capsules, tablets, suspensions, extended-release tablets, suppositories, and elixirs. The dosages given here are ones that are usually recommended for children. However, your doctor will determine the most appropriate dose and schedule for your child.

Aminophylline

- Children younger than 16 years: 1 to 2.5 mg per lb of body weight every 6 hours
- Children 16 years and older: 100 to 200 mg every 8 hours; for the sustained-release form, 200 to 500 mg daily in divided doses

Oxtriphylline

- Children 1 to 9 years: 2.8 mg per lb of body weight 4 times daily
- Children 10 years and older: 2 mg per lb of body weight 3 times daily; if using the sustained-release form, 400 to 600 mg every 12 hours

Theophylline

- Children younger than 1 year: consult your doctor
- Children 1 to 8 years: up to 10.9 mg per lb of body weight daily
- Children 9 to 11 years: up to 9 mg per lb of body weight daily
- Children 12 to 16 years: up to 8.1 mg per lb of body weight daily
- Children older than 16 years: up to 6 mg per lb of body weight daily, not to exceed 900 mg daily

It is very important to take xanthine bronchodilators exactly as prescribed, because even a small amount over the recommended dose can cause symptoms of overdose. Your doctor may check blood levels to determine the right amount of drug for your child.

Xanthine bronchodilators should be taken on an empty stomach at least 1 hour before or 2 hours after eating. If your child forgets a dose, give it as soon as you remember. However, if it is nearly time for the next dose, skip the one missed and resume the normal dosing schedule. Do not give a double dose.

TIME UNTIL THEY TAKE EFFECT
15 to 60 minutes

POSSIBLE DRUG, FOOD, AND/OR SUPPLEMENT INTERACTIONS
Tell your doctor if your child is taking any prescription or over-the-counter medications or any vitamins, herbs, or other supplements. Possible interactions with aminophylline may include the following:

- Medications that increase the effects of xanthine bronchodilators include flu vaccine, allopurinol, cimetidine, oral contraceptives, corticosteroids, ephedrine, erythromycin, interferon, quinolone anti-infectives, and thiabendazole.
- Many over-the-counter medications for colds, cough, allergy, sinus, or weight loss can cause a rise in blood pressure if taken with xanthine bronchodilators. Talk to your doctor before giving your child any of these drugs.
- Drugs that decrease the effects of xanthine bronchodilators include aminoglutethimide, barbiturates, charcoal, ketoconazole, rifampin, and phenytoin.
- Xanthine bronchodilators may interact with drugs used in anesthesia.
- Use of any product that contains caffeine (chocolate, colas, coffee, tea) should be discontinued while taking xanthine bronchodilators.
- High-carbohydrate and high-fat meals reduce the effects of xanthine bronchodilators.

- Avoid use of herbs such as ephedra, ginseng, and gotu kola when taking xanthine bronchodilators.

SYMPTOMS OF OVERDOSE
Symptoms may include difficulty sleeping, headache, loss of appetite, nausea, nervousness, restlessness, and vomiting, which may progress to abnormal heart rhythms, convulsions, and collapse. If overdose occurs, seek medical attention immediately and bring the prescription container with you to the hospital.

THINGS TO TELL YOUR DOCTOR
- Tell your doctor if your child has had allergic reactions to any medications in the past or if he or she is taking any medications now.
- Let your doctor know if your child has any of the following medical conditions: high blood pressure, heart rhythm disorder, thyroid disease, impaired kidney or liver function, seizures, stomach ulcers.
- Consult your doctor if your child is pregnant or becomes pregnant while taking xanthine bronchodilators. Although these drugs do not appear to cause birth defects, some infants born to mothers who take xanthine bronchodilators are nervous and irritable and gag when fed.

IMPORTANT PRECAUTIONS
- Do not stop using this drug suddenly without first consulting your doctor.
- Because these drugs can cause dizziness, make sure you know how your child reacts to them before he or she engages in potentially dangerous activities, such as riding a bike, driving a car, or operating machinery.
- Store xanthine bronchodilators in an airtight container away from moisture, heat, and direct light. Do not allow the liquid forms to freeze.

ZAFIRLUKAST—
see *Leukotriene Antagonist/Inhibitors*

APPENDIX:
DRUG CLASSIFICATIONS

☙

The following list presents the drugs discussed in this book, grouped by classification. Drugs are classified based on shared chemical characteristics, common side effects, and similarities in how they work in the body. In the "About This Drug" section of each entry in this book, we identify the drug(s) that have one or more class descriptors, such as "bronchodilator," "analgesic," or "muscle relaxant." Generally, if your child has a negative reaction to one drug in a specific class (e.g., bronchodilators), he or she likely will have a similar negative reaction to another drug in that class. You should talk to your doctor about any prescription or over-the-counter medications that you plan to give to your child.

Some drugs can be placed into more than one class. Aspirin, for example, is an analgesic (painkiller) and an antipyretic (fever reducer). It's important to note that because there is no universal list of drug class names, you may find different names for any given class in other books or information you read about drugs. For example, antibiotics are sometimes also referred to as anti-infectives, and narcotics can also be classified as opioids. We have included some of these alternative names in parentheses after the class name we have chosen to use.

Each of the generic drug names listed here is followed by a brand name in parentheses. In many cases, the brand name given is only one of several that are available for the given generic. Please refer to the main generic drug entry in this book for a more expanded list of available brand names.

Analgesics
acetaminophen (Tylenol)
acetaminophen + codeine (Tylenol with Codeine)
aspirin (Anacin)

Analgesic-Decongestant-Antitussive-(Antihistamine)
acetaminophen + pseudoepinephrine + dextromethorphan (Tylenol Cold Non-Drowsy)
acetaminophen + pseudoepinephrine + dextromethorphan + (chlorpheniramine) (TheraFlu Flu)

Anthelmintic Drugs (Antiparasitics)
mebendazole (Vermox)
permethrin (Nix)
pyrethrin + piperonyl butoxide (Tisit)
thiabendazole (Mintezol)

Antiacne Drugs
isotretinoin (Accutane)

Antiallergy Drugs
cromolyn sodium (Nasalcrom)
lodoxamide (Alomide)

Antianxiety Drugs
chlordiazepoxide (Lithobid)
lorazepam (Ativan)

Antiasthmatic Drugs
cromolyn sodium (Nasalcrom)
nedocromil sodium, inhalant (Tilade)

Anti-Attention Deficit/Hyperactivity Disorder (ADHD) Drugs
dexmethylphenidate (Focalin XR)
dextroamphetamine (Dexedrine)
dextroamphetamine + amphetamine (Adderall)
methylphenidate (Ritalin)

Antibiotics
(see also Cephalosporin Antibiotics, Penicillin Antibiotics, and Tetracycline Antibiotics)
azithromycin (Zithromax)
bacitracin (Bacticin)
clarithromycin (Biaxin)
clindamycin (Cleocin)
dirithromycin (Dynabac)
erythromycin (EryPed)
erythromycin + sulfisoxazole (Pediazole)
gentamicin, topical and ophthalmic (Garamycin)
loracarbef (Lorabid)
methenamine (Urex)
metronidazole (Flagyl)
neomycin + polymyxin B + gramicidin, ophthalmic (Ak-Spore Ophthalmic Solution)
neomycin + polymyxin B + hydrocortisone, otic (Ak-Spore HC Otic)
nitrofurantoin (Furadantin)
tobramycin (Tobrex)

Anticholinergics
ipratropium bromide (Atrovent)

Anticonvulsants
acetazolamide (Diamox)
carbamazepine (Tegretol)
gabapentin (Neurontin)
oxcarbazepine (Trileptal)
phenytoin (Dilantin)
primidone (Mysoline)
valproic acid (Depakote)

Antidepressants
(see also Selective Serotonin Reuptake Inhibitors [SSRIs] and Tricyclic Antidepressants)
bupropion (Wellbutrin)

Antidiabetic
insulin (various)

Antidiarrheal Drugs
attapulgite (Kaopek)
bismuth subsalicylate (Pepto-Bismol)
kaolin + pectin (Kao-Spen)
loperamide (Imodium)

Antidiuretics
desmopressin (Stimate)

Antieczema Drugs
pimecrolimus (Elidel)

Antiemetics
dolasetron (Anzemet)
granisetron (Kytril)
ondansetron (Zofran)
palonosetron (Aloxi)
trimethobenzamide (Tigan)

Antifungal Drugs
clotrimazole, topical (Lotrimin)
griseofulvin (Fulvicin)
ketoconazole (Nizoral)
nystatin (Mycostatin)

Antihistamines
azelastine, nasal (Astelin)
azelastine, ophthalmic (Optivar)
brompheniramine (Dimetapp Allergy)
cetirizine (Zyrtec)
chlorpheniramine (Aller-Chlor Oral)
cyproheptadine (Periactin)
desloratadine (Clarinex)
dimenhydrinate (Dramamine)
diphenhydramine (Benadryl)
emedastine (Emadine)
fexofenadine (Allegra)
hydrocodone + chlorpheniramine (Tussionex)
hydroxyzine (Anxanil)

loratadine (Alavert)
meclizine (Antivert)
nedocromil sodium, ophthalmic (Alocril)
promethazine (Phenergan)
triprolidine (Actidil)

Antihistamine-Decongestants
acrivastine + pseudoephedrine (Semprex-D)
azatadine + pseudoephedrine (Trinalin Repetabs)
brompheniramine + pseudoephedrine (Bromfed)
chlorpheniramine + pseudoephedrine (Novafed A)
dexbrompheniramine + pseudoephedrine (Dexaphen-SA)
fexofenadine + pseudoepehedrine (Allegra-D)
loratadine + pseudoephedrine (Claritin-D 12-Hour)
triprolidine + pseudoephedrine (Actifed)

Anti-inflammatory Drugs
nedocromil sodium, systemic (Tilade)

Antimanic Drugs
lithium (Lithane)

Antimetabolic Drugs
methotrexate (Folex)

Antipsychotic Drugs
clozapine (Clozaril)
haloperidol (Haldol)
olanzapine (Zyprexa)
risperidone (Risperdal)

Antipyretic (Fever-Reducing) Drugs
acetaminophen (Tylenol)
aspirin (Anacin)

Antispasmodic Drugs
oxybutynin (Ditropan)

Antitussives (Cough Suppressants)
dextromethorphan (Robitussin)
hydrocodone + chlorpheniramine (Tussionex)

Antiviral Drugs
acyclovir (Zovirax)
amantadine (Symmetrel)
rimantadine (Flumadine)

Benzodiazepine Drugs
chlordiazepoxide (Lithobid)
diazepam (Valium)
lorazepam (Ativan)

Bronchodilators
(see also Antiasthmatic Drugs and Xanthine Bronchodilators)
albuterol (Proventil)
ipratropium bromide (Atrovent)
metaproterenol (Metaprel)
salmeterol (Serevent)
terbutaline (Brethaire)

Cephalosporin Antibiotics
cefaclor (Ceclor)
cefadroxil (Cefadroxil)
cefdinir (Omnicef)
cefixime (Suprax)
cefpodoxime (Vantin)
cefprozil (Cefzil)
ceftibuten (Cedax)
cefuroxime (Ceftin)
cephalexin (Keflex)
cephradine (Velosef)
loracarbef (Lorabid)

Chelators
succimer (Chemet)

Corticosteroids, Nasal Inhalants
beclomethasone (Beconase)
budesonide (Rhinocort Aqua)
dexamethasone (Dexacort Turbinaire)
flunisolide (Nasalide)
fluticasone (Flonase)
mometasone (Nasonex)
triamcinolone (Nasacort)

Corticosteroids, Oral
betamethasone (Celestone)
cortisone (Cortone Acetate)
dexamethasone (Decadron)
hydrocortisone, systemic (Cortef)
methylprednisolone, systemic (Medrol)
prednisolone, systemic (Delta-Cortef)
prednisone (Deltasone)
triamcinolone (Aristocort A)

Corticosteroids, Oral Inhalants
beclomethasone (Beclodisk)
budesonide (Pulmicort Turbuhaler)
dexamethasone (Decadron Respihaler)
flunisolide (AeroBid)
fluticasone (Flovent)
triamcinolone (Azmacort)

Corticosteroids, Topical
alclometasone (Aclovate)
amcinonide (Cyclocort)
betamethasone (Teladar)
clobetasol (Cormax)
clocortolone (Cloderm)
desonide (DesOwen)
desoximetasone (Topicort)
dexamethasone (Decadron)
diflorasone (Florone)
fluocinolone (Fluonid)
fluocinonide (Lidex)

flurandrenolide (Cordran)
fluticasone (Cutivate)
halcinonide (Halog)
halobetasol (Ultravate)
hydrocortison (Delcort)
mometasone (Elcon)
prednicarbate (Dermatop)
triamcinolone (Kenalog)

Decongestants
oxymetazoline (Allerest 12 Hour)
phenylephrine, nasal (Neo-Synephrine)
phenylephrine, ophthalmic (Ak-Dilate)
pseudoephedrine (Sudafed)

Enzymes
pancrelipase (Viokase)

Expectorants
guaifenesin (Robitussin)

Insecticides
lindane (G-well)

Laxatives
psyllium (Metamucil)
sodium phosphate (Fleet Enema)

Leukotriene Antagonist/Inhibitors
montelukast (Singulair)
zafirlukast (Accolate)

Muscle Relaxants
baclofen (Lioresal)
dantrolene (Dantrium)

Narcotics (Opioids)
codeine
meperidine (Demerol)
morphine (MS Contin)

Nonsteroidal Anti-Inflammatory Drugs (NSAIDs)
ibuprofen (Advil)
ibuprofen + pseudoephedrine (Advil Cold and Sinus)

Penicillin Antibiotics (Anti-Infectives)
amoxicillin (Amoxil)
ampicillin (D-Amp)
cloxacillin (Cloxapen)
dicloxacillin (Dycill)
nafcillin (Unipen)
oxacillin (Bactocill)
penicillin V potassium (Veetids)

Selective Serotonin Reuptake Inhibitors (SSRIs) and Selective Norepinephrine Reuptake Inhibitors
atomoxetine (Strattera)
fluoxetine (Prozac)
fluvoxamine (Luvox)
sertraline (Zoloft)

Sulfa Drugs (Sulfonamides)
sulfadiazine (Microsulfon)
sulfamethoxazole + phenazopyridine (Azo Gantanol)
sulfamethoxazole + trimethoprim (Bactrim)
sulfasalazine (Azaline)
sulfisoxazole (Gantrisin)

Tetracycline Antibiotics (Anti-Infectives)
demeclocycline (Declomycin)
doxycycline (Doryx)
minocycline (Minocin)
oxytetracycline (Terramycin)
tetracycline (Tetracyn)

Thyroid Hormone Replacements
levothyroxine sodium (Synthroid)
liothyronine sodium (Cytomel)
liotrix (Thyrolar)
thyroid hormone (Armour Thyroid)

Tricyclic Antidepressants
    amitriptyline (Endep)
    clomipramine (Anafranil)
    desipramine (Norpramin)
    doxepin (Sinequan)
    imipramine (Tofranil)
    nortriptyline (Pamelor)
    trimipramine (Surmontil)

Vitamin Analogs
    calcitriol (Rocaltrol)

Xanthine Bronchodilators
    aminophylline (Phyllocontin)
    oxtriphylline (Choledyl)
    theophylline (Theobid)

INDEX

The following entries are classified according to these criteria:

- Generic names of drugs are listed in boldface.
- Brand names of drugs are listed in lightface, followed by the generic name in boldface.
- Italic type is used for the names of drug classifications.

A

K

L

M